HANDBOOK OF

Botulinum
Toxin Treatment

HANDBOOK OF
Botulinum Toxin Treatment

EDITED BY

Peter Moore

MB ChB MD FRCP
Senior Lecturer in Neurology, Liverpool University
Consultant Neurologist at
The Walton Centre for Neurology and Neurosurgery
Liverpool
UK

Markus Naumann

MD
Professor of Neurology
Department of Neurology
University of Würzburg
Würzburg
Germany

SECOND EDITION

Blackwell
Science

First published 1995
Second edition 2003
Reprinted 2005

Library of Congress Cataloging-in-Publication Data

Handbook of botulinum toxin treatment / edited by Peter Moore,
    Markus Naumann.—2nd ed.
        p. ; cm.
    Includes bibliographical references and index.
    ISBN 0–632–05957–5
    1. Botulinum toxin—Therapeutic use. 2. Spasms—Chemotherapy.
  3. Dystonia—Chemotherapy. 4. Strabismus—Chemotherapy.
  5. Eyelids—Diseases—Chemotherapy. I. Moore, Peter, MRCP. II. Naumann, Markus.
    [DNLM: 1. Botulinum Toxins—therapeutic use. QW 630.5.B2
  H236 2002]
  RC935.S64H36 2002
  615′.329364—dc21

2002011685

ISBN 0-632-05957-5

A catalogue record for this title is available from the British Library

Set in 9.5/13.5 Photina by SNP Best-set Typesetter Ltd., Hong Kong
Printed and bound in the United Kingdom by TJI Digital, Padstow, Cornwall

Commissioning Editor: Stuart Taylor
Managing Editor: Rupal Malde
Production Editor: Karen Moore
Production Controller: Kate Charman

For further information on Blackwell Publishing, visit our website:
http://www.blackwellpublishing.com

Contents

CONTENTS

List of Contributors

REINER BENECKE MD, *Universität Rostock, Gehslheimerstrasse 20, D-18147 Rostock, Germany*

STEFFEN BERWECK MD, *Children's Hospital Duisberg, Wedau Kliniken, Zu den Rehwiesen 9, D-47055 Duisberg, Germany*

ANDREW BLITZER MD, DDS, *New York Centre for Voice and Swallowing Disorders, 425 West 59th Street, New York NY 10019, USA*

MITCHELL F. BRIN MD, *University of California–Irvine, Irvine, California, USA & Allergan, Inc., 2525 Dupont Drive, Irvine, USA*

FABIO DANISI MD, *The Mount Sinai School of Medicine, 1 Gustave Levy Place, New York NY 10029-6574, USA*

DIRK DRESSLER MD, *Universität Rostock, Gehslheimerstrasse 20, D-18147 Rostock, Germany*

LESLIE J. FINDLEY TD, MD, MRCP, *Essex Neurosciences Unit, Oldchurch Hospital, Waterloo Road, Romford, Essex RM7 0BE, UK*

JEAN-MICHEL GRACIES MD PhD, *Neurology Department, Mount Sinai Hospital, New York NY 10024, USA*

H. KERR GRAHAM MD, FRCS (ED), FRACS, *Royal Children's Hospital, Department of Orthopaedics, Flemington Road, Parkville Victoria 3052, Australia*

HARALD HEFTER MD, *Heinrich-Heine Universität, Moorenstrasse 5, Dusseldorf 40225, Germany*

FLORIAN HEINEN MD, *Children's Hospital Duisburg, Wedau Kliniken, Zu den Rehwiesen 9, D-47055, Duisberg, Germany*

JOSEPH JANKOVIC MD, *Department of Neurology, Parkinson's Disease Center and Movement Disorders Clinic, Baylor College of Medicine, 6550 Fannin Street, Houston, Texas 77030, USA*

WOLFGANG JOST MD, *Deutsche Klinik für Diagnostik, Aukammallee 33, Wiesbaden 65191, Germany*

JOHN LEE FRCS, FRCOphth, FRCP, *Moorfields Eye Hospital, City Road, London EC1V 2PD, UK*

LIST OF CONTRIBUTORS

NICK LOWE MD, FRCP, FACP, Cranley Clinic, 19a Cavendish Square, London W1M 9AD, UK

CESARE MONTECUCCO MD, Centro CNR Biomembrane and Dipartmento di Scienze
Biomediche, Università di Padova, Via Colombo 3, 35121 Padova, Italy

PETER MOORE MB ChB FRCP MD, The Walton Centre for Neurology and Neurosurgery, Lower Lane,
Liverpool L9 7LJ, UK

JÖRG MÜLLER MD, Universitätsklinik für Neurologie, Anichstrasse 35, A-6020 Innsbruck, Austria

MARKUS NAUMANN MD, Neurologische Universitätsklinik, Josef-Schneider-Strasse 11,
D-97080 Würzburg, Germany

TURO J. NURMIKKO MD PhD, Pain Research Institute, Department of Neurological Science,
University of Liverpool, Lower Lane, Liverpool L9 7AL, UK

WERNER POEWE MD, Universitätsklinik für Neurologie, Anichstrasse 35, A-6020 Innsbruck,
Austria

ORNELLA ROSSETTO MD, Centro CNR Biomembrane and Dipartmento di Scienze Biomediche,
Università di Padova, Via Colombo 3, 35121 Padova, Italy

BIMSARA SENANAYAKE MBBS, MD, MRCP(UK), Essex Centre for Neurosciences, Oldchurch
Hospital, Waterloo Road, Romford, Essex RM7 0BE, UK

GEOFF SHEEAN MBBS, FRACP University of California San Diego Medical Centre, 200 West
Arbor Drive, San Diego CA 92103-8465, USA

DAVID M. SIMPSON MD, Mount Sinai School of Medicine, 1 Gustave Levy Place, New York
NY 10029-6574, USA

BORIS SOMMER MD, Rosenparkklinik, Heidelberger Landstraße 20, 64297 Darmstadt, Germany

LUCIAN SULICA MD, Department of Otolaryngology, Beth Israel Medical Center, The New York Eye
and Ear Infirmary 10 Union Square East, Suite 4J, New York NY 10003, USA

MADHAVI THOMAS MD, Department of Neurology, Parkinson's Disease Center and Movement
Disorders Clinic, Baylor College of Medicine, 6550 Fannin Street, Houston, Texas 77030, USA

KLAUS VIKTOR TOYKA MD, Neurologische Universitätsklinik, Josef-Schneider-Strasse II,
D-97080 Würburg, Germany

JEAN VERHEYDEN MD, New York Centre for Voice and Swallowing Disorders, 425 West 59th
Street, New York NY 10019, USA

JÖRG WISSEL MD, Kliniken Beelitz, Neurologische Rehabilitationsklinik, Paracelsugring 6a,
D-14547 Beelitz-Heilstätten, Germany

Foreword

To second edition

Botulinum toxin is the world's most powerful poison, and the story of how it has developed into an effective treatment for disorders related to excessive muscle contraction is a fascinating one. Drs Moore and Naumann, the editors of this *Handbook*, have updated the first edition and provide the reader with the history of this toxin, now turned into treatment. Whereas the first edition described the pioneering contributions of Alan Scott in investigating the use of botulinum toxin to treat strabismus, and also its usefulness in treating hemifacial spasm and the focal dystonias, such as blepharospasm and spasmodic torticollis, this new edition was sorely needed because the clinical indications have expanded far beyond these disorders. Spasticity and autonomic disorders have been benefited. Its use in eliminating wrinkles has gained notoriety in the popular press, and now the whole world is aware of botulinum toxin as a medical therapeutic agent. Moreover, in the first edition only botulinum toxin type A was obtainable commercially, and now the type B toxin is also available.

Drs Moore and Naumann have assembled a team of expert authors to write the chapters for this book. The chosen contributors are all leaders in the clinical application of botulinum toxin. Their experience has been put into clear writing, which will guide physicians on how to use this drug in their clinical practice. As a neurologist who evaluated botulinum toxin in the focal dystonias after Dr Scott showed its effectiveness for strabismus and blepharospasm, it is extremely gratifying to see how much our patients have benefited from this agent. Botulinum toxin injections have become the principal treatment of the various focal dystonias. These treatments are also of great benefit for those who suffer from more widespread dystonia, by using this agent to treat the parts of the body that are most troublesome to an individual patient.

No doubt we will see more imaginative usefulness of botulinum toxin over time, as investigators explore other potential clinical conditions that could benefit by a reduction of excessive muscle contractions. I applaud the editors for offering this *Handbook* to those clinicians already familiar with botulinum toxin and wish to become current with new uses, as well as those who are still new to this therapy and wish to learn as much as they can in a comprehensive manner. This volume will serve them well.

Stanley Fahn

To first edition

Botulinum toxin, the most lethal poison known to mankind, has recently provided hope and relief for thousands of ignored victims of a poorly understood group of neurological conditions characterised by uncontrollable, excessive and frequently painful muscular contractions. The injection of minute quantities of the toxin into the contorted muscles has been shown conclusively to improve, sometimes dramatically, the functional disability in these focal dystonias. Patients unable to see because of severe blepharospasm may regain their ability to read and drive, the strangulated embarrassing croak of laryngeal dystonia can be spectacularly abolished and the pain, depression and twisting of torticollis alleviated. The most remarkable results of all, however, have occurred in the treatment of hemifacial spasm, a distinct non-dystonic condition, which previously could only be treated by major brain surgery.

Dr Peter Moore's superbly edited handbook took its roots from a memorable workshop on botulinum toxin which he organised at the Maritime Museum in the Albert Dock, Liverpool, the city of my birth and a port still rich in inspiration, spirit and humour, despite an era of appalling social deprivation. The mode of action of botulinum toxin, the fascinating story of its introduction into clinical practice by the American ophthalmologist Alan Scott, and its multifarious applications in contemporary medical therapeutics, are all comprehensively covered by a galaxy of distinguished contributors. This compendium will be of value to all of those already committed botulinum toxin users who wish to refine their skills and knowledge, and also to those who are interested in embarking on a therapeutic technique, which while not curative, has helped reduce suffering and disability in large numbers of desperate patients.

I wish Dr Moore's book the resounding success it unquestionably deserves.

A.J. Lees

Preface

To second edition

Since publication of the first edition of this handbook seven years ago, knowledge and understanding of botulinum neurotoxins and their clinical applications have grown rapidly. There can be few drugs that span such a wide and still expanding range of indications and medical and surgical specialties.

Basic scientists have clarified the three-functional domain structure of clostridial neurotoxins. Clinical practice is much clearer in mature indications such as focal dystonia, and indications that were more exotic or were mere hypotheses are entering routine use in many more fields of medicine. These include cosmetic indications, spasticity in adults and children, autonomic glandular disorders such as focal hyperhidrosis, and sphincter diseases such as anal fissure and bladder overactivity. Botulinum toxin helps pain in some disorders and may prove useful in others. A second botulinum toxin serotype, type B, is now widely available and in clinical use, and its role is under active investigation. Also, the promise and success of these treatments have stimulated research in many related fields and improved our understanding of physiology and basic mechanisms of disease.

We have aimed this second edition at doctors and other professionals who need an overview combined with specific advice related to their specialty. General chapters provide essential background knowledge. In subsequent sections experienced clinicians describe each disorder, examine the place of and evidence for treatment with botulinum toxin, and give practical details on assessment and treatment, blending the science with the art of medicine—and making it clear which is which.

We would like to thank the contributors for all their hard work, the staff at Blackwell Publishing for their expert assistance, and our wives, Julia and Susanne, and families for their encouragement and patience, and often their practical help.

A. Peter Moore and Markus Naumann
Liverpool and Würzburg

To first edition

Over the last 15 years, the medical profession has been changing its mind about botulinum toxin. Research has transformed it from a dangerous and feared poison to a novel drug able to help and sometimes cure many conditions that were previously very difficult to treat. The toxin's most important property is its ability to cause prolonged focal muscle weakness without systemic toxicity, and Dr A. Scott was the first to demonstrate that botulinum toxin type A could safely and selectively weaken muscles in humans when he developed it in the early 1980s as a treatment for strabismus.

Botulinum toxin is arguably the safest and most effective new treatment in the management of movement disorders since the introduction of levodopa to treat Parkinson's disease over 20 years ago. Ophthalmologists are increasingly using it in squint and other ocular motility disorders. There is a steadily increasing range of new or potential indications in other fields, such as paediatrics, orthopaedics, ENT, rehabilitation medicine, plastic and cosmetic surgery, gastroenterology and urology.

Until recently, information about botulinum toxin has been scattered through many basic science and medical journals and textbooks, perhaps because so many specialties have been involved. This book was written to provide an overview of the science and development behind the clinical use of botulinum toxin, to inform the non-specialist on the opportunities opened up and conditions that may respond, and to give specific guidance on the techniques used.

The book opens with core chapters covering the history, basic science and general clinical principles of botulinum toxin use. Subsequent chapters review individual indications and alternative treatments, and set out practical details of toxin treatment, such as patient selection and assessment, anatomy, injection techniques, follow-up and side effects. These chapters are written by experienced clinicians who describe their own methods in detail and discuss alternatives.

There are many developments that seem set to improve existing treatment techniques and open new possibilities. For the future, the book discusses ways to improve our use of the toxin in already recognised indications. It aims to increase understanding of general principles, which will help in the assessment of new uses for both conventional botulinum toxin type A and other naturally occurring and newly engineered types of toxin.

I thank all the contributors for the time and effort they have put in to their chapters, and give especial thanks to my wife, Julia, for her patience and her moral—and practical—support in editing.

Peter Moore

PART ONE

General

CHAPTER 1

History and current applications of botulinum toxin — from poison to remedy

MARKUS NAUMANN, KLAUS VIKTOR TOYKA
& PETER MOORE

Introduction

Botulinum toxin (Bt) is a protein produced by the anaerobic bacterium *Clostridium botulinum*. It is the most potent toxin known. It was found to be the cause of botulism, a systemic food poisoning, at the end of the 19th century.

The earliest records of botulism go back probably to scripts in the Middle Ages and from the Roman Empire. However, the first accurate and complete description of the clinical symptoms of food-borne botulism was published between 1817 and 1822 by the German physician and poet Justinus Kerner (Fig. 1.1a) [1–3], who also developed the idea of a possible therapeutic use of Bt, which he called 'sausage poison' [4–7].

In 1820, Kerner published his first monograph on sausage poisoning [2]. In 1822, he summarized his work and his hypotheses on Bt in a second monograph (Fig. 1.1b) containing the clinical evaluation and summary of 155 cases of patients with botulism, including post-mortem studies, animal experiments and heroic experiments on himself [3]. Kerner deduced from the clinical symptoms and his experimental observations that Bt acts by interrupting signal transmission within the peripheral motor and the sympathetic and parasympathetic nervous systems, leaving sensory signal transmission intact. He accurately described all the muscular and autonomic symptoms and signs familiar to modern medicine.

In the final chapter of his 1822 monograph [3], Kerner discussed the possibility of using the toxin as a remedy for a variety of diseases. He concluded that small doses of the toxin would reduce excessive activity of the sympathetic nervous system. He suggested that St. Vitus' Dance would be a good indication, as at that time it was thought to be due to an overexcited sympathetic system. Other potential candidates were hypersecretion of body fluids, sweat or mucus and ulcers from malignant diseases. Some of his visions are now reality: although it is not useful for chorea, Bt has undoubtedly revolutionized the treatment of focal movement disorders such as dystonias, and a number of autonomic disturbances including focal hyperhidrosis and hypersalivation [8–11]. Kerner has earned his place as one of the intellectual founders of modern Bt therapy.

In 1870, the German physician Müller first used the term 'botulism' (from the Latin word *botulus* = sausage) to describe the effects of sausage poisoning.

The last major scientific step in the 19th century was the discovery of the guilty bacterium in 1895, when an outbreak of botulism followed a funeral ceremony in the Belgian village Ellezelles. Emille Pierre van Ermengem, a professor of microbiology

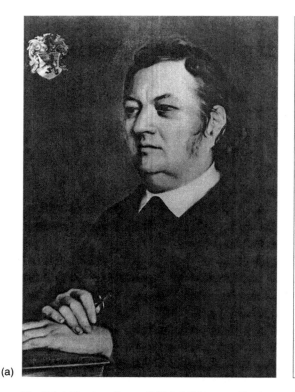
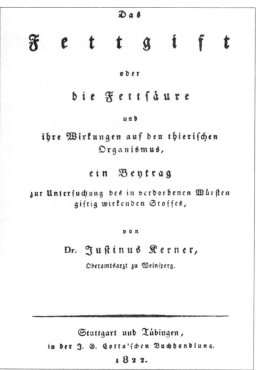

Fig. 1.1 (a) Justinus Kerner (1786–1862) painted by Ottavio d'Albuzzi (with permission of the Kerner Museum, Weinsberg, Germany). (b) Kerner's 1822 monograph.

in Ghent, examined the food and the victims of this food poisoning and isolated the anaerobic bacterium *Bacillus botulinus*—later called *Clostridium botulinum* [12]. He experimented on several animals. Subcutaneous injections and feeding with small fragments of ham provoked the typical symptoms of botulism. The bacteria isolated from food and the organs of victims were anaerobic and had numerous villi.

In the 1920s, Dr Hermann Sommer of the Hooper Foundation at the University of California made the first attempts to purify botulinum toxin type A (BtA), and his work paved the way for further studies on BtA and types B, C, D and E, at the military research institution Camp (Fort) Detrick, particularly during World War II. Bt was interesting to the military because of the toxin's potential threat as a biological weapon. Accordingly, a toxoid vaccine was produced and vaccination was available from the Centers for Disease Control (CDC) for researchers working with Bt and for military service men. In 1946, Dr Carl Lammanna first crystallized BtA, and later demonstrated that it was composed of toxic units bound to non-toxic proteins. Professor Edward Schantz at Fort Detrick supplied purified toxin to many researchers, and enabled a great deal of work on the structure and actions of the toxin [13]. In 1949, Burgen, Dickens and Zatman in London discovered that botulinum toxin type A blocked the release of acetylcholine at neuromuscular junctions [14]. A physiologist, Dr Vernon Brook, suggested in the 1950s that BtA might be used to reduce the activity of hyperactive muscles [15].

Dr Daniel Drachman pioneered the experimental use of Bt as a tool in research on the neurotrophic effects of acetylcholine transmission on skeletal muscles, and on the role of embryonic movement in joint development [16,17]. He first showed that local injection of Bt could be used to paralyze the injected muscle. Blockade of acetylcholine transmission by Bt resulted in a wide variety of atrophic changes in the morphology, physiology and biochemistry of the muscle, demonstrating the critical role of acetylcholine transmission in 'neurotrophic' maintenance of skeletal muscle properties. Drachman also found that paralysis of chick embryos with Bt led to joint abnormalities of clubfoot and arthrogryposis multiplex congenita, thus explaining the pathogenesis of those conditions in humans as due to any condition that causes immobilization of the embryo during joint development.

The first clinical use of this potent neurotoxin is credited to Dr Alan Scott of the Smith–Kettlewell Eye Research Foundation in San Francisco. By 1973, he demonstrated in animal experiments that it might help in the treatment of strabismus, and also suggested that it may be effective in blepharospasm. Scott first injected a patient with strabismus in 1977. In 1980 he published the results of the first clinical trial of BtA for strabismus. By 1982, he had also treated patients for nystagmus, hemifacial spasm, lid retraction, torticollis, and spasticity [18].

In 1992/1993, Giampietro Schiavo and coworkers demonstrated that tetanus and botulinum neurotoxins are metalloproteases specific for three proteins that form the core of the neuroexocytosis machinery [19–21]. They work by disrupting the ability of vesicles to attach to the cell membrane, thereby blocking acetylcholine release in cholinergic nerve terminals.

Following its initial success in treating strabismus, Bt has gone on to revolutionize the treatment of many neurological and ophthalmic diseases and has become part of treatment strategies in cosmetic, general, maxillofacial, orthopaedic and thoracic surgery, dermatology, otorhinolaryngology, pain clinics, paediatrics, rehabilitation medicine, and urology. Many studies confirmed the benefits of BtA for various forms of focal dystonia and spasticity in adults and children. Bt has become the first-line treatment for patients suffering from blepharospasm, hemifacial spasm, and cervical dystonia. It is superior to most medical treatment options for other forms of focal dystonias including oromandibular and limb dystonias. More recently, BtA has also proved highly effective in the treatment of localized autonomic disorders and in cosmetic indications. BtA is being tested in various pain syndromes such as migraine, tension type headache and back pain.

In 2001, another serotype of the neurotoxin —botulinum toxin type B (BtB) —was licensed in the US and European countries for cervical dystonia, and it will probably undergo testing for many of the other diseases currently treated with BtA. Other serotypes, such as types F and E, are currently being evaluated.

Although BtA has been licensed in some countries for blepharospasm, hemifacial spasm, focal spasticity in infantile cerebral palsy, and axillary hyperhidrosis and types A and B for the treatment of spasmodic torticollis, Bt is still not officially approved for most indications discussed in this book.

Table 1 summarizes the evidence for Bt treatment in various indications.

Table 1.1 Evidence for botulinum toxin treatment in various indications. This table is a guide only and represents a 'best fit' rather than a precise classification. The list is not exhaustive.

Indication	Inconclusive trial evidence, efficacy possible but not clear	Reasonable trial evidence, moderately effective	Conclusive evidence, effective treatment
Focal dystonias			
Blepharospasm			+++
Cervical dystonia			+++
Spasmodic dysphonia			+++
Meige syndrome		++	
Writer's cramp		++	
Foot dystonia		++	
Oromandibular dystonia		++	
Occupational cramps	+		
Axial dystonia	+		
Tremor			
Dystonic head tremor		++	
Essential head tremor		++	
Essential hand tremor	+		
Palatal tremor			+++
Hemifacial spasm			+++
Focal spasticity in adults			
Lower limb			+++
Upper limb			+++
Focal spasticity in children			
Lower limb			+++
Upper limb		++	
Ophthalmic indications			
Strabismus		++	
Sixth nerve palsy	+		
Nystagmus and oscillopsia	+		
Protective ptosis	+		
Autonomic indications			
Secretory disorders			
Focal hyperhidrosis			+++
Gustatory sweating			+++
Hyperlacrimation		++	
Siallorhea		++	
Urological indications			
DSD		++	
Hyper-reflexic bladder	+		
Urethrism	+		
Vaginismus	+		

Continued

Table 1.1 *Continued*

Indication	Inconclusive trial evidence, efficacy possible but not clear	Reasonable trial evidence, moderately effective	Conclusive evidence, effective treatment
Gastrointestinal uses			
Anal fissure			+++
Achalasia		++	
UOS	+		
Outlet constipation	+		
Anismus	+		
Sphincter of Oddi dysfunction	+		
Pain			
TTH		++	
Migraine	+		
Backaches	+		
Wrinkles		++	
Other unusual indications			
Tics	+		
Stiff person	+		
Rigidity	+		
Bruxism	+		
Myokymia	+		

DSD, detrusor-sphincter dyssynergia; TTH, tension-type headache; UOS, upper oesophageal sphincter.

The wider medical influence of botulinum toxins

The rapidly expanding medical potential of Bt has galvanized medicine in several other ways. It has provided an intellectual and financial stimulus, opening up a wide variety of fields. Bt has clarified our understanding of the aetiology and pathophysiology of diseases such as dystonia and spasticity. For instance, it is not so long ago that many clinicians considered dystonia to be a non-organic disease, and successful treatment with BtA helped to crystallize opinion and confirm dystonia as a physical rather than a psychiatric illness. Many patients have been extremely grateful for their new classification. Experiments on patients treated with BtA have yielded fascinating insights into the underlying neural mechanisms of dystonia and spasticity.

The financial muscle of the pharmaceutical industry has been drawn to these new fields and supports both basic and clinical research. Early investigators used a combination of science, imagination and intuition to broaden the scope of treatment with BtA, and to generate and test hypotheses in often small and uncontrolled studies. Their enthusiasm, combined with the discipline imposed by drug regulatory authorities, eventually led to more definitive randomized controlled trials (RCTs). For some disorders Bt was the first treatment subjected to these modern methods of scrutiny, and in turn it triggered re-evaluation of many older treatments. The challenge of rolling Bt out from research settings to routine use in health services has stimulated reviews and revision of much wider aspects of these services, especially for dystonia, spasticity and rehabilitation medicine.

References

1 Kerner J. Vergiftung durch verdorbene Würste. *Tübinger Blätter Naturwissenschaften Arzneykunde* 1817; **3**: 1–25.

2 Kerner J. *Neue Beobachtungen über die in Württemberg so häufig vorfallenden tödlichen Vergiftungen durch den Genuss geräucherter Würste.* Tübingen: Osiander, 1820.

3 Kerner J. *Das Fettgift oder die Fettsäure und ihre Wirkungen auf den thierischen Organismus, ein Beytrag zur Untersuchung des in verdorbenen Würsten giftig wirkenden Stoffes.* Stuttgart, Tübingen: Cotta, 1822.

4 Erbguth F, Naumann M. Historical aspect of botulinum toxin: Justinus Kerner (1786–1862) and the 'sausage poison'. *Neurology* 1999; **53**: 1850–3.

5 Erbguth F, Naumann M. On the first systematic descriptions of botulism and botulinum toxin by Justinus Kerner (1786–1862) (letter). *J History Neurosci* 2000; **9**: 218–20.

6 Grüsser OJ. Der 'Wurstkerner'. Justinus Kerners Beitrag zur Erforschung des Botulismus. In: Schott H, ed. *Justinus Kerner als Azt und Seelenforscher*, 2nd edn. Weinsberg, 1998: 232–257.

7 Grüsser OJ. Die ersten systematischen Beschreibungen und tierexperimentellen Untersuchungen des Botulismus. Zum 200. Geburtstag von Justinus Kerner am 18 September 1986. *Sudhoffs Arch* 1987; **10**: 167–87.

8 Naumann M, Jost W, Toyka KV. Treatment of disorders of the autonomic nervous system with botulinum toxin A. *Arch Neurol* 1999; **56**: 914–6.

9 Naumann M, Hofmann U, Bergmann I, Hamm H, Toyka KV, Reiners K. Focal hyperhidrosis: effective treatment with intracutaneous botulinum toxin. *Arch Dermatol* 1998; **134**: 301–4.

10 Naumann M, Zellner M, Toyka KV, Reiners K. Treatment of gustatory sweating with botulinum toxin. *Ann Neurol* 1997; **42**: 973–5.

11 Pasricha PJ, Ravich WJ, Hendrix TR, Sostre S, Jones B, Kalloo AN. Intrasphincteric botulinum toxin for the treatment of achalasia. *New Engl J Med* 1995; **322**: 774–8.

12 Van Ermengem EP. Über einen neuen anaeroben Bacillus und seine Beziehung zum Botulismus. *Z Hyg Infektionskrankh* 1897; **26**: 1–56.

13 Scott AB. Foreword. In: Jankovic J, Hallet M, eds. *Therapy with Botulinum Toxin.* New York: Marcel Dekker Inc., 1994: vii–ix.

14 Burgen A, Dickens F, Zatman LJ. The action of botulinum toxin on the neuromuscular junction. *J Physiol* 1949; **109**: 10–24.

15 Schantz EJ. Historical perspective. In: Jankovic J, Hallet M, eds. *Therapy with Botulinum Toxin.* New York: Marcel Dekker Inc., 1994: xxiii–vi.

16 Drachman DB. Atrophy of skeletal muscles in chick embryos treated with botulinum toxin. *Science* 1964; **145**: 719–21.

17 Drachman DB, Houk J. The effect of botulinum toxin on speed of muscle contraction. *Am J Physiol* 1969; **216**: 1435–55.

18 Scott AB, Rosenbaum A, Collins CC. Pharmacological weakening of extraocular muscles. *Invest Ophthalmol* 1973; **12**: 924–7.

19 Schiavo G, Poulin B, Rossetto O *et al.* Tetanus toxin is a zinc protein and its inhibition of neurotransmitter release and protease activity depend on zinc. *EMBO J* 1992; **11**: 3577–83.

20 Schiavo G, Benfenati F, Poulain B *et al.* Tetanus and botulinum-B neurotoxins block neurotransmitter release by proteolytic cleavage of synaptobrevin. *Nature* 1992; **359**: 832–4.

21 Schiavo G, Rossetto O, Catsicas S *et al.* Identification of the nerve terminal targets of botulinum neurotoxin serotypes A, D, and E. *J Biol Chem* 1993; **268**: 23:784–7.

The authors are grateful to Dr Daniel Drachman for his contribution to the chapter.

How botulinum toxins work

ORNELLA ROSSETTO & CESARE MONTECUCCO

Introduction

The identification of botulinum neurotoxin (Bt) as the sole cause of botulism, a disease first described by Kerner at the beginning of the 19th century [1], was made a little over a century ago by van Ermenghem through studying a case of food poisoning in Belgium [2]. This breakthrough followed advances in understanding and experimental techniques made while uncovering the infectious nature of tetanus, of the anaerobic and spore-forming bacterium *Clostridium tetani* and of tetanus neurotoxin (Tt) [3,4]. The bacterium producing Bt was characterized as *Clostridium botulinum*. *Clostridium barati* and *Cl. butyrricum* can also produce the toxin.

There are seven serotypes of Bt, designated BtA to BtG, each with different antigenic profiles and biochemical actions [5,6]. However, they all have a similar pharmacological effect. All the toxins bind to and enter inside peripheral cholinergic terminals, causing a sustained block of acetylcholine (ACh) release at the neuromuscular junction and in cholinergic autonomic nerves, with ensuing flaccid paralysis and autonomic symptoms. If the paralysis extends to respiratory muscles the patient dies of respiratory failure. Bt does not normally cross the blood–brain barrier.

Bt is produced under anaerobic conditions on a variety of organic substrates and it is usually introduced by eating contaminated foods (food botulism); less frequently intoxication follows germination of clostridial spores in the intestine of newborns (infant botulism) or in wounds (wound botulism) [6].

Food-borne botulism

This is the commonest form of botulism in man. If food is contaminated with *C. botulinum* spores they may germinate and form toxin. The disease follows ingestion of the preformed toxin. Food-borne botulism in humans occurs mainly with types A, B and E toxins with type F responsible for a minority of outbreaks [5,6]. So potent are the neurotoxins that ingestion of as little as 1–2 μg of toxin may prove fatal.

Fortunately, modern food preservation processes are very effective in preventing *C. botulinum* spore contamination, so that outbreaks are relatively rare in developed countries. In the period 1950–79, for example, only 215 outbreaks of food-borne botulism were recorded in the US [7]. In the UK botulism is extremely rare but poses a continuing threat — as was demonstrated by an outbreak involving hazelnut flavoured yoghurt in 1989 affecting 27 people [8]. New food processing techniques, such as the storage of food in modified atmospheres or under vacuum ('*sous vide*'), create an anaerobic environment without any competing microorganisms. There is still concern that spores of *C. botulinum* might grow under these conditions and produce toxin.

Wound botulism and infant botulism

Food-borne botulism is strictly an intoxication, but there are forms of botulism that result from direct infection by *C. botulinum*. Wound botulism is a very rare form of the disease in which *C. botulinum* contaminates, colonizes and produces toxin in wounds, a disease process analogous to that of tetanus [9].

Infant botulism is the third form of the disease, and is so called because infants of up to about 8 months old are particularly susceptible. *Clostridium botulinum* colonizes the intestinal tract, possibly after ingestion of food contaminated with spores. The colonizing bacteria in the gut produce toxin (mainly types A and B) which gives rise to a typical flaccid paralysis and the so–called *floppy baby syndrome*. Paediatricians are increasingly aware of it, and are reporting it more frequently so that it is now the most prevalent form of botulism in the US [10]. Botulism resulting from intestinal colonization may also occur in adults.

Treatment of botulism

Prophylaxis with toxoid vaccines is the only effective means of preventing the neuroparalytic effects of the toxins. Once affected, there is no known cure for the toxic paralysis of botulism. Although preparations of antitoxins are available, by the time clinical symptoms present they are usually ineffective, as the toxin has been irreversibly bound to cholinergic nerve terminals and internalized; within the cell it is not accessible to the antitoxin.

Antitoxin therapy using equine antitoxin is not recommended in infant botulism because of the risk of anaphylaxis, but antibiotics are useful in eliminating the basic enteric infection. Treatment otherwise consists of general supportive measures until the effects of the toxin are no longer apparent. In severe toxicity prolonged intensive care and respiratory support may be needed. Patients may recover completely, although it takes longer after BtA than after BtB or BtE poisoning [5,6].

Toxin formation, structure and action

The botulinum neurotoxins are proteins which all have similar molecular structures and molecular weights (MWs) of around 140–170 kDa. Some parts of the molecule are highly conserved, that is they are present in all forms of Bt with the implication that they are essential components of the molecule, and other parts are more variable. Within the bacteria the genes encoding for Bt are usually contained in mobile genetic elements such as phages and plasmids, whose acquisition converts a non-toxigenic strain into a toxigenic one [11]. Usually one bacterium harbours one toxin gene, but multiple toxin genes can occur [11]. Bt genes do not contain a secretion signal sequence and the protein neurotoxins only escape from the organism when it dies.

They escape as single polypeptide chains of 150 kDa that are only weakly toxic. They are later activated by a specific proteolytic cleavage within a loop containing a highly conserved disulphide bridge (S-S) [12]. This produces a much more potent di-chain molecule. There is a heavy-chain (H-chain) with MW 100 kDa, which is responsible for getting the toxin molecule to its target, a kind of homing device. The light-chain (L-chain), with MW 50 kDa, is the toxic portion of the molecule. The chains are joined primarily by the S-S bond and also interact via non-covalent associations (Fig. 2.1). The S-S bond is essential for neurotoxicity, and once in the cytosol of the neuron it is reduced to activate the ultimate toxic effect of Bt, by converting the L-chain into a proteolytic enzyme and releasing it [13].

How does botulinum toxin get into the body?

The Bts are naturally packaged as complexes with a variable number of accessory non-toxic proteins, including haemaglutinins, that protect the Bt molecule during its passage through the harsh acid conditions of the stomach. The complex dissociates at neutral pH values and the toxic portion passes through the intestine to the bloodstream by translocation across the intestinal epithelial monolayer [14]. Preparations of Bt used in human therapy are also complexed toxins so they will they resist damage and have a longer shelf life.

Mode of action (Fig. 2.2)

The botulinum neurotoxins are extremely potent agents that have specific toxicities ranging from 2×10^7 to 2×10^8 mouse median lethal doses per mg of protein. Their potency arises from a combination of highly specific and efficient homing devices and delivery mechanisms, and their ability to act as enzymes destroying essential proteins in a critical biochemical process. The evolutionary advantage of these toxins to the bacterium is obscure. Bt acts presynaptically by blocking the release of the neurotransmitter ACh, for instance at the neuromuscular junction. There are four stages involved in this inhibition [15–17] (Fig. 2.2).

1 Rapid, specific and irreversible *binding* to acceptors on the presynaptic nerve surface.

2 *Uptake* in which toxin enters the cell within a vesicle.

3 *Translocation* in which the toxin crosses the vesicle membrane and is released into the cytosol.

4 *Toxin activity* through proteolysis that disables the ACh release mechanism.

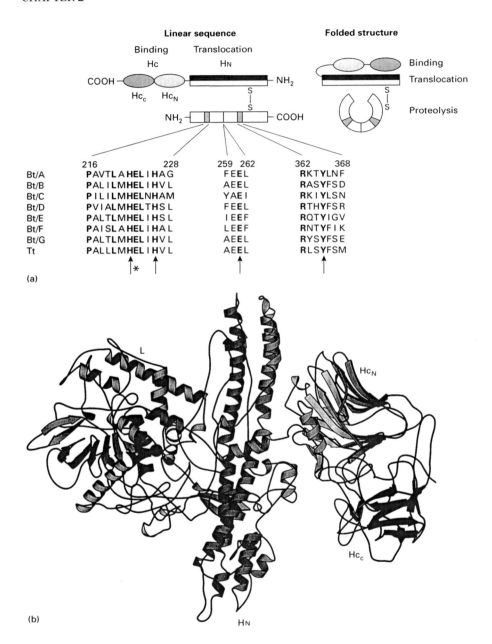

Linear sequence

Binding
Hc

Translocation
H_N

Folded structure

COOH — NH_2

Hc_c   Hc_N

NH_2 — COOH

Binding

Translocation

Proteolysis

	216	228	259	262	362	368
Bt/A	PAVTLA HEL I HAG		FEEL		RKTYLNF	
Bt/B	PAL ILMHEL I HV L		AEEL		RASYFSD	
Bt/C	P IL ILMHELNHAM		YAE I		RK IYLSN	
Bt/D	PVIALMHELTHS L		FEEL		RTHYFSR	
Bt/E	PALTLMHEL IHS L		IEEF		RQTYIGV	
Bt/F	PAISLA HEL IHAL		LEEF		RNTYF IK	
Bt/G	PALTLMHEL IHV L		AEEL		RYSYFSE	
Tt	PALLLMHEL IHV L		AEEL		RLSYFSM	

(a)

(b)

Binding

From the site of production or adsorption (intestine, wounds or injections), Bt diffuses in the body fluids to the presynaptic membrane of peripheral cholinergic terminals where it binds very specifically. It does not pass the blood–brain barrier. The H-chain of the toxin is responsible for the highly selective targeting of the toxin to cholinergic nerve terminals. It binds selectively and irreversibly to a small pool of high affinity acceptor molecules at the presynaptic membrane. The active receptor-binding domain is on the carboxyl terminal half of the H-chain [18,19], termed the Hc (Fig. 2.1). (Note: proteins have a 'C-terminus', or carboxyl end, and an 'N-terminus', or amino acid end, like the north and south poles of a magnet. Each section of linked proteins has its own C-terminus and N-terminus. The 'c' in Hc stands for carboxyl, not for chain.)

Detailed structure of binding domain

The H-chain Hc domain plays the major role in the remarkable specificity of Bt for cholinergic terminals, so-called neurospecific binding [20]. Additional regions may contribute. The binding domain is itself in two parts called subdomains, as shown in Fig. 2.1. Studies of crystals of BtA and BtB reveal that the N-terminal section (HcN) consists of 16 β-strands and four alpha-helices arranged in a jelly-roll motif, similar to that of carbohydrate binding proteins of the legume lectin family [21,22]. The amino acid sequence of this subdomain is highly conserved among Bts, suggesting a similar three-dimensional structure in each toxin subtype. On the other hand, the sequence of the C-terminal section of Hc (HcC) is poorly conserved. It folds to resemble trypsin inhibitors.

◀───

Fig. 2.1 The three-functional domain structure of clostridial (botulinum) neurotoxins (Bt).

(a) *Structure of active di-chain Bt.* The neurotoxins are composed of two polypeptide chains, the heavy-chain (H-chain) (100 kDa), and light-chain (L-chain) (50 kDa) held together by a single disulphide bridge (S-S). The disulphide bridge must be reduced within the target cell, and the L-chain separated from the H-chain before the toxic L-chain becomes fully active. *H-chain:* the C-terminus portion of the H-chain (domain Hc) binds the toxin specifically to cholinergic neurones. Structurally Hc can be further subdivided into two portions of 25 kDa, Hc_N and Hc_c. The N-terminus (H_N) is important for pore formation in the vesicle wall and for translocation of the L-chain from the endocytosed vesicle into the cytosol. *L-chain:* the L-chain L (50 kDa) is a zinc-endopeptidase responsible for the toxic intracellular activity of Bt. Segments which are similar (high homology) in different serotypes, and hence likely to be important, are in black. A short alpha-helix (216–228 in BtA) in the central part of the L-chain shows the highest homology and contains the zinc-binding motif of metallo-endopeptidases. Arrows (↑) indicate amino acids involved in the coordination of zinc or in the hydrolysis of the target protein (e.g. SNAP-25). * denotes the glutamic acid coordinating a water molecule responsible for the target hydrolysis.

(b) *The crystallographic structure of BtA.* This highlights the three functional domains. The L-chain contains both α-helix and β-strand secondary structures with the zinc (black: bold) and the zinc-binding motif (contained in the black alpha-helix) in the centre. The translocation domain (H_N) contains two long alpha-helices and a long loop interacting with the L-chain. Hc_N has two seven-stranded β-sheets arranged in a jelly-roll motif whereas the Hc_c contains a modified-trefoil folding.

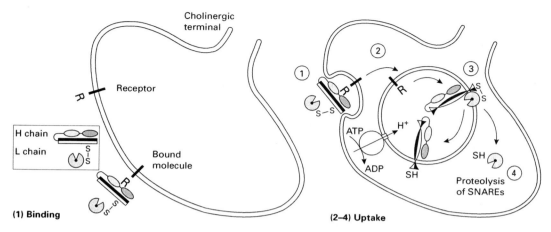

Fig. 2.2 Entry of Bt inside nerve terminals. (1) Bt binds to the presynaptic membrane at as yet unidentified receptors of peripheral cholinergic nerve terminals. (2) Binding is followed by internalization inside endocytic vesicles. (3) Bt separates from the acceptor molecule. An ATPase proton pump acidifies the vesicle lumen. At low pH, Bt changes conformation, inserts into the lipid bilayer of the vesicle membrane (pore formation) and passes (translocates) the L-chain into the cytosol. (4) Inside the cytosol the L-chain catalyzes the proteolysis of one of three SNARE proteins. Note that the active cleft of the L-chain (inside the loop) only becomes exposed at step 3. The acceptor molecule and H-chain remain attached to the vesicle wall. Reproduced with permission from [28].

The relative contribution of these two subdomains of Hc to the neurospecific binding is unclear. Experiments with the related Tt suggest that HcC plays a major role in the specific binding of toxin to cholinergic neurones, while HcN is important for subsequent toxin processing within the neuron, and its transport within the axon to reach the spinal cord [23].

Details of membrane acceptors

Studies using radio-iodinated toxins reveal hundreds per μm^2 of binding sites for BtA and BtB at rat neuromuscular junctions [24]. They consist of polysialogangliosides [25–27] together with as yet unidentified proteins of the presynaptic membrane [28]. The presence of lectin-like as well as protein binding subdomains in the Hc domain of Bt suggests that Bt binds strongly and specifically to the presynaptic membrane because of multiple interactions with both sugar and protein-binding sites [21,22]. BtB binds strongly to the synaptic vesicle protein synaptotagmin II, but only in the presence of polysialogangliosides [26], but the role of synaptotagmin II as *in vivo* receptor remains to be established.

Identification of the receptors for the various Bts would be a major advance and would probably help to improve therapeutic protocols. It might explain why there are rare patients who are insensitive to BtA treatment from the outset [29]. Some may carry anti-BtA antibodies following immunization in a subclinical episode of botulism, but this may not be the case for all. A variation in the structure/organization of the BtA presynaptic receptor would offer an alternative explanation.

Internalization: entry into the neurone (see Fig. 2.2)

Once bound to acceptors on the presynaptic nerve surface, a temperature and energy-dependent process actively takes the neurotoxin into the nerve terminal [30,31]. This probably resembles receptor-mediated endocytosis [15] with the toxin-acceptor complex becoming encapsulated in endosomes that migrate into the cytosol [32]. There is a close link between nerve stimulus—muscle contraction coupling and endocytosis at nerve terminals [33] and nerve stimulation facilitates intoxication by Bt [34]. Clinical trials are already attempting to exploit this mechanism to boost or focus the effect of the toxin using functional electrical stimulation.

Passage into the cytosol: translocation

Before it can act, the toxin must penetrate the hydrophobic barrier of the vesicle membrane (see Fig. 2.2) and escape into the cytosol [35]. A proton pump in the vesicle membrane actively acidifies the vesicle contents. The low pH alters the shape of the toxin and exposes hydrophobic patches. In turn these 'lead' the combined H- and L-chains through the hydrocarbon core of the membrane lipid bilayer, helping Bt to form low conductance ion channels and pass through to the cytosol [36–39]. The H-chain (H_N domain) is mainly responsible for this action.

Linking structure and function

The H_N domains of Bt are highly homologous and their predicted secondary structures are similar [16,21]. They feature two 100 Å-long antiparallel helices, similar to those of the colicins and influenza haemagglutinin which are known to interact with membrane proteins [21,22] (see Fig. 2.1B).

The precise mechanism of translocation is disputed, and there are two main theories.

1 The 'tunnel' model [40] proposes that the L-chain unfolds at low pH and permeates through a transmembrane pore made by the H-chain. Once exposed to the neutral pH of the cytosol, the L-chains refolds and is released from the vesicle by reduction of the inter-chain S-S bond (see Fig. 2.2). However, the Bt translocation domain is different from those of other pore-forming toxins. The long pair of alpha-helices with their triple helix bundle at either end bear more resemblance to some coiled-coil viral proteins [21,22] which do not translocate through pores but change structure at low pH and insert into membranes.

2   In a second model [41], as the vesicle internal pH decreases following the operation of the vacuolar-type ATPase proton pump, the toxin inserts into the lipid bilayer. It forms an ion channel that greatly alters electrochemical gradients, causing osmotic lysis of the toxin-containing acidic vesicle. Alternatively, the 'cleft' model envisages an H-channel opened laterally, with the L-chain crossing the membrane in contact with both the H-chain and the membrane lipids, rather than inside a wholly proteinaceous pore [17]. This accounts for the facts that the L-chain does contact the fatty acid chains of lipids during translocation [38], and the protein-translocating channel of the endoplasmic reticulum is open laterally to lipids. In this cleft model, the ion channel is a consequence of membrane translocation, rather than a prerequisite as predicted by the tunnel model.

Toxic activity

It is the L-chain which is the toxic portion of the botulinum neurotoxins [42]. When the L-subunit is injected directly into cells it blocks calcium-mediated exocytosis. This effect is not specific to cholinergic neurones (where it happens to block ACh release). BtA will, for instance, inhibit glutamate release when injected into glutaminergic neurones. The only reason the toxins are so specific in their natural di-chain form is that the H-chain binds selectively to cholinergic neurones and thus targets the L-chain precisely and selectively.

Normally, an action potential reaching the nerve ending triggers an influx of calcium ions that in turn stimulates release (exocytosis) of ACh-containing vesicles from active zones on the plasmalemma. The toxins do not affect the evoked influx of calcium. Instead, they selectively lyse proteins essential to the system that mediates fusion of synaptic vesicles with the outer cell surface membrane to enable exocytosis to take place.

Mechanisms of exocytosis

Exocytosis is the process of actively expelling specific cellular contents from the cell, in this case the ACh contained in vesicles in cholinergic nerve terminals. The molecular mechanisms that regulate exocytosis are highly conserved throughout evolution and occur at all levels of the secretory pathway. Within a nerve terminal a series of proteins must interact for fusion and exocytosis to occur. Three of these proteins, called vesicle-associated membrane protein (VAMP) [also known as synaptobrevin-2], synaptosomal associated protein of MW 25KDa (SNAP-25) and syntaxin link together as part of a protein complex, termed the SNARE (**SNA**p [**s**oluble **N**-ethyl-maleimide sensitive factor **at**tachment protein] **re**ceptor) complex, which brings the vesicle close to the target membrane [43] and helps the vesicle to fuse with the membrane [44]. The so-called SNARE proteins form the core of the neuroexocytosis machinery (Fig. 2.3).

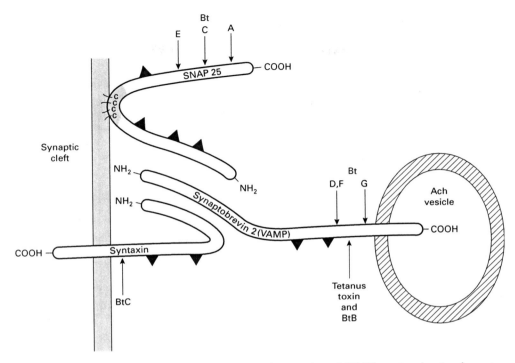

Fig. 2.3 Toxic action of botulinum neurotoxins by proteolysis of SNARE proteins, showing cleavage sites for Bt and for tetanus toxin. VAMP has a short C-terminal tail protruding in the vesicle lumen and a transmembrane segment, followed by a 60-residue long cytosolic part. This portion is highly conserved among isoforms and species, whereas the N-terminal portion is poorly conserved. Syntaxin is inserted in the plasma membrane and projects most of its mass in the cytosol. SNAP-25 is bound to the cytosolic face of presynaptic membrane via palmitoylated cysteine residues (c) located in the middle of the polypeptide chain and via interactions with syntaxin. Arrows indicate the sites of cleavage of Bt while the SNARE motifs required for Bt–substrate interaction are shown by filled triangles. Reproduced with permission from [28].

Action of botulinum toxin light-chains (Table 2.1)

The L-chains of Bts are remarkably specific proteases that recognize and cleave only these three proteins [16,28]. BtB, BtD, BtF and BtG cleave VAMP, each at different single sites [16,45]; BtA and BtE cleave SNAP-25 each at a single site whereas BtC cleaves both syntaxin and SNAP-25 [46–48]. Strikingly, tetanus toxin and BtB cleave VAMP at the same peptide bond (Gln76-Phe77) and yet they cause the 'opposite' symptoms of tetanus and botulism [45], conclusively demonstrating that the different symptoms of the two diseases derive from different sites of intoxication rather than from a different molecular mechanism of action.

Table 2.1 Target SNARE proteins of different botulinum toxins serotypes.

Toxin serotype	SNARE target	Cleavage site	Target localization*
A	SNAP-25	Gln197–Arg198	Presynaptic plasma membrane
B	VAMP/synaptobrevin	Gln76–Phe77	Synaptic vesicle
C	Syntaxin 1A	Lys253–Ala254	Presynaptic plasma membrane
	Syntaxin 1B	Lys252–Ala253	
D	VAMP/synaptobrevin	Lys59–Leu60	Synaptic vesicle
	Cellulobrevin	Unknown	All cells: vesicles of endocytosing/recycling system
E	SNAP-25	Arg108–Ile181	Presynaptic plasma membrane
F	VAMP/synaptobrevin	Gln58–Lys59	Synaptic vesicle
	Cellulobrevin	Unknown	All cells: vesicles of endocytosing/recycling system
G	VAMP/synaptobrevin	Ala81–Ala82	Synaptic vesicle

*Within neurone unless stated otherwise.
SNAP-25, synaptosomal associated protein of MW 25KDa; SNARE, soluble N-ethyl-maleimide sensitive factor attachment protein receptor; VAMP, vesicle-associated membrane protein.

Linking structure and activity

Botulinum toxin as an enzyme

Enzymes are biological catalysts of chemical reactions. That is they facilitate chemical reactions without themselves being destroyed. In theory, even one molecule of Bt L-chain in a nerve terminal could lead to the destruction or inactivation of all molecules of its target protein within the terminal, one at a time.

The N-terminal 50 kDa domain (L chain) acts as a metalloprotease, that is an enzyme (with a metal component) that splits protein. It links to the adjacent translocation domain on the H-chain (H_N, 50 kDa), which is in turn linked to the receptor-binding domain (see Fig. 2.1). There is little protein–protein interaction between the metalloprotease and the other parts of the molecule.

At the centre of a long cleft-shaped 'active site' in the metalloprotease there is a zinc atom coordinated via glutamic and two histidine residues of the highly conserved zinc-binding motif and by an additional glutamic residue (Glu262 of BtA and Glu268 of BtB) [49]. The Glu residue of the motif is particularly important because it coordinates the water molecule which actually performs the hydrolytic reaction of proteolysis. Its mutation leads to complete inactivation of these neurotoxins [50]. The active site of the L-chain faces the H-chain in the unreduced toxin, accounting for its lack of proteolytic activity, and becomes accessible to the target protein upon reduction of the interchain disulphide (S-S) bridge.

Bt proteolytic activity is zinc-dependent and heavy metal chelators such as ortho-phenantroline, which remove bound zinc, generate inactive apo-neurotoxins. Apo-neurotoxins can reacquire the active site metal atom when incubated in zinc-containing buffers [13]. The biochemical and structural properties of the Bt L-chains define them as a distinct group of metallo-proteases, of unknown evolutionary origin. It has not yet been traced in any of the other known families of these enzymes [13].

SNARE proteins

Once SNARE proteins link together in the SNARE complex they are resistant to Bt proteolysis [51], as one would expect as proteases only attack predominantly unstructured exposed loops. The molecular basis of the specificity of Bt for the three SNAREs is only partially known. The sequences flanking the cleavage sites in each protein do not show a conserved pattern that could account for such specificity. However, a nine residue long motif called the SNARE motif may be involved [52–54]. It is characterized by three carboxylate residues that alternate with hydrophobic and hydrophilic residues. As shown in Fig. 2.3, there are two copies (V1 and V2) of the motif in VAMP and syntaxin and four copies in SNAP-25. The various toxins interact with the SNARE motif in different ways [28].

There are numerous known isoforms of the three SNARE proteins and more will be identified as genome sequencing proceeds. Different SNARE isoforms coexist within the same cell [55], but only some of them are susceptible to proteolysis by Bt. Other SNARE proteins are resistant to Bt because of mutations at the cleavage site and/or in the regions involved in neurotoxin binding [16]. This could account for resistance to Bt in some toxin-naive patients.

Neurotoxicity of botulinum neurotoxins

Injection of Bt into a mammalian striated muscle causes several histological changes [56]. The first pathological sign is that synaptic vesicles accumulate by the cytosolic face of the plasma membrane [57]. This is the immediate consequence of the proteolytic cleavage of the SNARE proteins since synaptic vesicles are no longer able to fuse and discharge their neurotransmitter content. Hence they cluster in direct contact with the plasma membrane.

The nerve remains in anatomical contact with the muscle and there is no apparent loss of motor axons. The motor end plate enlarges, probably because of growth factors released by muscles. Sprouts develop from the end plate itself, from the terminal part of the axon and from adjacent nodes of Ranvier. They grow into the muscle [58,59], as documented in a recent remarkable dynamic analysis of the effect of BtA poisoning of nerve terminals in mice [60]. The number of motor end plates on a single muscle fibre increases, as does the number of fibres innervated by a single motor axon. Moreover, single muscle fibres may become innervated by more than one motor axon [56]. Acetylcholinesterase and ACh receptors spread from the neuromuscular junction to other regions of the muscle plasma membrane.

Following axonal sprouting and reformation of functional nerve–muscle junctions, the muscle eventually regains its normal size. In a second phase, sprouts eventually degenerate and the original end plate regains all its function with normal concentration of acetylcholinesterase and ACh receptors exclusively at the junctions [56,60]. The molecular aspects of this complex process are unknown.

Duration of action

The time to recovery after Bt paralysis varies for different types of nerve terminal and the type of Bt. The entire process typically requires 2–4 months at the human neuromuscular junction, but much longer (>1 years) at the autonomic nervous system [61]. We do not know why there is such a difference. BtA was the first serotype used for human therapy [62] and luckily it is the one that causes the longest-lasting effects in animal studies. The other Bt serotypes are very effective as paralysing agents, but recovery is more rapid, except that BtC is comparable to BtA [63,64]. This parallels the fact that botulism caused by BtA in humans is more dangerous than that caused by BtB and BtE [5], and observations at the rat neuromuscular junction [65–67].

We do not understand the biochemical and cellular basis of the different durations of action of the Bts. Several factors may contribute: (i) the lifetime of the L-chain in the cytosol; (ii) the turnover of the truncated SNARE proteins; (iii) secondary biochemical events triggered by the production of truncated SNARE proteins and/or the released peptides. Toxins may survive and be active in the cell for weeks [68–72]. In theory, toxin-mediated SNARE proteolysis will continue until the last molecule of L-chain is gone. In the laboratory, the truncated SNAP-25 generated by BtA or BtC persists for a long time in chromaffin cells and frog neuromuscular junctions and does indeed continue to interfere with exocytosis [72,73].

Morphology and electrophysiology of synapses poisoned with botulinum toxin

Morphological examination of synapses intoxicated *in vivo* or *in vitro* with Bt does not reveal major structural alterations. Synapses are not swollen, mitochondria, and large electron-dense vesicles are well preserved in terms of number, size and intraterminal distribution. The only consistent change is the increase in the number of synaptic vesicles close to the cytosolic face of the presynaptic membrane [57,74]. BtA poisoning of the frog neuromuscular junction causes the disappearance of the small membrane invagination normally detectable close to the active zones, which are believed to represent small synaptic vesicle fusion events [75].

Electrophysiology

Burgen *et al.* [76] conducted the first electrophysiological investigation of the effect of Bt on neuromuscular junctions in a rat hemidiaphragm preparation. Recent reviews [16,28,77] of Bt effects on a variety of different synaptic terminals suggest that for all serotypes:

(a)   Bt causes a major and persistent blockade of end plate potentials (EPPs) which is responsible for the impaired synaptic transmission at intoxicated synaptic terminals.

(b)   Bt greatly reduces the frequency, but not the amplitude, of evoked miniature end plate potentials (MEPPs). This implies that Bt reduces the number of vesicles capable of undergoing fusion and release, without affecting the ACh quantum (the amount of Ach in each vesicle).

(c)   Bt does not interfere with the processes of neurotransmitter synthesis, uptake and storage [25].

(d)   Bt affects neither the propagation of the nerve impulse nor calcium homeostasis at synaptic terminals [25].

(e)   Spontaneous MEPPs become less frequent, but they are not abolished.

(f)   Giant MEPPs remain just as frequent or even increase at intoxicated neuromuscular junctions.

BtC has been investigated only at central nervous system synapses with results comparable to those obtained with BtA [78], whilst no report is available for BtG.

SYNCHRONY OF QUANTAL RELEASE: TWO TYPES OF BOTULINUM TOXIN ACTION

BtA and BtE poison neuromuscular junctions so that the quantal release of ACh evoked by nerve stimulation remains synchronous. On the other hand, BtB, BtD and BtF desynchronize the quanta released after depolarization. Aminopyridines, by inhibiting potassium channels, indirectly increase the calcium level in the synapse and synchronize evoked neurotransmitter release in BtA and BtE poisoned terminals, leaving the release largely asynchronous in neuromuscular junctions treated with BtB, BtD and BtF [65]. Similar conclusions were reached with calcium ionophores. An increased calcium concentration within the synaptic terminal partially reverses the effect of BtA and BtC, but is relatively ineffective in BtE intoxicated synapses.

Conclusions

These extensive electrophysiological studies suggest that:

1   Bt acts upon components of the synaptic terminal that play essential roles within the neuroexocytosis machinery.

2 Bt types fall into two groups having different targets within the presynaptic terminal. On one side there are BtB, BtD and BtF and on the other side there are BtA, BtC and BtE; identification of their cytosolic targets has now fully substantiated this conclusion (see below).

3 The neurotoxin-impaired neuroexocytosis apparatus can still mediate some spontaneous residual synaptic activity, but with reduced efficiency. Less neurotransmitter is released and the overall process is slower.

Immunology of botulinum neurotoxins [25,79]

Clostridial toxins are large proteins and it is not surprising that they are immunogenic. Tetanus toxin, the cause of tetanus, is the other main clinically important clostridial toxin, and becomes a highly immunogenic vaccine (toxoid) after chemical inactivation with formaldehyde. Perhaps because botulism is much less dangerous than tetanus we know less about the immunogenic properties of Bt in humans—although this may change because of the potential of Bt both as a biological weapon and as a therapy.

General immunological properties of botulinum toxin

Formaldehyde also chemically inactivates Bt to give Bt toxoids that induce type-specific antibodies. Animals, particularly horses, produce high titres of specific antisera when inoculated with native Bt. Anti-Bt antisera can prevent toxicity and speed recovery from botulism, provided that they are injected very soon after poisoning [79]. Many protective anti-Bt antibodies target the Hc binding domain [80–84]. Because it is difficult to prepare complete Bt in heterologous systems, researchers are trying to express and clone the Hc domain of Bt. Purified recombinant Hc domain is non-toxic, competes with Bt for binding and induces the formation of antibodies which prevent neurotoxicity [20]. These various types of antibotulism vaccines have not been extensively studied in humans, but it is clear clinically and in the laboratory that at least BtA is immunogenic. A few patients develop protective antiBtA antibodies, particularly when large therapeutic toxin doses are injected in anatomical regions rich in lymph nodes such as the neck (private communication). Switching to other Bt serotypes may help, particularly with BtB (NeuroBloc®/MYOBLOC™) or BtC [62].

Measuring anti-Bt antibodies [79,84–86]

This is discussed in more detail in Chapter 3. There are two main assay types.

(a) Immunochemical methods that detect the formation of antigen-antibody complexes.

(b) Biological tests of the ability of an antibody or an antiserum to prevent toxicity of native Bt.

Type (a) assays detect both protective and non-protective antiBtA antibodies, with many false positives [85] and sometimes poor sensitivity. Biological assays detect only protective antibodies and do reflect the functional response to Bt. Traditionally, biological assays are performed by injecting groups of mice with the toxin or with varying ratios of toxin-antisera mixtures and watching for symptoms of botulism. These tests are time-consuming and there is growing general concern about using laboratory animals in toxicity tests. More recently, assays with isolated nerve-muscle preparations use fewer animals and give a more quantitative result [20,85]. *In vitro* methods using neurones in culture are not yet reliable enough.

Acknowledgements

Work described in the authors' laboratory is supported by Telethon-Italia grant 1068 and by EU contract BMH4-97 2410.

References

1 Kerner J. Vergiftung durch verdorbene Wurste. *Tubinger Blatter Naturwissenschaften Arzneikunde* 1817; **3**: 1–25.

2 Emergem EV. Ueber einen neuen anaeroben *Bacillus* und seine Beziehungen zum Botulism. Z *Hyg Infekt* 1897; **26**: 1–56.

3 Faber K. Die Pathogenie des Tetanus. *Berl Klin Wochenschr* 1890; **27**: 717–20.

4 Tizzoni G, Cattani G. Uber das Tetanusgift. *Zentralbl Bakt* 1890; **8**: 69–73.

5 Smith LD, Sugiyama H. *Botulism: the organism, its toxins, the disease.* Springfield, IL: CC Thomas Publishers, 1988.

6 Hatheway CL. Botulism. The present status of the disease. *Curr Top Microbiol Immunol* 1995; **195**: 55–75.

7 Feldman RA, Morris JG, Pollard RA. Epidemiologic characteristics of botulism in the United States. In: Lewis GE, ed. *Biomedical Aspects of Botulism.* New York: Academic Press, 1981: 271–84.

8 O'Mahoney M, Mitchell E, Gilbert RJ *et al.* An outbreak of food-borne botulism associated with contaminated hazelnut yoghurt. *Epidemiol Inf* 1990; **104**: 389–95.

9 Stephen J, Pietrowski RA. *Bacterial Toxins.* Walton-on-Thames, Surrey: Nelson, 1981: 1–8.

10 Arnon S. Infant botulism. In: Borriello SP, ed. *Clinical and Molecular Aspects of Anaerobes.* Petersfield, Hants: Wrightson Biomedial Publishing Ltd, 1990: 41–8.

11 Popoff MR, Marvaud JC. Structural and genomic features of clostridial neurotoxins. In: Alouf JE, Freer JH, eds. *The Comprehensive Sourcebook of Bacterial Protein Toxins,* 2nd edn. London: Academic Press, 1999: 174–201.

12 Das Gupta BR. Structures of botulinum neurotoxin, its functional domains and perspectives on the crystalline type A toxin. In: Jankovic, J, Hallett, M, eds. *Therapy with Botulinum toxin.* New York: Marcel Dekker, 1994: 15–39.

13 Schiavo G, Montecucco C. Tetanus and botulism neurotoxins: isolation and assay. *Meth Enzymol* 1995; **248**: 643–52.

14 Maksymowych AB, Simpson LL. Binding and transcytosis of botulinum neurotoxin by polarized human colon carcinoma cells. *J Biol Chem* 1998; **273**: 21950–7.

15 Simpson LL. The origin, structure and pharmacological activity of botulinum toxin. *Pharmacol Rev* 1981; **33**: 155–88.

16 Schiavo G, Matteoli M, Montecucco C. Neurotoxins affecting neuroexocytosis. *Physiol Rev* 2000; **80**: 717–66.

17 Montecucco C, Papini E, Schiavo G. Bacterial protein toxins penetrate cells via a four-step mechanism. *FEBS Lett* 1994; **346**: 92–8.

18 Shone CC, Hambleton P, Melling J. Inactivation of *Clostridium botulinum* type A by trypsin and purification of two tryptic fragments. Proteolytic action near the cross-terminus of the heavy subunit disrupts toxin-binding activity. *Eur J Biochem* 1985; **151**: 75–82.

19 Kozaki S, Ogasawora J, Shimate Y, Kamata Y, Sakaguchi G. Antigenic Structure of *Clostridium botulinum* type B neurotoxin and its interaction with gangliosides, cerebrosides and free fatty acids. *Infect Immun* 1987; **55**: 3051–6.

20 Lalli G, Herreros J, Osborne SL *et al.* Functional characterization of tetanus and botulinum neurotoxins binding domains. *J Cell Sci* 1999; **112**: 2715–24.

21 Lacy DB, Stevens RC. Sequence homology and structural analysis of the clostridial neurotoxins. *J Mol Biol* 1999; **291**: 1091–104.

22 Swaminathan S, Eswaramoorthy S. Structural analysis of the catalytic and binding sites of *Clostridium botulinum* neurotoxin B. *Nat Struct Biol* 2000; **7**: 693–9.

23 Halpern JL, Loftus A. Characterization of the receptor-binding domain of tetanus toxin. *J Biol Chem* 1993; **268**: 11 188–92.

24 Black JD, Dolly JO. Interaction of ^{125}I-labelled botulinum neurotoxins with nerve terminals. II. Autoradiographic evidence for its uptake into motor nerves by acceptor-mediated endocytosis. *J Cell Biol* 1986; **103**: 535–44.

25 Habermann E, Dreyer F. Clostridial neurotoxins, handling and action at the cellular and molecular level. *Curr Top Microbiol Immunol* 1986; **129**: 93–179.

26 Nishiki T, Tokuyama Y, Kamata Y *et al.* The high-affinity binding of *Clostridium botulinum* type B neurotoxin to synaptotagmin II associated with gangliosides GT1b/GD1a. *FEBS Lett* 1996; **378**: 253–7.

27 Halpern JL, Neale EA. Neurospecific binding, internalization, and retrograde axonal transport. *Curr Top Microbiol Immunol* 1995; **195**: 221–41.

28 Rossetto O, Seveso M, Caccin P, Schiavo G, Montecucco C. Tetanus and botulinum neurotoxins: turning bad guys into good by research. *Toxicon* 2001; **39**: 27–41.

29 Jankovic J, Hallett M. *Therapy with Botulinum Toxin.* New York: Marcel Dekker, 1994.

30 Black JD, Dolly JO. Interaction of ^{125}I-labelled botulinum neurotoxins with nerve terminals. *J Cell Biol* 1986; **103**: 521–34.

31 Dolly JO, Black J, Williams RS, Melling J. Acceptors for botulinum neurotoxin reside on motor nerve terminals and mediate its internalization. *Nature* 1984; **307**: 457–60.

32 Niemann H. Molecular biology of clostridial neurotoxins. In: Alouf JE, Freer JH, eds. *Sourcebook of Bacterial Protein Toxins.* London: Academic Press, 1991: 303–48.

33 Cremona O, De Camilli P. Synaptic vesicle endocytosis. *Curr Opin Neurobiol* 1997; **7**: 323–30.

34 Hughes R, Whaler BC. Influence of nerve-endings activity and of drugs on the rate of paralysis of rat diaphragm preparations by *Clostridium botulinum* type A toxin. *J Physiol (London)* 1962; **160**: 221–33.

35 Blasi J, Chapman ER, Link E *et al.* Botulinum neurotoxin selectively cleaves the synaptic protein SNAP-25. *Nature* 1993; **365**: 160–3.

36 Shone CC, Hambleton P, Melling J. A 50 kDa fragment from NH$_2$-terminus of the heavy subunit of *Clostridium botulinum* type A neurotoxin forms channels in lipid vesicles. *Eur J Biochem* 1987; **167**: 175–80.

37 Simpson LL, Coffield JA, Bakry N. Inhibition of vacuolar adenosine triphosphatase antagonizes the effects of clostridial neurotoxins but not phospholipase A2 neurotoxins. *J Pharmacol Exp Ther* 1994; **269**: 256–62.

38 Montecucco C, Schiavo G, Dasgupta BR. Effect of pH on the interaction of botulinum neurotoxins A, B and E with liposomes. *Biochem J* 1989; **259**: 47–53.

39 Hoch DH, Romero Mira M, Ehrlich BE *et al.* Channels formed by botulinum, tetanus, and diphtheria

toxins in planar lipid bilayers: relevance to translocation of proteins across membranes. *Proc Natl Acad Sci USA* 1985; **82**: 1692–6.

40 Boquet P, Duflot E. Tetanus toxin fragment forms channels in lipid vesicles at low pH. *Proc Natl Acad Sci USA* 1982; **79**: 7614–8.

41 Beise J, Hahnen J, Andersen Beckh B, Dreyer F. Pore formation by tetanus toxin, its chain and fragments in neuronal membranes and evaluation of the underlying motifs in the structure of the toxin molecule. *Naunyn Schmiedebergs Arch Pharmacol* 1994; **349**: 66–73.

42 de Paiva A, Dolly JO. Light-chain of botulinum, neurotoxin is active in mammalian nerve terminals when delivered by liposomes. *FEBS Lett* 1990; **277**: 171–4.

43 Sutton RB, Fasshauer D, Jahn R, Brunger AT. Crystal structure of a SNARE complex involved in synaptic. *Nature* 1998; **395**: 347–53.

44 Chen YA, Scales SJ, Patel SM, Doung YC, Scheller RH. SNARE complex formation is triggered by Ca^{2+} and drives membrane fusion. *Cell* 1999; **97**: 165–74.

45 Schiavo G, Benfenati F, Poulain B *et al.* Tetanus and botulinum B neurotoxins block neurotransmitter release by proteolytic cleavage of synaptobrevin. *Nature* 1992; **359**: 832–5.

46 Blasi J, Chapman ER, Yamasaki S, *et al.* Botulinum neurotoxin C1 blocks neurotransmitter release by means of cleaving HPC-1/syntaxin. *Embo J* 1993; **12**: 4821–8.

47 Blasi J, Chapman ER, Link E *et al.* Botulinum neurotoxin A selectively cleaves the synaptic protein SNAP-25. *Nature* 1993; **365**: 160–3.

48 Schiavo G, Santucci A, Dasgupta BR *et al.* Botulinum neurotoxins serotypes A and E cleave SNAP-25 at distinct COOH-terminal peptide bonds. *FEBS Lett* 1993; **335**: 99–103.

49 Schiavo G, Poulain B, Rossetto O *et al.* Tetanus toxin is a zinc protein and its inhibition of neurotransmitter release and protease activity depend on zinc. *EMBO J* 1992; **11**: 3577–83.

50 Li L, Binz T, Niemann H, Singh BR. Probing the mechanistic role of glutamate residue in the zinc-binding motif of type A botulinum neurotoxin light-chain. *Biochemistry* 2000; **39**: 2399–405.

51 Hayashi T, McMahon H, Yamasaki S *et al.* Synaptic vesicle membrane fusion complex: action of clostridial neurotoxins on assembly. *EMBO J* 1994; **13**: 5051–61.

52 Rossetto O, Schiavo G, Montecucco C *et al.* SNARE motif and neurotoxins. *Nature* 1994; **372**: 415–6.

53 Pellizzari R, Rossetto O, Lozzi L *et al.* Structural determinants of the specificity for synaptic vesicle-associated membrane protein/synaptobrevin of tetanus and botulinum type B and G neurotoxins. *J Biol Chem* 1996; **271**: 20 353–8.

54 Vaidyanathan VV, Yoshino K, Jahnz M *et al.* Proteolysis of SNAP-25 isoforms by botulinum neurotoxin types A, C, and E. domains and amino acid residues controlling the formation of enzyme-substrate complexes and cleavage. *J Neurochem* 1999; **72**: 327–37.

55 Bock JB, Scheller RH. SNARE proteins mediate lipid bilayer fusion. *Proc Natl Acad Sci U S A* 1999; **96**: 12 227–9.

56 Borodic GE, Ferrante RJ, Perace LB, Alderson K. Pharmacology and histology of the therapeutic application of botulinum toxin. In: Jankovic, J, Hallet, M, eds. *Therapy with botulinum toxin*. New York: Marcel Dekker, 1994: 119–57.

57 Neale EA, Bowers LM, Jia M, Bateman KE, Williamson LC. Botulinum neurotoxin A blocks synaptic vesicle exocytosis but not endocytosis at the nerve terminal. *J Cell Biol* 1999; **147**: 1249–60.

58 Angaut Petit D, Molgo J, Comella JX, Faille L, Tabti N. Terminal sprouting in mouse neuromuscular junctions poisoned with botulinum type A toxin. morphological and electrophysiological features. *Neurosci* 1990; **37**: 799–808.

59 Comella JX, Molgo J, Faille L. Sprouting of mammalian motor nerve terminals induced by *in vivo* injection of botulinum type-D toxin and the functional recovery of paralysed neuromuscular junctions. *Neurosci Lett* 1993; **153**: 61–4.

60 de Paiva A, Meunier FA, Molgo J, Aoki KR, Dolly JO. Functional repair of motor end plates after

botulinum neurotoxin type A poisoning: Biphasic switch of synaptic activity between nerve sprouts and their parent terminals. *Proc Natl Acad Sci USA* 1999; **96**: 3200–5.

61 Naumann M, Jost WH, Toyka KV. Botulinum toxin in the treatment of neurological disorders of the autonomic nervous system. *Arch Neurol* 1999; **56**: 914–6.

62 Schantz EJ, Johnson EA. Botulinum toxin. The story of its development for the treatment of human disease. *Perspect Biol Med* 1997; **40**: 317–27.

63 Eleopra R, Tugnoli V, Rossetto O, Montecucco C, De Grandis D. Botulinum neurotoxin serotype C. A novel effective botulinum toxin therapy in human. *Neurosci Lett* 1997; **224**: 91–4.

64 Eleopra R, Tugnoli V, Rossetto O, De Grandis D, Montecucco C. Different time courses of recovery after poisoning with botulinum neurotoxin serotypes A and E in humans. *Neurosci Lett* 1998; **256**: 135–8.

65 Molgo J, Dasgupta BR, Thesleff S. Characterization of the actions of botulinum neurotoxin type E at the rat neuromuscular junction. *Acta Physiol Scand* 1989; **137**: 497–501.

66 Sellin LC, Kauffman JA, Dasgupta BR. Comparison of the effects of botulinum neurotoxin types A and E at the rat neuromuscular junction. *Med Biol* 1983; **61**: 120–5.

67 Kauffman JA, Way JF Jr, Siegel LS, Sellin LC. Comparison of the action of types A and F botulinum toxin at the rat neuromuscular junction. *Toxicol Appl Pharmacol* 1985; **79**: 211–7.

68 Habig WH, Bigalke H, Bergey GK *et al.* Tetanus toxin in dissociated spinal cord cultures. Long-term characterization of form and action. *J Neurochem* 1986; **47**: 930–7.

69 Marxen P, Bigalke H. Tetanus and botulinum A toxins inhibit stimulated F-actin rearrangement in chromaffin cells. *Neuroreport* 1991; **2**: 33–6.

70 Bartels F, Bergel H, Bigalke H *et al.* Specific antibodies against the Zn^{2+}-binding domain of clostridial neurotoxins restore exocytosis in chromaffin cells treated with tetanus or botulinum A neurotoxin. *J Biol Chem* 1994; **269**: 8122–7.

71 Keller JE, Neale EA, Oyler G, Adler M. Persistence of botulinum neurotoxin action in cultured spinal cord cells. *FEBS Lett* 1999; **456**: 137–42.

72 O'Sullivan GA, Mohammed N, Foran PG, Lawrence GW, Oliver Dolly J. Rescue of exocytosis in botulinum toxin A-poisoned chromaffin cells by expression of cleavage-resistant SNAP-25. Identification of the minimal essential C-terminal residues. *J Biol Chem* 1999; **274**: 36897–904.

73 Raciborska DA, Charlton MP. Retention of cleaved synaptosome-associated protein of 25 kDa (SNAP-25) in neuromuscular junctions: a new hypothesis to explain persistence of botulinum A poisoning. *Can J Physiol Pharmacol* 1999; **77**: 679–88.

74 Osen Sand A, Staple JK, Naldi E *et al.* Common and distinct fusion proteins in axonal growth and transmitter release. *J Comp Neurol* 1996; **367**: 222–34.

75 Pumplin DW, Reese TS. Action of brown widow spider venom and botulinum toxin on the frog neuromuscular junction examined with the freeze-fracture technique. *J Physiol Lond* 1977; **273**: 443–57.

76 Burgen ASV, Dickens F, Zatman LJ. The action of botulinum toxin on the neuromuscular junction. *J Physiol (London)* 1949; **109**: 10–24.

77 Humeau Y, Doussau F, Grant NJ, Poulain B. How botulinum and tetanus neurotoxins block neuro-transmitter release. *Biochimie* 2000; **82**: 427–46.

78 Capogna M, McKinney RA, O'Connor V, Gahwiler BH, Thompson SM. Ca^{2+} or Sr^{2+} partially rescues synaptic transmission in hippocampal cultures treated with botulinum toxin A and C but not tetanus toxin. *J Neurosci* 1997; **17**: 7190–202.

79 Middlebrook JL, Brown JE. Immunodiagnosis and immunotherapy of tetanus and botulinum neurotoxins. *Curr Top Microbiol Immunol* 1995; **195**: 89–122.

80 Atassi MZ, Dolimbek BZ, Hayakari M *et al.* Mapping of the antibody-binding regions on botulinum neurotoxin H-chain domain 855–1296 with antitoxin antibodies from three host species. *J Prot Chem* 1996; **15**: 691–700.

81 Oshima M, Hayakari M, Middlebrook JL, Atassi MZ. Immune recognition of botulinum neurotoxin

type A. Regions recognized by T cells and antibodies against the protective HC fragment (residues 855–1296) of the toxin. *Mol Immunol* 1997; **34**: 1031–40.

82 Rosenberg JS, Middlebrook JL, Atassi MZ. Localization of the regions on the C-terminal domain of the heavy-chain of botulinum A recognized by T lymphocytes and by antibodies after immunization of mice with pentavalent toxoid. *Immunol Invest* 1997; **26**: 491–504.

83 Kubota T, Watanabe T, Yokosawa N *et al*. Epitope regions in the heavy-chain of *Clostridium botulinum* type E neurotoxin recognized by monoclonal antibodies. *Appl Env Microbiol* 1997; **63**: 1214–8.

84 Pless DD, Torres ER, Reinke EK, Bavari S. High-affinity, protective antibodies to the binding domain of botulinum neurotoxin type A. *Infect Immun* 2001; **69**: 570–4.

85 Goschel H, Wohlfarth K, Frevert J, Dengler R, Bigalke H. Botulinum A toxin therapy. Neutralizing and non-neutralizing antibodies: therapeutic consequences. *Exp Neurol* 1997; **147**: 96–102.

86 Dressier D, Dimberger G, Bathia KP *et al*. Botulinum toxin antibody testing: comparison between the mouse protection assay and the mouse lethality assay. *Mov Disord* 2000; **15**: 973–6.

CHAPTER 3

General and clinical aspects of treatment with botulinum toxin

PETER MOORE & MARKUS NAUMANN

General and clinical aspects

Since botulinum toxin (Bt) became available for clinical use in the late 1980s there has been a steady stream of new indications and involvement of new specialities. Botulinum toxin A (BtA) is now a recognized treatment for a wide spectrum of conditions characterized by relative overactivity of one or a few muscles, and the recently launched type B toxin (BtB) may follow suit. Since the first edition of this book, triallists have also harnessed the autonomic effects of BtA to treat hypersalivation and excessive sweating. Some indications for BtA/BtB treatment are now fully licensed, and advances in techniques and new uses are still appearing regularly. There has been a pattern of anecdotal reports of benefit in a new indication followed by multiple small, uncontrolled or open studies, and eventually controlled and blinded trials appear and are duly summarized in systematic reviews, for instance in the Cochrane Library [1,2]. This process has been fastest in easily defined situations, such as cervical dystonia and focal hyperhidrosis, and much slower in more complex fields such as rehabilitation.

Evaluate potential new uses cautiously. It is easier to demonstrate technical efficacy such as weakening of overactive muscles than to prove real benefit for the patient. The literature contains many anecdotal reports of successful treatment in small numbers of patients. Uncritical initial enthusiasm creates an atmosphere inhibiting or delaying adequate controlled trials in a new indication. Some reports inevitably prove unfounded, and the benefits claimed turn out to be illusory—not least because intramuscular treatment with a potent neurotoxin is likely to have a significant placebo effect [3].

Side-effects are generally transient and acceptable, but some may be dangerous, and licensing authorities have hesitated to allow unrestricted use of the toxin. Factors that may have delayed licensing include a lack of long-term animal and human toxicity studies. The perceived high cost of Bt treatment has undoubtedly slowed wider acceptance, and this perception will only change if well-conducted pharmacoeconomic studies are sufficiently persuasive. However, purchasers should realize that in many situations a single injection session every 3 or 4 months may replace or reduce the daily dose of other medications and reduce nursing costs, with better symptom control or fewer side-effects. Therefore, Bt treatment may well be cost effective.

Expert panels began to disseminate guidelines to acceptable practice a decade ago [4,5], although these are not currently reinforced by any legislation. Strictly speaking, a large amount of expert practice with Bt remains 'off-licence' and unproven. Where relevant we tell patients and carers that treatment with Bt is off-licence or is experimental, and they must accept this. We always obtain signed consent before starting any course of Bt treatment. Any doctors wishing to treat patients for unlicensed indications should clarify the legal position in their country and institution. However, the fact that an indication is licensed does not absolve the doctor from blame if complications occur.

Principles of clinical use

We nowadays use Bt in a wide variety of conditions in which there is focal muscle overactivity and in some autonomic disturbances (see Chapter 1). In clinical use, we usually inject Bt intramuscularly into carefully selected muscles or glands. Its effect is concentrated in the injected muscles/glands so that it is possible to generate highly focal weakness or suppression of glandular secretion.

Bt takes effect gradually after several days to weeks, and causes clinically detectable weakness and muscle atrophy for 2–4 months in most situations, sometimes rather longer. It wears off gradually. The degree and to some extent duration of weakness are dose-dependent. Until recently it was thought that the concentration of Bt was less critical [6], but new evidence suggests that for BtA (Dysport®) at least there may be an optimum concentration [7]. The weakened muscles always recover if left long enough. Repeat injections follow the same course though biological tolerance can occur.

Bt is rarely a cure. It is a symptomatic treatment and is likely to need repeating at regular intervals. Fortunately, unless toxin neutralizing antibodies intervene, muscles continue to respond just as well to BtA after multiple injections over several years [8]. In some conditions, such as focal dystonias, it may be sufficient treatment; in others it is one component of a wider programme of treatment which clinicians should not neglect. For instance, in spasticity the best effects of Bt treatment may only obtain when it is combined with physiotherapy and splinting—and vice versa [9,10].

Main mechanism of action (Fig. 3.1)

Bt works by causing chemical denervation of structures served by peripheral cholinergic neurones. It selectively inactivates these nerve terminals by blocking the release of acetylcholine. Its most important effect is at the neuromuscular junction (see Chapter 2) where it causes muscle weakness and atrophy. Bt also influences autonomic function by blocking sympathetic and parasympathetic ganglion cells, and postganglionic parasympathetic and cholinergic sympathetic neurones. Bt does not kill neurones; rather, it produces a temporary and ultimately reversible blockade of cholinergic transmission.

Injecting Bt directly into overactive muscles produces controlled, selective and temporary weakness. The lower motorneurone is the final common pathway transmitting excess efferent activity to the muscle, and the source of the excess traffic is different in each disorder treated. *True* overactivity may originate from central nervous system disease as in focal dystonia or spasticity, or from cranial nerve or peripheral nervous system disease. Sometimes there is merely *relative* overactivity with failure to suppress contraction of the antagonists of a paralysed muscle (e.g. in sixth nerve palsy). Occasionally there is *no* muscle overactivity and Bt is given to block normal function, for instance to produce a protective ptosis.

In most situations Bt acts mainly by causing muscle paralysis and clinical improvement correlates best with the degree of weakness induced [4]. In some disorders other mechanisms may be important, either directly or indirectly.

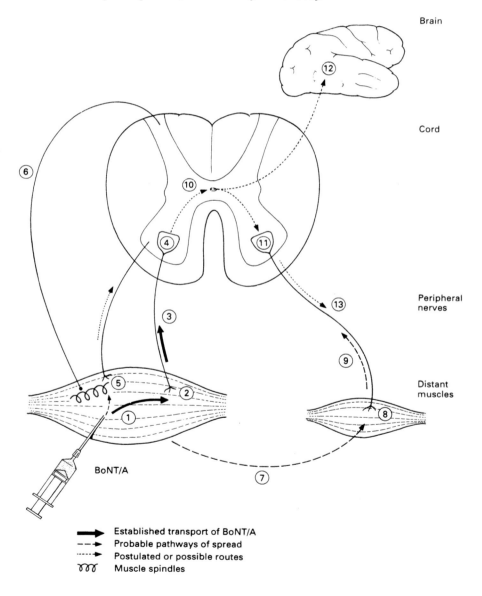

Other possible mechanisms of action

At the molecular level

Bt acts at the molecular level by selectively cleaving proteins involved in the SNARE (**SNA**p [**s**oluble **N**-ethyl-maleimide sensitive factor **a**ttachment protein] **rec**eptor) complex. The SNARE complex is essential for the release of synaptic vesicles from the nerve terminal. It orchestrates docking and fusion of vesicles to the presynaptic membrane. Different toxin serotypes cleave different proteins within the complex. BtA cleaves SNAP-25, and BtB damages synaptobrevin (see Chapter 2). The most obvious effect is on 'regulated' exocytosis, the calcium-dependent release of synaptic vesicles in response to electrical depolarization.

Although SNARE proteins are concentrated in the plasma membrane of the nerve terminal they are found elsewhere in the cell. Thus, theoretically, Bt could act directly

◀—————————————————————————————————

Fig. 3.1 Botulinum toxin (Bt): where it goes and what it does. The Bts do not normally cross the blood–brain barrier.

Established pathway: Bt is injected into the muscle and diffuses (1) to the synapse between nerve and muscle where it is taken up into the cholinergic nerve terminal (2). It is transported axonally (3) to the ipsilateral anterior horn cell (4). The figure does not show the analogous Bt flows to cholinergic autonomic nerve terminals.

Probable pathways: (a) Bt diffuses through muscle to the intrafusal gamma-efferent motor nerve terminal (5) within the muscle spindle. (b) Diffusion through the muscle fascia and haematogenous spread (7) carry Bt to distant muscles (8) where it is scavenged by cholinergic neurones and presumably carried proximally by axonal transport (9).

Possible or postulated pathways: Trans-synaptic passage within the spinal cord (10) to the contralateral anterior horn cells at the same segmental level (11) and rostral or caudal spread to other segments or even the brain (12). Anterograde axonal spread to distant muscles (13) has also been suggested.

Point on diagram	Location of toxin	Proposed mechanism of action
(2)	Cholinergic nerve terminal (muscle or autonomic)	Weakness Direct blockade of cholinergic stimulation of secretion
(3)	Cholinergic axon	? Other, e.g. axon growth
(4)	Anterior horn cell	? Other
(5)	Gamma-efferent nerve terminal (spindles)	Reduce reflexes (6)
(8)	Distant NMJ and spindles	? Weakness ? Reduce reflexes
(10)	Spinal cord	? Reduce reflexes
(12)	Brain	? Alter central program indirectly ? Neuronal plasticity

NMJ, neuromuscular junction.

through mechanisms other than blockade of regulated acetylcholine release and could impair other cell functions. For instance, SNAP-25 also plays a part in 'constitutive' exocytosis. This differs from regulated exocytosis in being independent of electrical depolarization, and is used by cells for protein secretion (e.g. of growth factors) and for insertion of newly formed protein components into the plasmalemma [11]. Blocking expression of SNAP-25 has been shown to impair axonal growth in chick retinal neurones [12], although this may involve a different isoform of SNAP-25.

Effects on nearby and distant motorneurones

Bt spreads through tissue planes to adjacent muscle fibres and *nearby* muscles, presumably by diffusion. In theory, Bt is more poisonous to neuromuscular junctions serving the most actively contracting fibres, so that if only part of a muscle complex is involved in involuntary activity, that section is more likely to be affected [13], a kind of autofocusing.

There is strong evidence from single-fibre electromyography (EMG) of systemic spread of a small amount of toxin to *distant* muscles, with widespread abnormalities of jitter following focal BtA injections [14,15]. In health BtA does not cross the blood–brain barrier and thus haematogenous spread to the central nervous system is unlikely. There is no evidence that BtA has any direct central actions in human use, but after intramuscular injection there is rapid retrograde axonal transport of BtA to ipsilateral spinal anterior horn cells [16], and BtA is also found in the corresponding contralateral spinal cord segment. This raises the possibility of *trans*-synaptic transfer within the cord and passage to other spinal segments. Anterograde axonal transport of toxin within the lower motorneurones might then affect their presynaptic function [17]. However, the time course of EMG changes is compatible with spread either via intra-axonal transport and cord transfer, or haematogenous spread and highly efficient scavenging and uptake of BtA at the distant neuromuscular junction [17]. Subsequent anterograde passage of toxin could thus take it to spinal cord structures contralateral to the injected site.

Alteration of reflex and central activity

Patients with focal dystonias may find their involuntary movements are completely suppressed by Bt and yet the equivalent voluntary action is in part preserved. Spasticity may subside in muscles far away from those injected. The benefit seems out of proportion to the induced weakness [18]. What mechanisms could explain this? Would they contribute to benefits seen in other conditions?

First, Bt toxicity may focus on the most active cholinergic neurones (see above). This would preferentially weaken the most affected fibres, with significant preservation of strength in other fibres. Second, there could be direct or indirect changes to reflex or other central activity, either through alteration of traffic in stable circuits or changes in the circuitry itself via neuronal plasticity.

How could Bt affect the gain of reflexes? *Indirectly*, weakening a muscle will alter the length-tension relationships seen in both active and passive contraction and this could alter reflex gain. Reduction in the power and amplitude of involuntary movements is likely to reduce pain and other sensory stimuli that commonly reinforce excessive reflex activity.

Bt could *directly* alter reflex gain through its peripheral action if it produced differential weakening of intrafusal (spindle) and somatic muscle fibres. The γ-motorneurone efferents to muscle spindles are cholinergic and are blocked by BtA in the same way as the α-motorneurones to somatic muscle fibres [19]. This should act to diminish muscle spindle afferent output, which in turn would reduce α-motorneurone drive. Blocking muscle afferents with lidocaine (lignocaine) does indeed reduce vibration-induced dystonia [20].

In rats, injection of BtA into the masseter reduces muscle spindle afferent discharge from jaw muscles even before there is any detectable weakness [21]. A similar decrease in afferent discharge and stretch sensitivity was found in extraocular eye muscles [22]. Thus BtA may act in part by changing the sensitivity of the reflex arc. It is possible that remote spread of small amounts of toxin to distant muscle spindles contributes to this effect even with no detectable distant weakness.

The transfer of BtA to the spinal cord suggests a theoretical possibility of a direct central action to decrease motorneurone excitability or enhance presynaptic inhibition. Animal studies have shown that injecting BtA directly into the spinal cord can alter cord function. It blocks the recurrent cholinergic inhibition of motorneurones that is mediated by Renshaw cells [23], a change that would *increase* reflex muscle activity. However, this is a highly unphysiological method of applying BtA and the distribution of toxin within the cord is unlikely to reflect 'naturally' occurring spread of BtA.

There may be other, disease-specific, mechanisms of action. The action-specific provocation of many focal dystonias and the obvious value of sensory tricks in stabilizing dystonic movements suggest factors that Bt might influence. Bt could modulate reflex activity evoking these clinical features. Clinical studies of the effect of BtA on reflex abnormalities in focal dystonia have indeed uncovered evidence that BtA induces central changes, but have not clarified whether this is a direct or indirect effect. For instance, BtA may reduce the amplitude of central components of the long-loop reflex in cervical dystonia [24]. Bt sometimes alters the patterns of muscle activation, with recruitment of new muscles to replace those weakened by Bt, probably by central reprogramming [25]. In dystonia there is abnormal cocontraction of agonist and antagonist muscles, often attributed to failure of reciprocal inhibition, and there are abnormalities of intracortical inhibition. BtA can normalize both reciprocal inhibition [26] and intracortical inhibition [27]. Transcranial magnetic stimulation shows that in dystonia there is enlargement of the cerebral cortical areas representing individual muscles, and after BtA these areas temporarily become more normal, also compatible with an increase in cortical inhibition [28].

Prolonged benefit

In most situations any benefit from Bt lasts only as long as the muscle paralysis. Occasionally there is much more prolonged benefit, suggesting that other mechanisms are operating. Dystonias may die down for a year or more: this may be due to a coincident remission. Following acute correction of squint, binocular fusion mechanisms may be sufficiently powerful to maintain binocular vision even when the toxin-induced weakness has cleared, especially if there is even a partial recovery of lateral rectus function (see Chapter 16).

Early treatment of spasticity could in theory break a cycle of spasm, pain, fibrosis and contracture and influence remodelling of central circuits. It certainly assists physiotherapy by making it easier to manipulate limbs and retrain antagonists, and allows more comfortable and better tolerated splinting. In children with spastic diplegia the timely use of BtA may tide a child over a period of evolving spastic deformity and contracture and prevent the development of unfavourable patterns of muscle activity (see Chapter 11).

There is evidence that peripheral mechanical factors such as the compliance of the muscle-tendon complex may be important contributors to spasticity [29]. In early studies using the hereditary spastic rat, Cosgrove injected BtA into the gastrocnemius muscle of infant rats *before* they developed spasticity. They showed convincingly that BtA blocked the development of the expected biomechanical changes of spasticity, of overall shortening of the muscle-tendon unit and of increase in the tendon : muscle ratio [30]. Note that this experiment was in growing rats and perhaps informs human paediatric practice more than adult medicine, but it does suggest the possibility of a therapeutic window early in the development of spasticity, even in adults.

Temporary weakness may be an advantage in dystonia

Dystonia is probably caused by abnormal execution of motor programs, and this idea is consistent with the results from surgical series. When muscles are weakened by nerve root section the dystonia sometimes recurs after an interval, perhaps because the brain adapts and provokes the movement through different muscles. One of the strengths of treatment with Bt may lie in the very fact that it wears off, and the fluctuating course may prevent adaptation of the motor program. In addition, when repeat injections are given there is the opportunity to modify the pattern of injection to paralyse newly recruited muscles.

Recovery from botulinum toxin poisoning

The fate of the toxin molecule within the cell is not known. Recovery of function within nerve terminals presumably depends on the rate at which the toxin is cleared from or metabolized by nerve endings, and the rate at which the nerve cells replace damaged

SNARE proteins [31]. New SNARE protein must be synthesized in the cell body and transported down the axon to the nerve terminals.

Single injection cycle

Although acetylcholine release is blocked, the nerve terminals and neuromuscular junctions do not disappear [32–35]. New motor nerve axon terminals begin to sprout within 2–4 days and form synaptic contacts [36, 37] within 1–2 weeks, reaching a peak at 5–10 weeks [35, 38]. By day 28 the sprouts, but not the parent terminals, can activate the muscle. They contain the necessary SNARE proteins and are clearly functional synapses [39]. Over the next 4 weeks the parent terminals begin to recover and the sprouts regress and become less active. At three months the parent terminals look and may be functioning normally again [39].

Repeated injection cycles

The morphological effects of repeated injections of BtA have been studied in human orbicularis oculi. BtA produced cumulative changes in the pattern of innervation. The relative abundance of sprouts increased with the total number of injections, with a profusion of unmyelinated axonal sprouts that ended blindly. Individual motor axons innervated an increased number of muscle fibres. Thin, unmyelinated axonal collaterals were in contact with muscle end plates. There were multiple end plates on individual muscle fibres and a greater range of end plate sizes. The axonal sprouts seemed able to form new end plates and single muscle fibres may become innervated at separate sites by more than one axon [40]. The muscle fibres themselves eventually recover if BtA injections cease, and they do not show permanent histological changes [41].

Repeated BtA treatments also produce cumulative histological changes in *distant* muscles. The effects of these presumably low doses may focus more on some fibre types than others, as shown by fibre atrophy in muscle biopsies from vastus lateralis after 2–4 years treatment for cervical dystonia. BtA increased the frequency of atrophic type IIB fibres, and reduced the size of type IIA fibres [42]. After periorbital injections in humans, the low doses of BtA reaching extraocular muscles appeared to affect fibres controlling static alignment (which are served by single neurones) more than those serving saccades. After a higher dose in systemic botulism all fibre types were affected [43].

Health and safety

Terminology and doses: a health warning

It is essential that clinicians using Bt are aware that there has been much confusion over doses and units of potency of Bt, and sometimes over the names of the manufacturers and the commercially available preparations. Many patients, relatives, administrative and paramedical staff and even doctors remain dangerously muddled.

In the early literature it was usual to quote doses in nanograms of toxin-haemagglutinin complex. When a second preparation of toxin became available attempts were made to standardize on a unit of biological potency. The standard unit of potency used for all three preparations is now derived from a biological mouse assay. In this assay 1 iu, or mouse unit (mu, or U), of Bt is the amount that kills 50% of a group of mice when injected intraperitoneally (LD50 or mouse lethality test).

Unfortunately, the mouse unit assays used by the manufacturers of the three commercially available formulations of Bt seem to produce incompatible results, as shown in Table 3.1 (below). These differences may reflect species differences, the use of different bioassay procedures or differences in diffusion or other formulation characteristics.

Dose equivalence: potency, side-effects and antibody generation

There is considerable variation in response to Bt in many disorders, with some patients deemed to need seven times as much as others [44], some patients unable to tolerate the optimal dose, and others whose best dose depends heavily on optimal muscle selection and hence the experience of the injector. This heterogeneity is one factor that has made it difficult to compare different Bt preparations to establish potency and adverse effect ratios.

Some observers have challenged the whole concept of clinically usable ratios [45,46], and simply recommend that clinicians switching patients between preparations should establish where the current dose lies within the range for the particular indication being treated and use an equivalent dose for the alternate product [46]. Nevertheless, this still implies a ratio, and a ratio is an attractive concept to drug companies wishing to persuade clinicians that their preparation is more cost effective, and convenient for clinicians who are converting patients for whatever reason. The danger is that ratios may give false reassurance of clinical dose equivalence. In addition, the tests used ignore smooth muscle and autonomic effects.

In vitro or animal studies to compare potencies of different formulations of Bt are interesting [45,47], though it may be hazardous to apply the results to human use of Bt [46,48]. In humans, expert opinion gave valuable early clues, but anecdotes and small or uncontrolled studies risk misleading results. Controlled studies to compare the preparations have mainly followed a strategy of picking a potency ratio, testing it in a clinical trial (usually in cervical dystonia), and when no statistical difference is found, implying dose equivalence at that ratio [49–52]. Unfortunately, such conclusions are an abuse of the null hypothesis and the strategy has inevitably 'demonstrated' equivalence for a wide range of ratios.

In comparisons between Botox® and Dysport® such chosen ratios vary between 1 : 1 [53] and 1 : 8 [54]. Occasional studies suggest that one preparation is superior at the chosen ratio, generating more weakness or lasting longer [55,56]. These types of

Table 3.1 Comparison between available preparations of Botulinum toxin (Bt). Note that all preparations contain some human albumen. Dose equivalences are approximate and remain under review. Simplistic use of conversion factors can be dangerous: see text for details, pp. 35–40.

Preparation	Botox®	Dysport®	Neurobloc®/ MYOBLOC™
Serotype	A	A	B
Manufacturer	Allergan Ltd (US)	Ipsen (UK) (formerly Porton and then Speywood)	Elan/Athena (US)
Relative potency per mu*	3–5	1	0.01–0.02
Equivalent dose (mu)*	1	3–4	50–100
Contents of one vial (mu)	100 mu	500 mu	2500; 5000; 10 000 mu
1 ng toxin- haemagglutinin	20 mu	40 mu	100 (70–130) mu
Protein load/dose†	5 ng in 100 mu	12.5 ng in 500 mu	100 ng in 10 000 mu
Presentation	Powder Reconstitute with 0.9% saline	Powder Reconstitute with 0.9% saline	Liquid 5000 mu/mL Can be diluted with 0.9% saline
Shelf life unopened (from the date of manufacture)	24 months	12 months	21 months
Stored at	2–8°C	2–8°C	2–8°C or room temperature
Shelf life opened/reconstituted, if aseptic technique	4 h	8 h	4 h
Refrigerate at	2–8°C	2–8°C	2–8°C or room temperature

Data from manufacturers except: *Authors' estimate. †Manufacturer's recommended dose for cervical dystonia.

comparison do not generate confidence intervals for ratios of potency, risk of side-effects or development of antitoxin antibody, nor can they examine factors that might influence the ratios for individual patients. Meta-analysis is impossible, so opinion is swayed by the number of trials reporting a particular ratio—which depends on the number of trials performed at that ratio.

Occasional open label studies have compared Botox® and Dysport® doses required to optimize benefit over several injections and reported Botox® : Dysport® equivalence ratios of 1.0 : 2.86 [57] and 1.0 : 5.3–6.0 [58].

It remains possible that the ratios vary between patients and depend also on the condition being treated, toxin dilution, etc. Overall, however, at equipotent doses the two preparations of BtA have qualitatively and quantitatively similar clinical efficacies and side-effects. For the common indications of cervical dystonia, hemifacial spasm and blepharospasm the Botox® : Dysport® ratio is probably between 1 : 3 and 1 : 5. To date the manufacturers have adjusted their prices so that effective treatment costs are similar.

The relative clinical potency of BtB is under active investigation, and the ratio given in Table 3.1 derives from expert opinion and from indirect comparisons in cervical dystonia using mainly historical controls. It is only an approximate guide, and the quoted ratio may turn out not to apply to all the diseases likely to be treated with BtB. Direct randomized controlled comparisons are under way using a format similar to the comparisons between BtA toxins. Just as for the early comparisons between BtA preparations, experts exploring off-label indications for BtB will provide more or less scientifically based estimates of the dose ranges in these other disorders, to be tested in more formal studies. Non-experts should beware that simple conversions using a dose ratio are risky.

At the time of writing (2002) the Movement Disorder Society is considering creating a website containing dose recommendations for different muscles and diseases. The aim would be to show the latest consensus on doses, and it would provide an excellent independent resource available world-wide. The American WeMove organization has posted Elan's guidelines for BtB doses based on expert recommendations, and will no doubt update this regularly (http://www.wemove.org).

When reading the literature clinicians must take great care to establish which preparation is under discussion as it could be disastrous to use the wrong dose schedule. At least one study using Dysport® has used the term 'Botox' as a generic term for BtA [59]. Similar misuse of the convenient word 'Botox' is widespread, and is sloppy and dangerous. It will probably be applied even to BtB. In practice many clinics become familiar with one preparation so that confusion is less likely. Unfortunately, other clinics use all three preparations, giving plenty of scope for errors. It is particularly important that clinicians (and patients) switching preparations or moving to other clinics understand the issue. In this book contributors make it clear which preparation they have been using. They quote doses for that preparation and give conversion factors or doses where possible, or refer to published guidelines.

Safety considerations for staff and patients

Vials of Bt available for clinical use contain relatively low quantities of toxin, and physicians probably do not need immunization with botulinum toxoid [60]. The toxin is not infectious, inflammable or volatile, but in theory mists or aerosols may form and cause dangerous exposure. In practice this does not seem to be a problem. It would be interesting to know whether experienced injectors develop antitoxin antibodies and become re-

Table 3.2 Botulinum toxin A/B (BtA/B) preparations: approximate dose and toxicity comparisons. For Dysport® the animal toxicity and human food poisoning data are calculated as three times the Botox® doses. Figures for NeuroBloc® are for 2002, and may evolve.

	BtA Botox®	BtA Dysport®	BtB NeuroBloc®
Primate — systemic injection			
LD50 (mu/kg)	30–40	90–120	
Lethal dose (mu/kg)			2400
Human — food poisoning			
Mild (mu)	3500	10000	
Severe (mu)	3000–30000	30000–90000	
Human — systemic injection			
Maximum tolerated dose*			
Adults 70 kg (mu)			135000
Children 36 kg (mu)			60000
Cervical dystonia			
Typical dose (mu)	100–200	350–700	7500–15000
For 70 kg person, approximately equivalent to (mu/kg)	1.5–3.0	5.0–10.0	100–200
Ratio of typical cervical dystonia doses: LD50 or lethal dose	12–33	10.5–21.0	12–24
Maximum recommended dose (adults)			
Per session (mu)	400	1200	25000
Per injection site (mu)	50	150	4000

*Maximum tolerated doses are extrapolated from adult and juvenile cynomolgus monkey toxicity studies [61].

sistant — good in that they would be protected from accidental exposure in the clinic or to food poisoning, bad if they developed a disorder requiring treatment with Bt! The manufacturers recommend that spills can be inactivated with 0.5% sodium hypochlorite (bleach). It is safe to dispose of needles, syringes and small amounts of unused toxin in 'sharps' boxes.

It is difficult to establish doses of Bt likely to cause various degrees of systemic toxicity, as there are many variables such as the precise Bt formulation, method of exposure to the toxin, and species differences. Table 3.2 sets out comparisons between the clinically available toxin types, derived from the studies discussed below. One further study in mice examined safety margins for Botox®, Dysport®, a preparation of BtB (not NeuroBloc®/MYOBLOC™), and one of botulinum toxin type F (BtF). Efficacy was measured using the digit abduction scoring (DAS) assay in which mice are suspended briefly by the tail to elicit a startle response in which the animal abducts its hind digits more or less completely. The safety margin was calculated as the ratio of the median effective dose for reducing digit abduction, and median lethal dose. The ratio (standard deviation) for BtF was 16.7 (3.9), for Botox® 13.9 (1.7), Dysport® 7.6 (0.9) and BtB 4.8 (1.1) [45]. Note that the ratio for these muscles in mice may differ from the equivalent ratio in men.

Botulinum toxin A

For BTA, 3000–3500 mu of BtA (Botox equivalent) may be enough to cause human food poisoning [62,63]. Studies on adult primates suggest that the human LD50 for systemic injection may be 30–40 mu/kg [64] or 39 mu/kg [65] body weight or 2500–3000 mu for an adult of average weight. Assuming a conversion factor of three, equivalent LD50 doses for Dysport® are 120 mu/kg body weight or 7500 mu for an average adult. Typical cervical dystonia doses are 100–200 mu Botox® and 350–700 mu Dysport®. Tsui and O'Brien recommend a maximum dose per session of 400 mu Botox® (1200 mu Dysport®) [65], although 5000 mu Dysport® has been used [66].

Botulinum toxin B

In adult cynomolgus monkeys the lowest dose producing systemic signs is 1440 mu/kg, and the approximate lethal dose of NeuroBloc® is 2400 mu/kg. Juvenile monkeys tolerate similar doses/kg [61]. Note that this appears to be a different measure to the LD50 used for BtA preparations. Although species differences may make such comparisons risky, these doses are 16.8-fold higher than the therapeutic dose of 10 000 mu used for cervical dystonia in a typical 70 kg person [61]. Treatment of human cervical dystonia with doses up to 15 000 mu (214 mu/kg) NeuroBloc® was 'safe and well-tolerated', with adverse effects similar to those for therapeutic doses of BtA [67].

Storage and reconstitution of botulinum toxin

Botulinum toxin A

BtA is currently available in vials of 100 mu (Botox®) or 500 mu (Dysport®). Pure toxin is inherently unstable and it is prepared commercially as a freeze-dried toxin-haemagglutinin complex to improve storage. In this form it has been claimed to be stable for up to 4 years when frozen, for months when refrigerated and for weeks when stored at room temperature [68]. Freeze-dried toxin is stable enough to be transported by ordinary delivery [69].

The manufacturers recommend that BtA should be reconstituted in normal (0.9%) saline and used within 4–6 h, and that remaining toxin should be discarded. BtA will still work if dissolved in sterile water but this causes intense short-lived pain at the site of injection. Clinicians usually minimize waste of toxin by treating several patients in a clinic, but this is not always possible and there are particular logistical problems when very small doses are required, most obviously in the treatment of spasmodic dysphonia using doses of 5–10 mu (Dysport®) or 2.5 mu (Botox®).

The perceived high cost of BtA has prompted some clinicians to refreeze unused reconstituted toxin to preserve it for future use. Early clinical observation did not reveal any drop in potency using this approach [70]. However, failure to identify loss of activity could have arisen from difficulty quantifying the clinical effects of BtA, and from the then 30% vial to vial variation in the potency of freeze-dried BtA (Botox®) [69]. Later animal studies using the LD50 mouse bioassay showed a 69.8% loss of potency when BtA (Botox®) was reconstituted in normal saline, immediately frozen (−70°C) and then assayed 2 weeks later. Statistically significant degradation in potency occurred after refrigerator storage (−6°C) for 12 h but not after 6 h [69]. This suggests that reconstituted toxin should not be frozen for later use because its potency is unpredictable. In addition, there was theoretical concern that the loss of activity associated with refreezing and thawing might reflect structural changes that could also make BtA more immunogenic. Greene subsequently argued that *in vitro* experiments may not reflect clinical practice, and reiterated his experience that frozen/thawed reconstituted toxin remained effective for several weeks [71]. Our advice is to follow the manufacturers' recommendations.

Botulinum toxin B

BtB (NeuroBloc®/MYOBLOC™) is a liquid formulation currently available in vials containing 2500 mu, 5000 mu and 10 000 mu at a standard concentration of 5000 µ/mL. It does not need to be reconstituted. When stored at 2–8°C there is no significant loss of activity for up to 30 months, and at room temperature (25°C) it lasts at least 9 months [72]. The vial does not contain sterilizing or antibiotic agents, and once breached it should be discarded after a few hours. The range of vial sizes will reduce waste. If appropriate, clinicians can dilute NeuroBloc®/MYOBLOC™ as much as six-fold using normal saline [72], but cannot generate more concentrated solutions. NeuroBloc®/MYOBLOC™ is slightly acidic (pH 5.6).

Effects of dose, concentration and precision of injection

The doses and techniques of injection in current use have largely been derived by trial and error. There are differences in treatment and assessment protocols between centres, and technical problems such as accuracy of diagnosis or muscle identification, crude rating scales and the inherent variability of conditions, such as dystonia and spasticity, make it difficult to compare many of their results directly.

At present we cannot reliably predict the exact dose and concentration of Bt needed to produce the desired weakness in a particular muscle. Factors that might influence the necessary dose and concentration include the density of neuromuscular junctions, placement of Bt near the motor end plates within the muscle, spread of toxin along and between tissue planes, and whether single or multiple point injections are used. There may be individual genetic or acquired susceptibilities including residual weakness or antibodies against Bt from previous injections. The best dose for a muscle may vary depending on the underlying disorder; for instance, forearm muscles need noticeably smaller doses to treat writer's cramp than spasticity. On a broader scale the clinical effectiveness of Bt depends on the selection and paralysis of appropriate muscles or muscle groups. Some conditions may respond best to selective and accurate and well focused injections, in others diffuse infiltration or a degree of diffusion of Bt may be an advantage.

Animal studies

The effects of location, dose and concentration of BtA on muscle paralysis were examined in rat tibialis anterior muscle using a technique that physiologically traced BtA activity. 'Paralysis' was quantified by electrically stimulating the nerve to the muscle and then staining sections of the muscle for glycogen. Fibres not paralysed by BtA stained negative as they were able to contract and utilize their glycogen. Fibres still staining for glycogen represented regions of sufficient BtA action to prevent muscle contraction. The technique did not measure the degree of weakness. Injections directly into the motor endplate region were the most effective, and injections only 0.5 cm from the end plate region produced 50% less paralysis. The region of 'paralysis' was doubled by a 25-fold increase in dose (constant volume) or a 100-fold increase in volume (constant dose) [6]. This study used microlitre volumes of injectate and the results may not be applicable to clinical injections of larger volumes, which intuitively might physically disrupt tissues and permit easier spread. Indeed there is ultrasound evidence that this occurs in clinical practice.

In another study, spread of toxin effect from single point injections was assessed using acetylcholinesterase staining, muscle fibre diameter (atrophy) and fibre diameter variability [73]. BtA produced a gradient of denervation in the muscle, and both the magnitude of denervation and the volume of muscle affected were dose dependent. Small doses (1–5 mu Oculinum®/Botox®) produced a limited denervation field with a graduated biologic effect inversely related to the distance from the point injection, and large doses (10 mu) affected the whole of the injected muscle. For small doses the linear spread of denervation was greater within the injected muscle than in adjacent muscles at an equivalent distance from the point of injection.

There are probably limits to the amount of Bt that individual muscles can take up. There will be no further muscle relaxation or functional gain if the Bt dose exceeds the 'saturation capacity' of a muscle, and systemic side-effects perhaps become more likely. Doses should not exceed 50 mu Botox® or 250 mu Dysport® per injection site, and 100 mu Botox® or 500 mu Dysport® per muscle.

If we can establish diffusion fields for injected and adjacent muscles it may become possible to predict optimal patterns of injection, concentration and dose for individual muscles and thus weaken target muscles with minimal spread to other muscles. Muscles with fibres arrayed in parallel may be more effectively weakened by multiple injections transversely across the muscle belly, whilst muscles with fibres arranged longitudinally may require a spread of injections along their length.

Clinical studies

It is a general impression that higher doses of toxin produce more weakness. Women and lightweight patients may need smaller doses to reduce the risk of side-effects [74]. In keeping with the results of the animal experiments the concentration of BtA and the volume of injection seem to be less critical, although higher volumes may be associated with greater diffusion and spread of toxin.

The importance of precise muscle selection and accurate placement of injections is still disputed for some conditions, but is critical in others. Treatment with Bt has proved to be remarkably robust, with some benefit often accruing even when operators are not certain which muscles to inject, or find they have injected the wrong muscles. One reason why precision may not always be essential is that muscle fascia reduce the spread of toxin by only 23% [75], so toxin can easily diffuse through muscle boundaries and injections delivered into approximately the right place will often still work. Perhaps autofocusing contributes. A more powerful explanation may be the direct effect of Bt in damping peripheral stretch reflexes [21,22] (see p. 32).

There may be an optimum concentration for some Bt preparations. *In vitro* and human experiments showed that lowering the concentration of Dysport® made it more potent, unit for unit, until the human albumen content fell too low (albumen protects the toxin from adsorption onto glass and plastic surfaces). This study suggested that reformulating Dysport® with more albumen might allow the use of lower concentrations and doses, with reduced risk of side-effects and antibody formation, and could deliver a Botox® : Dysport® potency ratio of 1 : 1. Dysport® also worked faster at lower concentration, perhaps because of more rapid diffusion to end-plate zones [7].

Single versus multipoint injections

In many conditions Bt effectively weakens the target muscle with a single injection. It is possible that multiple injections per muscle would produce more uniform weakening of the target muscle with less spread to adjacent muscles and less risk of side-effects [73]. It is also possible that multiple punctures allow toxin to leak out again more easily. However, in one study in 49 patients with torticollis, multiple injections per muscle gave better relief of pain and postural deformity, and a greater range of motion and general activity than did single point injections. Cervical muscle hypertrophy and the degree of involuntary movement improved equally with the two techniques [76].

Predicting the response to botulinum toxin

The delayed onset and prolonged effects of Bt can make it difficult to predict the optimum dose and even whether focal weakness will be useful. One approach to predicting the clinical response to Bt has been to use intramuscular succinylcholine, which can safely produce selective muscle weakness lasting several hours [77]. Local anaesthetics are also able to weaken muscle after intramuscular injection but they cause more sensory blockade than Bt and succinylcholine, making them less reliable as predictive tests because dystonia may be influenced by many sensory factors [78]. Although local anaesthetic might allow an accurate forecast of the degree of weakness, this still may not reflect the clinical benefit from Bt.

Which patients and which muscles?

It is easier to define the principles of selection than to issue a precise menu of indications. Any patient with persistent and relatively focal muscle overactivity may benefit, almost independently of the cause, and many with intermittent spasms or tics, occasionally even tremor. The associated reduction in pain can be as useful as improvement in posture or involuntary movements. Muscle hypertrophy may itself interfere with function or look unsightly as in masseteric hypertrophy, making Bt-induced atrophy desirable. Correction of cosmetic defects can restore a recluse to normal social life: examples include facial asymmetry, involuntary grimacing, or limb distortions.

Susceptible muscles range from the largest to the smallest. Knee extension spasms may stop after injection into quadriceps (but beware loss of the 'spastic prop' in ambulant patients). Interestingly, spasms may subside after much smaller doses than would be needed to relieve other facets of spasticity. Palatal myoclonus or spasmodic dysphonia can be abolished by BtA in the soft palate and vocal cord muscles, respectively.

The autonomic effects can also be harnessed. There is growing use of cutaneous BtA for focal hyperhidrosis, and salivary gland injections for sialorrhea. In experienced hands a certain amount of imagination can pay dividends.

How are muscles selected for botulinum toxin injection?

In theory, correct muscle selection and accurate injections will produce the best results with minimum use of Bt, making treatment more effective and cheaper, allowing injection of more muscles and reducing the risk of antibody formation [79]. Muscle selection can be straightforward provided the clinician has a good understanding of local functional anatomy and muscle dynamics. Different disorders warrant different strategies. In ophthalmology, the pattern of ocular movements determines the muscles for injection. In the focal dystonias and spasticity, initial muscle selection is based first on clinical factors and sometimes supported by EMG. The response to previous injections of Bt often guides subsequent injections. Care is required because the pattern of active muscles, or even the direction of the dystonic movement, may change.

Clinical criteria for selection of individual muscles vary between diseases. For instance, in dystonia they include:

1 The patient's and relatives' descriptions of the movement and the tricks employed to compensate for it. For example, patients with torticollis often prefer to sit on the side of a group that enables them to face into it.

2 The primary involuntary movement and the most likely agonist muscles, as decided by observation. However, it is sometimes difficult to decide which is the primary involuntary movement and which is merely compensatory. Clues are that patients generally find it easier to attain and maintain a voluntary posture in the direction of the primary involuntary movement, and that the *geste* usually turns the posture away from it. A few patients overcompensate, effectively producing a paradoxical resting posture counter to the true abnormal posture. Residual weakness from a previous injection cycle may trick the observer, classically with a dropped shoulder after trapezius injection for cervical dystonia. Ask the patient which is the shoulder that rises involuntarily.

3 Muscles which are painful, tender or hypertrophied.

4 Agonist muscles which are visibly or palpably contracting simultaneously with the involuntary movement. Take care to avoid selecting antagonists that may be cocontracting.

5 In writer's cramp there may be mirror movements of the affected hand while the patient tries to write with the other hand. These movements may reflect important elements of the underlying dystonia.

The value of electromyography

1 *For muscle selection.* Some units use EMG to help in muscle selection, employing multichannel recordings to study the patterns and amplitudes of muscle activation and to decide whether particular muscles are triggering symptoms, being recruited (cocontraction), or even antagonizing the primary involuntary contraction. In spasticity, EMG may help to distinguish actively contracting muscles from those resisting stretch because of passive changes in muscle viscosity, or even contracture. Muscles without a clear EMG burst when stretched may not respond usefully to Bt. The pattern of activation is less helpful because any stimulus tends to produce widespread cocontraction.

In many focal dystonias EMG is not routinely required and results are adequate without it. In a randomized prospective study in patients with cervical dystonia, EMG-assisted muscle selection and injection did not increase the number of patients showing some improvement, nor did the frequency of side-effects differ. However, EMG was found to increase the magnitude of benefit and the number of patients showing marked improvement [80]. Some clinics use EMG-guided muscle selection routinely because particular movements can be produced by different patterns of dystonic muscle activation (see Chapter 4).

If pain becomes a more widely accepted indication for Bt treatment, it may prove important to show abnormal EMG activity in muscles considered for injection (see Chapter 17).

2 *For accurate injections.* Even if not used for muscle selection, EMG can aid accurate placement of Bt. EMG is especially useful when target muscles are difficult to palpate, for instance in orbital muscles or obese patients. Once muscles have been selected, either clinically or by EMG, EMG with special hollow combination EMG/injection needles can help to confirm needle placement in the chosen muscle using various activation procedures, or simply to prove that the needle is in muscle and not other tissue when Bt is injected. This can be essential in obese patients. Portable EMG equipment is available, either as a full system giving visual and sound confirmation of needle placement, or simpler, more portable and cheaper audio-only. The latter can be very helpful but tricky to use for reinjections. To an inexperienced electromyographer the sound from an EMG needle in a previously treated muscle is similar to that from a distant untreated muscle. This is not just a theoretical problem as previously treated muscles may remain atrophic at the time of retreatment and can be more difficult to locate.

3 *To identify denervated muscle fibres.* EMG may identify muscle fibres still denervated from previous injection cycles. If there is severe denervation it may be worth injecting other parts of the muscle or using the patient's 'allowance' of Bt in other muscles. This is a difficult judgement because muscles that are recovering will still give an abnormal EMG signal but may nonetheless need reinjection.

Such theoretical benefits must be balanced against the increased complexity of treatment when EMG is used. EMG is clearly required in some situations, but it can be time consuming and expensive in itself, so that overall costs may not fall and clinics might treat fewer patients.

4 *To monitor effects of treatment.* Quantitative EMG using turns analysis gives objective data, and in one study in cervical dystonia, summed scores from a variety of treated and untreated muscles decreased after Bt injections [81]. In a double blind study EMG changes mirrored clinical outcome measures [82]. It is possible such techniques can help to optimize doses and other technical niceties, but Bt treatment is usually symptomatic, and ultimately clinical outcomes are likely to remain more important.

Muscle selection and injection placement

Most experienced clinicians have evolved their own techniques for muscle selection and accurate injection placement for the common indications. Some disorders such as blepharospasm or hemifacial spasm present little difficulty in muscle selection, and variations in treatment revolve around Bt dose and concentration, or patterns of placement of injections. Although EMG can be very helpful, a simpler technique will suffice in many cases. Make the muscle belly stand out visibly or palpably using isometric counter force or repetitive movements. If the needle is placed in the belly of the muscle and the muscle then gently activated or stretched passively, the differential movement of muscle and skin tilts the needle and syringe and confirms its position inside the muscle fascia [83]. This is most helpful in long limb muscles such as hamstrings, gastrocnemius, long finger flexors, etc., and much less use in wrist pronators and neck muscles. With experience, the position of the needle tip can sometimes be gauged by the resistance to movement of the needle and the pressure required to inject the toxin. If the needle tip appears to be in place the force required to inject will diminish if the patient can relax the muscle, providing further confirmation of needle position.

Some clinics reserve EMG assistance for muscle selection or injection placement in patients who respond poorly to freehand injections, who are obese or badly deformed, or have abnormal muscle anatomy. EMG may be essential when injecting small, delicate, deep or closely packed structures, such as extraocular, laryngeal or many of the forearm muscles.

Image guidance

In some conditions it is worth using ultrasound, endoscopy, X-ray screening or computer tomorgraphy (CT), or magnetic resonance imaging (MRI) to ensure accurate delivery of injections to preselected targets. Examples include salivary gland, laryngeal, sphincter of Oddi and psoas injections.

Matching the dose to the patient

Experience has generated 'standard' doses that work for most patients and provide a good starting point. However, individual sensitivities to Bt vary, and doses recommended by the manufacturers and in this book are guidelines only. Larger doses will produce more intense and prolonged benefits and side-effects. In general, large, hypertrophied or highly active muscles need bigger doses [74], and small or lightweight patients need smaller doses. Treatment of dystonia needs smaller doses than spasticity in the same muscles. With experience it is possible to modify the initial dose accordingly. Assess the effects after each injection session, in order to optimize the dose next time.

Reduce the dose when there is:

1 Pre-existing weakness, for example from previous toxin injections or neuromuscular disease, such as Bell's palsy, motorneurone disease, myasthenia gravis [84] or Lambert–Eaton syndrome [85]. However, BtA given after denervation surgery is reported to be less effective. It is not clear whether this was related to the degree of further weakness induced by BtA or to some other factor [86]. An excessive effect from Bt may warn clinicians of a serious underlying disorder such as myasthenia gravis.

2 Increased hazard should side-effects occur, as in pregnancy or chronic bronchitis. Note that Bt treatment is not recommended in pregnancy and during lactation.

3 Special susceptibility to side-effects. Bruises or other local tissue damage can alter diffusion of the toxin, generally allowing it to spread more easily. Nearby placement of Bt, or large doses even at a distance could aggravate pre-existing dysphagia or strabismus or precarious sphincter control.

In some situations we use a cautious strategy with modest doses on the first injection session, titrating upwards if the effect is inadequate. This works well when there is a risk of inconvenient weakness, such as in occupational dystonias, e.g. writer's cramp, musician's cramp, or our recent favourite, slot-car racer's trigger finger (Scalextric®). The disadvantage is that it may take several sessions over 3–6 months to find the optimum compromise. In other situations we prefer to give a fuller dose and reduce it if there are problems. This is appropriate when a more rapid effective response is needed, and where undue collateral weakness is unlikely to matter, as commonly occurs in spasticity in a limb unlikely to be functionally useful even if the spasticity is abolished.

After the injections

Enhancing the response to botulinum toxin

Focusing botulinum toxin induced weakness

There are many clinical factors that could influence focusing. These include: the particular preparation used; the dose, volume and concentration of Bt; the site, distribution, accuracy, force or rate of injection; genetic or other patient factors such as general health and specific systemic or local pathology (bruising, oedema or infection allow Bt to spread); events after the injections, such as local massage, muscle activity and temperature.

In the laboratory, BtA is more avidly taken up by active muscles, possibly because nerve activity increases recycling of the vesicle membrane at the nerve terminal [87,88]. In the dystonias or spasticity this could concentrate the induced weakness in the most active muscles or muscle fibres, a kind of autofocusing. For a short time after the injection it may be possible to amplify the effect by encouraging or provoking contraction of the target muscles through active exercise or functional electrical stimulation via a motor nerve. Small studies have indeed suggested that functional electrical stimulation can enhance the paralytic effect of BtA in dystonia [89], and in poststroke leg [90] and arm [91] spasticity. Note that in theory direct muscle stimulation might be less effective as it would not always stimulate the motor nerve and hence nerve terminal activity.

One study in monkeys examined local and 'distant' spread of Bt. Botox® was injected into the abductor pollicis brevis (APB) muscle of one hand, NeuroBloc®/MYOBLOC™ into the other hand. EMG compound muscle action potential (CMAP) changes were recorded in APB, in the first dorsal interosseous (1st DIO), an adjacent muscle, and adductor digiti minimi (ADM), a 'distant' muscle in the same hand. For equivalent weakening of APB, NeuroBloc®/MYOBLOC™ caused less weakness of the nearby and the distant muscle [92]. Even within this animal model there were differences in the relative effects of the two preparations in adults as compared to juveniles, which emphasizes the risk of extrapolating the results to humans.

Stabilizing botulinum toxin induced weakness

In some conditions it would be useful to be able to delay or stop recovery of muscle strength after a perfect injection. Two methods have been suggested. Firstly, chimeric toxin molecules might be designed to kill motorneurones rather than temporarily paralyse them. Animal studies of muscle toxins such as ricin, linked to antibodies, show that they can destroy and weaken muscle. In theory, specially designed antibodies could target either Bt light chains or other toxins to muscles recovering from Bt toxicity as these muscles may have special patterns of receptor expression. Such drugs could 'freeze' a satisfactory primary response to Bt [93]. Secondly, drugs such as aminoglycoside and macrolide antibiotics which enhance neuromuscular blockade could theoretically be used to potentiate and thus prolong the toxin-induced weakness. However, this has never been studied.

In other situations, such as in spasticity, appropriate physical therapy and splinting may enhance and prolong the benefit of toxin-induced weakness, but do not truly prolong the weakness.

Maximizing the benefit: stretch muscles and promote antagonist activity

The weakened target muscles stretch more easily. In spasticity, a programme of positioning, stretching and splints during the period of toxin induced weakness is practical and probably helps to maintain or increase muscle length. Take care with vigorous stretching as it is easier to strain the weakened muscles. The muscle relaxation also frees and permits retraining of antagonists, usually by physical therapists. Once the BtA target muscle weakens, functional electrical stimulation of the antagonists might help but is currently unproven. In theory the opportunity to learn motor skills could stimulate beneficial neuronal plasticity and longer-term benefit (see Chapter 10). However, these physical therapies rarely seem useful in dystonia.

Measuring the effects of botulinum toxin

Disease severity and benefit from treatment are difficult to measure in many of the conditions treated with Bt. It is relatively easy to chart improvement in ocular alignment using standard techniques, but even in such apparently straightforward situations the benefit to the patient may not correlate with simple mechanical measures—in this instance cosmetic benefit or development of binocular fusion may be much more important.

It is helpful to classify the disease severity and response to treatment using the World Health Organization (WHO) International Classification of Impairments, Disabilities and Handicaps (ICIDH-2 [94]). In its earlier incarnation [95], the most important concept was that any illness could be considered at four levels: pathology, impairment, disability and handicap [96]. ICIDH-2 uses body structure and function, activities, participation and considers 'contextual factors' such as the patient's environment and attitudes. Whilst global scores combining two or more of these elements can be valuable, it may be better to keep them separate. Unfortunately there are many scales which do not distinguish between them.

Body structure (formerly pathology) and function (impairment)

These have been combined in ICIDH-2. 'Structure' covers the damage or abnormal process occurring within an organ system. In some circumstances Bt may improve underlying pathology or prevent further problems. A protective ptosis might prevent or allow resolution of underlying eye disease and strabismus is sometimes cured by Bt. Treatment of severe spasticity may minimize secondary complications such as bedsores. The patient is aware of 'function', the direct neurophysiological consequence of the underlying structure or pathology, measured as the severity of sweating in hyperhidrosis, degree of rotation or tilt in torticollis, the duration of periods of functional blindness in blepharospasm, or the angular misalignment of visual axes in a sixth nerve palsy. Function or impairment is the equivalent of symptoms and signs or the immediate consequence of pathology as perceived by the person [96]. The main importance of impaired body function is that it restricts activity.

Scoring systems that use *objective* criteria are often available. Unfortunately, many are only applicable in the laboratory or the clinic, and few are suitable for patients or relatives to apply at home. This is true of most clinical scales used for rating the severity of dystonia, such as the Tsui scale for cervical dystonia. Laboratory measurements may use video imaging with clinical ratings or computer-aided analysis such as in gait analysis. Movement transducers include goniometers, accelerometers and optical or electromagnetic tracking systems. Changes in electrical resistance, or moisture sensitive chemicals, can measure the area affected by, and the severity of, sweating. Whilst such devices are very helpful in technical analyses and may be useful for clinical trials it is easy for clinicians to fixate on such objective measures and forget that Bt is essentially a symptomatic treatment. Some scales such as the Toronto Western Spasmodic Torticollis Rating Scale (TWSTRS) or the Cervical Dystonia Scale combine objective and subjective measures.

Activities (formerly disability)

The patient's primary complaint often relates to any activity the patient is unable to perform. Patients with writer's cramp are unable to write, spasmodic dysphonia prevents effective speech, hemifacial spasm may be a cosmetic disaster. Disability is the personal nuisance caused by the impaired body function [96]. It is much harder to measure the severity of these problems, and scales more often use subjective items. There are generic scales such as the SF36, which allow comparisons between different disorders, and more disease specific scales may soon be available.

Participation (formerly handicap)

Some of the above scales also reflect participation in society or 'life situations', and any restrictions due to the disease that limit or prevents the fulfilment of a role that is normal for that individual. Examples include inability to attend school, divorce or loss of a job through illness.

Subjective scales

Subjective scales may be extremely helpful in trials and in clinical practice. They can include predefined categories and definitions of severity. More flexibly, the clinician and patient/carer can agree on the goals of treatment, and score only changes relevant to the individual. They can include problems at one or more levels of the ICIDH-2 classification. Some scales can combine benefits and adverse effects into an overall picture. We use a generic measure of quality of function/activities/participation, modified from Brin *et al.*'s original version [97]. It is shown in Fig. 3.2 and discussed in more detail below. There are also self-rating scales that are more dedicated to particular conditions, such as torticollis, or which measure changes in quality of life [98] and psychopathology [99].

Baseline and follow-up assessments

Write a clear baseline description of the clinical problem, and score its severity using as objective and repeatable a scale as possible. Only then can you monitor the response. Some disorders have established rating scales such as the TWSTRS [100] or the Tsui [101] scales for torticollis, and these can be sensitive to Bt-induced changes. Unfortunately some other conditions are much harder to monitor, and the huge variety of clinical problems makes it difficult to devise satisfactory scales. Modified Ashworth scores may be useful in spasticity, but can only rate the impairment crudely. They may not reflect clinically important benefit, for instance when severe poststroke fisting relaxes enough to prevent palmar trauma and skin infection, but the Modified Ashworth score does not change.

Remember that Bt is mainly a symptomatic treatment, so the patient's and carer's opinions are usually more important than the doctor's 'objective' assessment. Quality-of-life studies are therefore particularly important in measuring the benefit from Bt treatment. It can be very helpful to agree treatment goals specific to

How effective are your injections?
Global Clinical Rating Scale

Name _____ Condition treated _____

CURRENT PERCENT OF NORMAL FUNCTION

	(No function, very bad)	(Normal function, very good)

Week
___/___/___ start 0--5--10--15--20--25--30--35--40--45--50--55--60--65--70--75--80--85--90--95--100
___/___/___ 1 0--5--10--15--20--25--30--35--40--45--50--55--60--65--70--75--80--85--90--95--100
___/___/___ 2 0--5--10--15--20--25--30--35--40--45--50--55--60--65--70--75--80--85--90--95--100
___/___/___ 3 0--5--10--15--20--25--30--35--40--45--50--55--60--65--70--75--80--85--90--95--100
___/___/___ 4 0--5--10--15--20--25--30--35--40--45--50--55--60--65--70--75--80--85--90--95--100
___/___/___ 5 0--5--10--15--20--25--30--35--40--45--50--55--60--65--70--75--80--85--90--95--100
___/___/___ 6 0--5--10--15--20--25--30--35--40--45--50--55--60--65--70--75--80--85--90--95--100
___/___/___ 7 0--5--10--15--20--25--30--35--40--45--50--55--60--65--70--75--80--85--90--95--100
___/___/___ 8 0--5--10--15--20--25--30--35--40--45--50--55--60--65--70--75--80--85--90--95--100
___/___/___ 9 0--5--10--15--20--25--30--35--40--45--50--55--60--65--70--75--80--85--90--95--100
___/___/___ 10 0--5--10--15--20--25--30--35--40--45--50--55--60--65--70--75--80--85--90--95--100
___/___/___ 11 0--5--10--15--20--25--30--35--40--45--50--55--60--65--70--75--80--85--90--95--100
___/___/___ 12 0--5--10--15--20--25--30--35--40--45--50--55--60--65--70--75--80--85--90--95--100
___/___/___ 13 0--5--10--15--20--25--30--35--40--45--50--55--60--65--70--75--80--85--90--95--100
___/___/___ 14 0--5--10--15--20--25--30--35--40--45--50--55--60--65--70--75--80--85--90--95--100
___/___/___ 15 0--5--10--15--20--25--30--35--40--45--50--55--60--65--70--75--80--85--90--95--100
___/___/___ 16 0--5--10--15--20--25--30--35--40--45--50--55--60--65--70--75--80--85--90--95--100

1. **How soon did you feel some effect?** _____days/weeks after
2. **How long did this last?** _____days/weeks
3. **Over how long did it wear off?** _____days/weeks
4. **For how long had it worn off completely?**_____days/weeks

5. **Did you experience any side effects?**
   If yes, please describe below:

Side effects	Start	End	Duration (days)	Severity
1				
2				
3				
4				

OVERALL EFFECT (please complete at the end of the observation period)

6. **What was the effect of your injection?**

Major deterioration	Moderate deterioration	Minor deterioration	No effect	Minor benefit	Moderate benefit	Major benefit

7. **How did it compare to your previous injection/treatment?**

Much worse	Worse	Slightly worse	Same	Slightly better	Better	Much better

Fig. 3.2 Generic measure of quality of function/activities/participation (modified from [97]).

the patient in advance and to concentrate on monitoring those goals. Spasticity is an excellent example of a complex situation where benefit must be monitored in a broader sense.

We also use a generic diary (Fig. 3.2) for all patients starting on Bt treatment and for later cycles in any patient where we anticipate difficulties. The patient or carers can fill it in once a week. If there are several problems, or if adjusting the muscle selection or dose in the next injection cycle, prime the scorer to use different coloured inks for each problem or cycle. This allows direct comparison of the perceived benefit from each. It permits finer tuning, and retains the patient's sense of participation. Most patients or relatives are capable of using this scale and it can provide a more continuous picture of the changes following Bt treatment than the snapshot afforded by measurements made in the clinic. It measures change relative to a baseline and it may be useful to 'calibrate' it by using more objective measures.

Until the pattern of response is clear, clinicians may need to see the patient 3–6 weeks after each injection, at the time of anticipated maximal response. Once everyone is satisfied of benefit such intensive monitoring becomes unnecessary, so if a pattern is established after a few sessions we rely on patients, carers or therapists to tell us when a repeat injection is needed. Keep any diary forms completed early on as they give an excellent and personalized measure of baseline severity and responsiveness to Bt injections.

Patterns of response and timing of repeat injections

Both the onset of weakness and the recovery of muscle power are gradual, but symptom relief and recurrence can occur either abruptly or gradually. Symptom relief may take from one day to several weeks to appear, and its relationship to the development of objective weakness has not been systematically explored. The duration of BtA-induced weakness is typically around three months in striated muscles. BtB is similar, but it is not yet clear whether there is a systematic difference in its duration of action. With BtA or BtB there is considerable variation, from a few weeks to six months or more, depending on the dose and on individual susceptibility. Symptom relief is generally for a shorter period than objective weakness as there comes a point at which the involuntary muscle activity becomes troublesome again. In some patients the pattern of response is erratic, others show more consistent benefit and side-effects.

The response to each Bt injection is usually clear cut. Occasionally patients whose first few treatments resulted in dramatic swings between improvement and then loss of benefit report that repeated treatments are producing diminishing returns. This may be because the toxin is no longer effective, but often it seems that patients have reached a relatively steady state maintained by the intermittent treatment. These patients remain much better than their baseline severity (the *plateau* effect), and if repeat injections are postponed for long enough they invariably deteriorate. When there is doubt it can be helpful to defer injections for 6 months or more.

Strategy for repeat injections

Ideally, aim to keep patients symptom free. In practice most will cycle through periods of relative relief following each injection, followed by gradual deterioration to a point when further injections are appropriate. Symptom relief is generally shorter lived than objective weakness as there comes a point at which the involuntary muscle overactivity becomes troublesome again. The timing of repeat injections should as far as possible allow for response variability and duration of side-effects. All concerned with the patient learn to anticipate an injection wearing off and compensate for the time lag of benefit after a repeat injection.

Where possible, maintain a minimum 3-monthly interval. There may be pressure to repeat injections frequently, and clinics should avoid booster injections as they increase the risk of developing toxin-neutralizing antibodies [102]. However, if doses large enough to give sufficient symptom relief over a long period always produce significant short-term side-effects it may be necessary to settle for more frequent injection with a lower dose of Bt. Occasional patients fail to benefit from frequent modest doses and are obliged to endure the side-effects of larger doses. It is usually better to aim for incomplete but acceptable benefit than to attempt absolute control that requires excessive toxin use. Sometimes it is difficult to uncover the real reason behind patient pressure for reinjection: one patient with leg adductor spasticity eventually said that less than excellent control of spasms prevented sexual intercourse.

Many patients like to have their next appointment for review and usually treatment at a prearranged interval, especially if their response is fairly predictable. Those with an unpredictable or long-lasting response may prefer self-referral when their last injections are wearing off. Bt clinics should attempt to accommodate both: although patient-initiated appointments may be difficult to fit in, this strategy generally acts to reduce the number of injection sessions.

Failure to respond

When patients respond to Bt treatment and reach their treatment goals as hoped, follow-up and decisions about further treatment are usually straightforward. Sometimes, unfortunately, Bt does not work as planned. *Primary* failure to respond is defined as complete biological failure of the toxin, with no muscle atrophy, weakness or EMG changes, or autonomic effects. It is extremely rare. *Secondary* failure may occur if there is a relative or complete non-response to Bt after a detectable response from a previous Bt treatment. Similar problems may contribute to either type of failure. It is important to distinguish true failure of the biological effect of Bt from failure of the biological effect to help the patient, which may occur for many reasons.

Clinically, secondary non-responders are patients with:

1 A history of at least two successful injections (i.e. score improvement of at least 20%

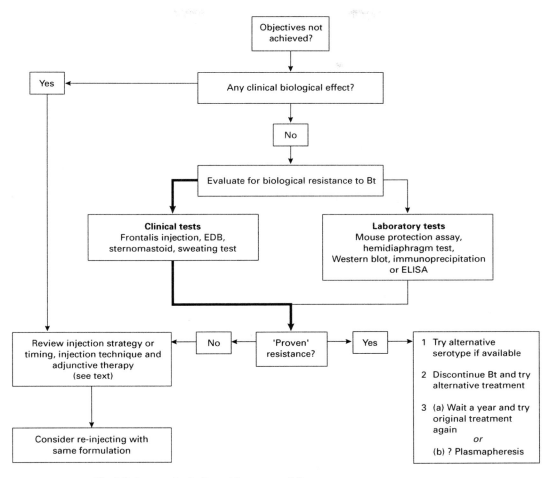

Fig. 3.3 Strategy for dealing with treatment failure.

and/or atrophy of injected muscles combined with EMG abnormalities such as denervation potentials) and/or complaints of typical Bt related adverse events.

2 No objective treatment effect or worsening of the severity score and no typical therapy-related adverse events in two subsequent treatment sessions. Some definitions require failure despite an increase in dose.

Why has botulinum toxin failed this patient? What can I do next?

Figure 3.3 illustrates one strategy for dealing with treatment failure. However, consider first whether the treatment really has failed. Is there failure of the toxin, or has there been an error? Mistakes may be:

1 Administrative. Who gave the injection? How experienced or overworked were they? Could there have been a simple administrative mistake such as writing in the wrong notes, entering the wrong date, muscle injected or dose. Was there a failure to communicate that prevented necessary adjunctive treatment?

2 Selection errors include poor selection of patients, muscles for injection or goals. Muscles with a fixed contracture will not improve, or the clinician or patient may have been too optimistic.

3 Errors in injecting Bt include using the wrong dose or preparation of Bt, incorrect transport, primary storage or reconstitution. It is easy in the hurly burly of a clinic for a clinician to mistake a used vial of BtA for an unused one. Once more saline is inserted there is no way to be sure. If a reconstituted vial is incorrectly labelled there is potential for error and confusion with other vials if it is stored even for a few minutes. This applies just as much to BtB as clinicians can and often do dilute the supplied liquid. When was that vial that you (or someone else) retrieved from the refrigerator originally opened or reconstituted? Label any vial for storage with your initials, the volume of dilution, and a use-by time.

Consider whether the dose was split between too many muscles, or was simply too small, and whether the injection itself was satisfactory. Were there clinical or technical problems such as obesity, difficulty locating the chosen muscles or using EMG or imaging? It can be useful to record any such technical difficulties to help in the subsequent outcome assessment.

4 Assessment errors are common. One trap is the patient who complains at reinjection time that the last injections are not working. Careful questioning often reveals that Bt worked perfectly well and the patient has forgotten that it is expected to wear off. Some patients respond well at first, only to complain of a diminishing response with subsequent treatments. Surprisingly often this is because they have forgotten the original severity of their symptoms, and the previous injection has not completely worn off. The next injection thus makes a less impressive difference, though most patients accept that they remain better than their baseline. Alternatively, perhaps that enthusiastic response to the first injection cycle was a placebo response.

Some patients report failure of the toxin because side-effects have spoilt the benefits, or the patient has gone through a bad patch in the middle of a period of good relief. Also, because injections sometimes takes several weeks to work, patients complain that the reinjection has made them worse when the deterioration is in fact due to the previous injections still wearing off. Review the original response diaries, and discuss them with the patient. When in doubt, postpone injections for a few months. Gradual decline of symptom control may persuade all concerned that Bt was helping. Remember that coincident pathology or an increase in severity of the underlying condition may overwhelm any benefit from Bt.

Even if the desired weakness does arise it may prove to be unhelpful, for instance when spastic muscles have additional contracture, weakening the muscle may not allow it to lengthen. Too much weakness may be counterproductive, as when a spastic knee extensor prop is abolished causing the leg to give way.

Anticipate problems by educating patients in what to expect and how to report the results, perhaps by charting a weekly visual analogue score. Prime them to remember key points. Keep good records of the baseline state, such as a recognized scale score, video or still photography or a diagram. Remember it may be another clinician that assesses your patient next time.

5 Expecting too much. Failure to ensure delivery of adjunctive treatment such as physiotherapy, positioning or splinting for spasticity, prisms for diplopia, or ptosis props may lead to inadequate benefit. There may be a change in the pattern or severity of muscle involvement, the underlying disease may deteriorate, a new disorder may appear or the patient's drug regime may have changed.

6 Other unavoidable factors. Some injection cycles are spoiled by unrelated emotional or social turmoil or physical illness, and the next cycle proves satisfactory again. Even after a series of good responses in consecutive injection cycles an injection may fail to help for no obvious reason or may produce unexpected adverse effects. There is significant variability in the active contents of vials of Bt, so we often simply recommend another try with the patient's usual dose, unless the side-effects were intolerable or dangerous. If consecutive cycles give inadequate benefit then increase the dose. There are no undisputable grounds for recommending a particular percentage increase. Most clinics suggest increases of 10–30% depending on the clinical picture. Larger changes can be appropriate.

Antibodies and biological failure of the toxin

After an unpredictable number of injection cycles Bt may start to work less well. Despite increasing doses there are diminishing benefits and side-effects that raise the possibility of true biological secondary failure due to neutralizing antibodies, i.e. antibodies that prevent the toxin from working. This is a major problem because it eventually entails stopping treatment, with little likelihood of future benefit from that toxin serotype. The antibodies are not in themselves dangerous, but they are long-lasting and even when they subside they are easy to reactivate. We do not know whether biological changes such as down-regulation of acceptor protein on nerve terminals could cause resistance that is not antibody-mediated.

Bt preparations contain the active toxin plus several other proteins. Antibodies may develop against any component. Only antibodies against the toxin itself are neutralizing, and antibodies against nonessential parts of the toxin-haemagglutinin complex may not neutralize it. Although Bt serotypes are antigenically distinct they are large molecules with significant homology between serotypes so that antibodies to one serotype such as BtA might still cross react with another, such as BtB. So far, the cross-reacting antibodies detected have been non-neutralizing [72], and in clinical practice many patients who have antibodies to BtA do respond to BtB. The reverse may also hold but has not been tested.

If Bt is not working it is sometimes helpful to test for antibodies. Unfortunately, there are no perfect clinical or laboratory tests. Equivocal results occur, and may be due to low titres of neutralizing antibodies. In general, the tests trade sensitivity for specificity. Tests that detect non-neutralizing antibodies tend to be very sensitive and may make good screening tools, but tests that are specific for neutralizing antibodies, such as the mouse protection assay (MPA), correlate better with clinical response. Some of the more common tests are described below:

Clinical tests. There are several clinical tests for biological failure of Bt, developed for use with BtA but likely to work just as well for BtB once appropriate doses are established. They are useful for assessing clinical non-responders. Remember that these tests only demonstrate failure of the injection to work. Even though antibodies are the most likely culprits, the tests do not prove that the failure is due to antibodies.

1 Frontalis antibody test (FTAT) [103]. This is easy to perform in the clinic, and cheap if there is some spare toxin available. Warn patients about the possibility of facial asymmetry that may last some weeks or months. Rarely, ptosis or diplopia may occur. If they are happy to proceed, inject Botox® 2×7.5 mu or Dysport® 2×20 mu into the forehead about 3 cm above the lateral canthus of one eye. If the toxin is biologically active it will paralyse or greatly reduce forehead wrinkling around the injection site 1–3 weeks later. Ask the patient to raise the eyebrows: an asymmetric response shows that the toxin was effective and antibodies are unlikely. This test is usually easy to interpret, but like the edrophonium test for myasthenia gravis, it can occasionally give equivocal results. Ensure the patient can wrinkle the forehead before giving the test injection.

2 Extensor digitorum brevis (EDB) test using EMG [104]. This test is more cumbersome but also more objective. Measure the amplitude of the compound muscle action potential (CMAP) of EDB using supramaximal peroneal nerve stimulation before and two weeks after injection of 50 mu Botox® or 200 mu Dysport®. If the toxin is biologically active, the CMAP should fall to <50% of the baseline value and there will usually be clinical evidence of atrophy and weakness. A <20% decrease in CMAP suggests that neutralizing antibodies are present; 20–50% decrease is equivocal.

3 Sweating test [105]. Inject 5 mu Botox® (0.25 mL) or 20 mu Dysport® (0.25 mL) intradermally into the skin of the back, upper arm, upper leg or even forehead (see FTAT). 5–10 days after injection, the Minor's iodine starch test will reveal an anhidrotic spot of about 2.5 cm diameter if antibodies are absent. Injecting the forehead combines the frontalis test with the sweating test in a single session and may be more informative.

Laboratory tests

1 Enzyme-linked or sphere-linked immunosorbent assay (ELISA or SLIDA).
These *in-vitro* tests are fairly sensitive but results do not correlate well with clinical resistance, as they do not distinguish neutralizing from non-neutralizing antibodies.

2 Immunoprecipitation assay (IPA) [106]. More recently developed, this *in vitro* assay also does not distinguish neutralizing from non-neutralizing antibodies, but is sensitive and more specific for predicting clinical response than the ELISA/SLIDA. It can detect low titres of antibody, which may be useful for prognosis and warn clinicians to minimize the risk of encouraging antibodies.

3 Mouse protection assay (MPA), mouse neutralization assay (MNA) or mouse lethality assay (LD50 test) [103]. Slow and relatively expensive, these are standard commercially available *in vivo* tests in which patient's serum is incubated with a dose of toxin that is lethal to mice. The serum is then injected into mice. If neutralizing antibodies are present the mice live, if not the toxin remains active and they die. Although the tests are not very sensitive, a positive result is a good predictor of clinical resistance.

4 Western blot assay (WBA). This is also commercially available. It is less cumbersome and does not use animals, but is a little less specific than the mouse protection assay [103].

5 Mouse hemidiaphragm-phrenic nerve bioassay. This *in vitro* test uses only one mouse per sample and produces quantitative results in a few hours. It correlates well with the extensor digitorum brevis test [107], and is more sensitive and possibly more reproducible than the mouse protection assay [108].

PREVALENCE OF ANTIBODIES

The true prevalence is unclear because of the difficulties defining secondary non-response, technical problems with antibody tests, and variations in dose and concentration of Bt, frequency of exposure and potential predisposing factors. Clinic surveys are usually retrospective and suffer from unknown selection and attrition bias, especially as patients who stop treatment may be lost to follow up. Individual clinicians and patients evolve their own compromises in the trade-off between larger doses with a good response, and smaller doses with a lower risk of antibodies. These compromises invalidate historical comparisons and controls. Such factors make it difficult to compare quoted rates of antibody formation for the various commercial preparations of Bt, which vary between about 2.5% [44,109,110] and 15.3% [111] in cervical dystonia. Rates appear to be much lower or negligible in hemifacial spasm and blepharospasm [112], perhaps a function of the lower doses.

RISK FACTORS

Most surveys suggest that risk factors for antibody development include high doses, injection cycles of less than 3 months or use of interim booster injections. Note that this is potentially a circular argument as patients with antibodies are more likely to receive such treatments, and we would need a prospective randomized controlled comparison of these factors to be certain. Other possible risk factors might be unlucky genes, or unknown drug or disease adjuvants. One survey reported that antibody-positive patients were younger at the onset of dystonic symptoms than those continuing to respond ($P = 0.007$) [44].

The relative clinical risk of neutralizing antibodies with the available commercial preparations remains uncertain, and there are competing claims. For reasons discussed above, *in vitro* and animal *in vivo* studies inform but cannot decide the debate as they use theoretical arguments about protein immunogenicity, load and dose equivalence. They may not translate to clinical practice. Ideally, we need evidence from controlled clinical trials that ensure equivalent exposure to Bt. There is no clinically proven difference between the various preparations currently available.

STRATEGIES TO PREVENT ANTIBODIES

It is risky to transfer results from *in vitro* or animal studies to humans, or to assume that a theoretical advantage in the laboratory will translate to a practical clinical advantage. However, immunological theory does complement the results from clinical surveys, and suggests rational strategies to prevent antibodies. These aim to minimize exposure to the antigen, and include reducing the protein load per effective dose, making the proteins less immunogenic, and restricting the dose and frequency of injections.

Thus the new formulation of Botox® in 1997 contained less protein, and the proteins in NeuroBloc® are said to be less immunogenic because they are not lyophilized. For their part, clinicians act as goalkeepers and should resist pressures to over treat. Key requirements are:

1 Wait as long as possible between injections; at least 10 and preferably 12 weeks [113].

2 Avoid booster injections [113].

3 Use the smallest possible doses [113]. This is easier with correct muscle selection and good injection technique.

4 Where patients have Bt for several indications, try to synchronize treatment cycles and give injections for all of the indications in a single session to avoid multiple exposures. If one indication requires most of the dose consider not treating it in order to preserve the long-term response for the other indications.

5 Do not expose the patient to different toxin types unnecessarily, either sequentially or simultaneously.

DEALING WITH TREATMENT FAILURE DUE TO ANTIBODIES

1 Before high titres develop, simply increasing the dose of Bt or frequency of injections may deliver sufficient clinical benefit, at the risk of consolidating antibody formation.

2 Wait a while. After a year or more without Bt treatment, some patients lose their resistance to BtA, at least at first. Note that repeating clinical tests such as the frontalis or the sweat test risks reactivating antibodies.

3 Recent anecdotal reports suggest that plasma exchange can remove antitoxin antibodies in some patients, temporarily restoring sensitivity to BtA [114]. This is unlikely to prove a practical option for long-term management of most patients, as plasma exchange would probably need to be performed before every injection session. One group tried intravenous immunoglobulin in a single patient but it did not help [115].

4 Switch to an antigenically distinct preparation if the response failure is due to antibodies. BtB can weaken muscles in some patients with torticollis who have become resistant to BtA [116]. We do not yet know if the inverse is true. No doubt clinicians and drug companies will test, both informally and in trials, a variety of strategies such as rotating or mixing serotypes in attempts to reduce the risk of antibody formation. It is worth remembering that only a few patients develop antibodies now, and mixing or rotating Bt serotypes could just as easily have the opposite effect of increasing antibody formation, whatever the theoreticians may say.

STOPPING BOTULINUM TOXIN TREATMENT

It is important to not persist with useless injections, whether failure is due to antibodies or to other factors. Bt treatment is expensive and time consuming, it can have side-effects, and sometimes other treatments are ignored or deferred because the patient is receiving Bt. If in doubt, and with the patient's consent, repeated $n = 1$ trials comparing active and placebo injections may give the answer.

How to proceed in cases with secondary non-response

After checking and excluding causes of secondary treatment failure not linked to antibodies, discuss alternative treatments with the patient. For instance, these include injections of another serotype of Bt, surgical treatments (mainly relevant for cervical dystonia patients) or injections of phenol (suitable for patients with spasticity). We usually prefer to inject another serotype such as BtB as it is technically the easiest approach, with a relatively low risk. Anecdotally, repeated plasmaphereses or immunoadsorption may remove antibodies against BtA, allowing successful reinjection. As this procedure is time consuming and may be very costly it should be reserved for special indications only [114].

Side-effects of botulinum toxin

Some side-effects are trivial, some are deemed to be worth suffering for the sake of the benefits of treatment, and others are recognized as too unpleasant or potentially dangerous to be ignored, such as severe dysphagia after lingual injections or treatment for torticollis. However, there are often ways of minimizing the side-effects, by prevention, symptomatic relief, or perhaps in future by reducing the paralytic effect of the toxin.

Immediate side-effects of Bt are largely due to excessive weakness of the target muscles, unintentional spread of toxin and paralysis to adjacent muscles, or to local autonomic dysfunction. There is no compelling evidence that distant effects are clinically important at standard doses.

It is difficult to specify a dangerous absolute dose of Bt because the side-effects and the therapeutic index vary widely with the site of injection. In a given situation the incidence and severity of side-effects is likely to be dose related, and the effects of single/multipoint injections, and volume and concentration of toxin are still being examined.

Patients new to the toxin generally receive a 'standard' dose, often modified empirically in the light of muscle mass and risk factors. For instance, in one study of BtA treatment in torticollis, complications were more likely in women and in patients of low body weight. It is usually possible to balance benefits and side-effects in individuals after a few treatment sessions. Dosage flexibility is one of the major safeguards, and must take into account any local factors such as recent toxin injections and previous surgery, and also systemic diseases which might exaggerate the effect of the toxin.

Long-term problems include resistance to further BtA or BtB injections. This may be real and due to toxin-neutralizing antibodies [117] or proliferation of new axon terminals [40], or only apparent, caused perhaps by an undetected change in the pattern of dystonic muscle activation (see Chapter 4) so that the pattern of injections becomes suboptimal. If BtA is still capable of inducing weakness there will usually be detectable muscle atrophy or immediate side-effects. Bt antibodies are discussed in more detail above. Neither local nor distant effects have been examined in long-term animal studies simulating the human situation with repeated sublethal doses of Bt.

Prevention of side-effects

There will be no side-effects if Bt is not used. The initial decision to treat is influenced by knowledge of alternative treatments and their side-effects, and the presence of other problems such as pregnancy. If treatment is to proceed then good technique and knowledge of special risks are the next important factors: for example injections into some muscles such as the sternomastoid or genioglossus are more likely to provoke dysphagia. It is necessary to get the timing of subsequent treatments right, and to be prepared to hold off, or use a smaller dose or even abandon Bt if necessary.

Antitoxin

Antitoxin is often mentioned as a possible counter to side-effects. If an overdose is given and the situation is immediately realized it may be worth giving antitoxin as it can still neutralize Bt not bound to the plasma membrane. However, antitoxin will not help after a day or so, and will certainly be useless by the time delayed side-effects are apparent. By this time the toxin has been internalized and is not accessible to antitoxin, and it has already blocked acetylcholine release. Treatment of adverse events is symptomatic, to tide the patient over until natural recovery occurs. As the most commonly available antitoxin preparations are of equine origin their use also carries a risk of anaphylaxis.

Minimizing the impact of side-effects

Warn patients and family practitioners of possible side-effects as some are otherwise alarming and may trigger unnecessary investigation or treatment. Patients will tolerate even quite unpleasant side-effects if they have been warned about them in advance and know that they will pass off. Tell them also that if side-effects do occur it is often possible to minimize or avoid them next time by modifying the injections. The peak is usually at 2–4 weeks postinjection, and adverse effects usually wear off long before the clinical benefit disappears. The same dose and pattern of injections can produce variable results, with side-effects cropping up even after several apparently identical and successful injections.

There is no systematic information on the effect of therapeutic Bt in general anaesthesia. In theory, patients could be more sensitive to muscle relaxants. It seems sensible to warn patients to tell their anaesthetist preoperatively, though in practice no problems have been reported.

Although the clinical aim is to produce a controlled and temporary focal weakness, there is commonly some spread to nearby muscles, sometimes enough to provoke more widespread *local* weakness. Whether this matters depends on the clinical situation. Troublesome dysphagia may follow Bt treatment for torticollis, but even quite marked unintentional weakness of hand muscles after forearm injections for spasticity may have no adverse effects in a limb that is anyway useless.

SOME SITE-SPECIFIC PROBLEMS: INJECTION AROUND THE EYES

Tell patients about possible difficulty with eye closure and instruct them about the dangers of foreign bodies in the eye. They should take protective measures and avoid risky situations. It may be helpful to tape the eye shut overnight. The GP should be consulted if problems develop, and should be primed to prescribe methylcellulose or antibiotic eyedrops if required.

An eye patch is helpful for diplopia, or temporary prisms may prove useful. Toxin-induced paralytic ptosis may be controlled using a spectacle mounted ptosis prop such as the Lundie Loop*. This can be obtained either through local opticians or ophthalmology departments or by mail. It must be adapted to the patient's anatomy individually to avoid local skin or corneal lesions. In a few patients this device allows larger doses of toxin to be used, with longer benefit. Patients should understand that the loops will only counter passive ptosis and will not overcome returning blepharospasm. Baggy eyelids may develop and contribute to an apparent ptosis. They may require a blepharoplasty.

LIMB, NECK AND OROMANDIBULAR INJECTIONS

Splints may help excessive limb weakness, though they are rarely necessary. Vigorous muscle stretching exercises after limb injections for spasticity can lead to soft tissue or

---

*In the UK, Lundie Loops can be fitted to spectacle frames sent to: Mr J. Lundie, 48 Tawe Park, Glanrhyd, Ystrad-glynais, Powis SA9 1GU. Tel: 0639 849988.

even joint damage as the weakened muscle is less able to resist the stretch. Neck weakness may cause inconvenience in a few situations such as rising from bed, but here trick movements suffice and a collar is rarely needed. A few patients complain of undue lolling movements of the head when driving. Sometimes these are enough to induce travel sickness and a collar may then be helpful. Rarely, there is a mild vertigo after neck injections, perhaps due to decoupling or resetting of vestibular-proprioceptive reflexes [118]. It usually resolves spontaneously. Masseter and temporalis muscles seem fairly resistant to excessive weakness, even when obviously atrophied, and it is unusual for patients to complain of difficulty chewing.

Dysphagia is potentially the most dangerous side-effect and can occur after neck, laryngeal or oro-mandibular injections. Ask patients with torticollis about dysphagia before treating them with Bt as over half of them may have pre-existing dysphagia [119]. Although the usual advice is to regard pre-existing dysphagia as a risk factor [74], if it is due to dystonia it might in theory be improved by Bt.

In early studies using large doses of BtA, dysphagia occurred as a side-effect after up to 90% of treatments for cervical dystonia. The incidence depends on the dose, muscles injected, the experience of the operator, and patients' expectations and thresholds for reporting symptoms. Dysphagia may be more likely in women, in thin patients, and following sternomastoid injections [117]. As experience has been gained, reported series have used lower doses and reported a much lower incidence (for example, 10%–28% [120,121] of patients or 5% of visits [122]. About 50% experience dysphagia at some time during their therapy over multiple injection cycles [44].

Dysphagia is mainly due to spread of muscle weakness or to autonomic dysfunction. It is usually mild, often no more than a feeling of a dry throat, and patients cope by taking care, sitting in an optimal posture when eating or drinking, chewing thoroughly and washing food down with a drink. In moderate dysphagia they may need to modify the diet to softer food which is more easily chewed or swallowed. In severe dysphagia the risk of aspiration with pneumonia or choking is real, and very rarely hospitalization and nasogastric feeding may be needed. One problem is the patient who derives considerable benefit from toxin injections and plays down any dysphagia, knowing that complaints may lead to lower doses and thus less benefit. The doctor can usually negotiate an acceptable compromise between benefits and adverse events. Patients with pre-existing lung disease are most at risk, and in the UK one patient with severe chronic bronchitis has died from bronchopneumonia following BtA injection for cervical dystonia [123].

Systemic side-effects

Serious systemic side-effects could be related to spread of toxin or an immunological reaction and are rare at standard doses. Treatment is usually symptomatic, combined with reassurance that side-effects wear off. Long-term adverse reactions have not been reported [4].

A feeling of general fatigue may develop, without objective weakness. Although widespread single-fibre EMG abnormalities such as increased jitter do occur after localized BtA administration, the magnitude of the increased jitter does not correlate with the dose of BtA [14]. Other EMG changes such as postexercise facilitation do not occur in muscles distant from the injection site [15]. In one double blind study more patients complained of lassitude after injection with placebo [101]. Treatment with BtA may unmask serious underlying neuromuscular disease, such as Lambert–Eaton myasthenic syndrome [85]. However, BtA has been deliberately used to treat torticollis in a patient with myasthenia gravis, and proved effective and safe [124].

Gallbladder dysfunction leading to cholecystectomy has been reported and attributed to autonomic side-effects of the toxin [125]. In theory any of the autonomic disorders found in botulism could occur, such as paralytic ileus, gastric dilatation and hypotension [126]. Mildly abnormal cardiovascular reflexes have been demonstrated following BtA treatment for craniocervical dystonia and hemifacial spasm [127].

Immunological reactions

Systemic anaphylaxis has not been reported after many hundreds of thousands of injections world-wide. Allergic reactions can, however, occur, and have been held to constitute an absolute contraindication to further injections [128]. Rare patients develop 'localized anaphylactic reactions' or persistent localized rash [129] The tolerance to BtA which occasionally develops is due in some patients to the formation of toxin-neutralizing antibodies. This is discussed in more detail above. Other systemic side-effects have included brachial plexopathy, which may be immune mediated [130,131] and an influenza-like illness. These do not preclude further treatment with Bt [132]. Repeat injections may be trouble free.

Pregnancy and breast feeding

There is little information on the effects of therapeutic doses of BtA on pregnancy. In animal studies of Botox® using pregnant mice and rats, there were no abortions or teratogenic effects with doses up to 4 mu/kg. Doses of 8 and 16 mu/kg, which are much higher than those licensed for clinical use, were associated with reduced fetal body weight and/or delayed ossification of the hyoid bone, which may be reversible. In rabbits, the species most sensitive to BtA, daily Botox® injections of 0.125 mu/kg/day for days 6–18 of gestation, and 2 mu/kg for days 6–13, produced severe maternal toxicity, abortions and/or fetal malformations [133].

There is one report of treatment given to three women known to be pregnant and six treated inadvertently during an unsuspected pregnancy. One woman gave birth prematurely but this was not thought to be related to BtA treatment [134]. Another two women treated inadvertently during pregnancy delivered normal healthy babies [135]. One who received a total of 1280 mu Dysport® in three separate courses at weeks 3, 5 and 8 of pregnancy had an uneventful pregnancy [information supplied by Ipsen]. Questionnaire replies from 396 American physicians using BtA reported 12 who had injected Botox® into a total of 16 pregnant patients, 10 in the first trimester, three in the second trimester and one unknown. The dose ranged from 1.25 to 300 mu. Two women had miscarriages, 13 had normal deliveries and one delivered twins. All the newborns appeared healthy [136]. Pooling these results gives 30 reported births after exposure to therapeutic BtA in pregnancy, with normal deliveries in 27, two miscarriages and one premature birth.

One woman who contracted systemic botulism in the 5th month of pregnancy became almost completely paralysed, with only fetal movements detectable. She needed a tracheostomy and respiratory support for 2 months before recovering. She had a normal spontaneous term delivery of a healthy child.

In the absence of further information, the general advice is to avoid treatment with Bt during pregnancy. It is not known whether treatment during breast feeding is safe: if we consider treatment is essential our policy is to ask the patient to suspend breast feeding for 2 days after injection with Bt. After this time Bt is likely to be fixed in the tissues.

Children

Children are prone to the same side-effects as adults. There is now increasing experience with relatively large doses and so far no special side-effects have emerged (see Chapter 11). The theoretical possibility that Bt might alter cell functions such as axonal growth (see Chapter 2) makes careful monitoring important.

Reducing excess paralytic effect of the toxin

There have been no advances in this area since the first edition of this book. Blocking the initial steps of binding, internalization and transport is not likely to be useful, as these all occur before side-effects have appeared. However in future it might prove possible to accelerate SNARE protein recovery or nerve terminal regeneration, or to overcome established muscle paralysis. Side-effects are usually due to spread of a small amount of toxin, with a less intense loss of power than in the target muscles, and there may be a penumbra with limited damage which is capable of responding to an imperfect toxin antagonist.

Drugs elevating intracellular calcium

A number of agents which alter calcium handling in nerve terminals reduce the activity of the toxin *in vitro*, though some are only helpful in the early stages of poisoning, and others are themselves poisonous. Some, such as calimycin, Black Widow spider venom and lanthanum, increase *resting* calcium levels within the nerve terminal and increase spontaneous quantal release in BtA-poisoned muscles [87]. Others enhance calcium flow during *depolarization,* and in this group the most promising drug is 3, 4-diaminopyridine (DAP) [137]. DAP has been successfully used to treat the Lambert–Eaton syndrome [138] in which there is a similar presynaptic blockade of acetylcholine release. In animal studies DAP strongly antagonizes the effects of BtA in the early stages of poisoning [139] and can delay the onset of paralysis [140]. *In vitro* studies show less effect in established BtA poisoning, and in a double blind study on a single patient with type A botulism it did not alter muscle strength, respiratory function or the EMG compound muscle action potential [141]. Neither was there consistent benefit from DAP in a double blind placebo controlled study in six patients with side-effects of treatment with BoNT/A, although some patients did appear to improve [142].

Recovery by faster nerve regeneration

It may be possible to speed up regeneration of nerve terminals. In animal models of BtA-induced paralysis further damage to the motor nerve, such as a crush lesion, may stimulate faster end-plate regeneration [143]. The mechanism of this effect is uncertain, but duplicating it pharmacologically could prove useful. For instance, Black Widow spider venom destroys presynaptic nerve terminals and can induce regeneration and restoration of synaptic contact after only a few days. It significantly shortens the recovery from paralysis following BtA [32]. In addition, a more normal pattern of reinnervation is established, as opposed to recovery after BtA alone when many ectopic endplates are formed [32].

Running a botulinum toxin service

Many Bt clinics have developed piecemeal, run by interested specialists as part of their wider service. Ophthalmologists and neurologists were the first to exploit Bt and run clinics in most major cities. The wide range of specialities now using Bt in other fields has led to diverse clinic profiles, and clinicians who are setting up new clinics should review the options and adapt to their local circumstances. There are some points that affect most services:

1 The cost of Bt has led many clinicians to use it in a dedicated service to minimize waste.

2 Bt clinics rarely get smaller. Local demand is likely to grow, and as most of the disorders treated require regular repeat treatments, clinicians can rapidly find themselves spending more time and resources running a Bt service. It is essential to plan for this, and especially to establish systems to cope with the workload and the costs.

3 Where appropriate, guidelines advise using Bt in the context of a wider clinical service. Good examples are management of adult spasticity with Bt in the setting of a rehabilitation unit with a multidisciplinary approach [9], or childhood spasticity in a child development centre with access to neurology, orthopaedics, physiotherapy and orthotics, etc. [10].

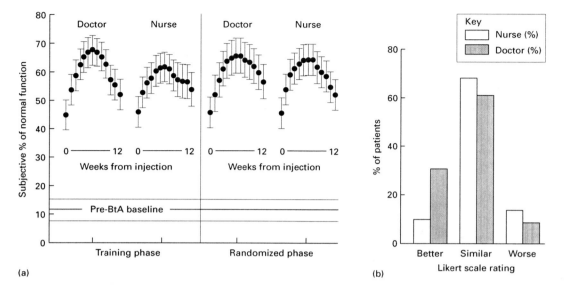

Fig. 3.4 Randomized, open, crossover trial comparing injections given by trained nurse or by doctor, to patients with hemifacial spasm, blepharospasm or cervical dystonia, and a stable response to previous injections [146]. (a) Mean (95% CI) weekly scores for subjective percentage of normal function for four injection cycles of 12 weeks: 0 = no function or very bad; 100 = normal function or very good. In the training phase, nurse cycle followed doctor cycle. Injector sequence was then randomized for second phase. (b) Likert Scale rating of subjective BtA effectiveness in randomized phase of trial. Y-axis is the percentage of patients reporting each grade of effect.

4 Users must have appropriate general training in their speciality and specific training in the use of Bt. General training includes understanding the diagnosis and differential diagnosis, investigations and choice of treatment. Specific training should cover the pharmacology, physiology, biochemistry, benefits and adverse effects of Bt, relevant dynamic anatomy, short- and long-term strategies for using Bt, monitoring outcomes and when to stop treatment. There are specific training guidelines in some situations [144].

Delegating injections

Some conditions are straightforward to treat and suitably trained delegates can be effective and safe. It does not always have to be the doctor giving the injections, though we advise doctors to control and monitor delegates closely. Clinics in the UK are using specialist nurse practitioners to deliver some Bt treatments, and two randomized controlled trials have shown that for selected patients this practice is indeed effective and safe, as a home care service [145], and in a hospital-based clinic [146]. Figure 3.4 shows patients' own ratings of the effects of Bt injections over four successive injection cycles in the latter study. Patients had cervical dystonia, blepharospasm or hemifacial spasm, with a stable and predictable response in at least the three previous injection cycles. In

Table 3.3 Advantages and disadvantages of botulinum toxin.

Advantages	Disadvantages
Often simple, given in outpatients, focused	Can be complex, requiring experience
Side-effects few and short-lived	Wears off, has to be repeated
Flexible—can 'chase' involuntary activity	Potentially expensive, funds not identified
Reduces need for systemic drugs	Logistical—organizing a clinic
Easily integrated with other treatment	Long-term commitment
Benefits independent of cause of abnormality	Inadequate for widespread disease
	Discomfort of multiple injections

this trial, the first injections were given by the doctor, the second cycle injections by a nurse trained and supervised by the doctor. In the third and fourth cycles patients were randomized in an open crossover study to nurse- or doctor-given injections. The main outcome measure was a visual analogue score recorded weekly by the patient at home, with 0 = very bad, cannot imagine being worse, and 100 = very good, no problem. At the start of the trial, patients gave a score for their recall of the original severity of their problem, before receiving their very first BtA injection (visual analogue scale baseline 0). The area under the curve (AUC) represented the patient's own perception of cumulative benefit over the 3-month cycle (Fig. 3.4a). Patients also completed two seven-point Likert scales just before each attendance, rating: (a) the effect of the trial injection (major deterioration: major benefit); and (b) comparing it with their previous injection (much worse: much better) (Fig. 3.4b). In the randomized phase of the study there was no statistically significant difference in any of these outcomes between the nurse- and the doctor-given injections.

Conclusions

We continue to improve our understanding of when and how to use Bt. Table 3.3 gives some of the advantages and disadvantages. It can be deceptively simple—and often is quite straightforward—but Bt can also raise complex questions which experts struggle to answer convincingly. Anyone using Bt will use it more effectively if they understand the issues outlined in this chapter.

References

1 Ade-Hall R, Moore A. A systematic review of controlled trials of the use of botulinum toxin type A for the treatment of leg spasticity in cerebral palsy. The Cochrane Library 2000: Q1.

2 Costa J, Ferreira J, Sampaio C. Botulinum toxin A for the treatment of cervical dystonia: a systematic review. *Mov Disord* 2000; **15**: 29.

3 Moore A, Blumhardt LD. A double blind trial of botulinum toxin 'A' in torticollis, with one year follow up. *J Neurol Neurosurg Psychiatry* 1991; **54**: 813–6.

4 Therapeutics and Technology Subcommittee of the American Academy of Medicine. Assessment: the clinical usefulness of botulinum toxin A in treating neurologic disorders. *Neurology* 1990; **40**: 1332–6.

5 Williams A. Consensus statement for the management of focal dystonias. *Br J Hosp Med* 1993; **50**: 655–9.

6 Shaari CM, Sanders I. Quantifying how location and dose of botulinum toxin injections affect muscle paralysis. *Muscle Nerve* 1993; **16**: 964–9.

7 Bigalke H, Wohlfarth K, Irmer A, Dengler R. Botulinum A toxin. Dysport® improvement of biological availability. *Experimental Neurology* 2001; **168**: 162–70.

8 Sloop R, Cole D, Patel M. Muscle paralysis produced by botulinum toxin type A injection in treated torticollis patients compared with toxin naive individuals. *Mov Disord* 2001; **16**: 100–5.

9 Barnes M, Bhakta B, Moore P *et al. The Management of Adults with Spasticity using Botulinum Toxin: a Guide to Clinical Practice. Consensus Document from a Panel Discussion.* Byfleet, Surrey: Radius Healthcare, 2001

10 Graham H, Aoki K, Autti-Rämö I *et al.* Recommendations for the use of botulinum toxin type A in the management of cerebral palsy. *Gait Posture* 2000; **11**: 67–9.

11 De Camilli P. Exocytosis goes with a SNAP. *Nature* 1993; **365**: 387–8.

12 Osen-Sand A, Catsicas M, Staple JK *et al.* Inhibition of axonal growth by SNAP-25 antisense oligonucleotides *in vitro* and *in vivo. Nature* 1993; **364**: 445–8.

13 Hallett M, Glocker F, Deuschl G. Mechanism of action of botulinum toxin. *Ann Neurol* 1994; **36**: 449–50.

14 Lange DJ, Brin MF, Warner CL, Fahn S, Lovelace RE. Distant effects of local injection of botulinum toxin. *Muscle Nerve* 1987; **10**: 552–5.

15 Olney RK, Aminoff MJ, Gelb DJ, Lowenstein DH. Neuromuscular effects distant from the site of botulinum neurotoxin injection. *Neurology* 1988; **38**: 1780–3.

16 Wiegand H, Erdmann G, Wellhoner HH. [125]Labelled botulinum A neurotoxin: pharmacokinetics in cats after intramuscular injection. *Naunyn-Schmiedebergs Arch Pharmacol* 1976; **292**: 161–5.

17 Garner CG, Straube A, Witt TN, Gasser T, Oertel WH. Time course of distant effects of local injections of botulinum toxin. *Mov Disord* 1993; **8**: 33–7.

18 Hallett M. How does botulinum toxin work? *Ann Neurol* 2000; **48**: 7–8.

19 Rosales RL, Arimura K, Takenaga S, Osame M. Extrafusal and intrafusal muscle effects in experimental botulinum toxin A injection. *Muscle Nerve* 1996; **19**: 488–96.

20 Kaji R, Rothwell JC, Katayama M *et al.* Tonic vibration reflex and muscle afferent block in writer's cramp. *Ann Neurol* 1995; **38**: 155–62.

21 Filippi GM, Errico P, Santarelli R, Bagolini B, Manni E. Botulinum A toxin effects on rat jaw muscle spindles. *Acta Otolaryngologica Stockholm* 1993; **113**: 400–4.

22 Manni E, Bagolini B, Pettorossi VE, Errico P. Effect of botulinum toxin on extraocular muscle proprioception. *Doc Ophthalmol* 1989; **72**: 189–98.

23 Hagenah R, Benecke R, Wiegand H. Effects of type A botulinum toxin on the transmission at spinal Renshaw cells and on the inhibitory action at 1a inhibitory interneurones. *Naunyn-Schmiedebergs Arch. Pharmacol* 1977; **299**: 267–72.

24 Naumann M, Reiners K. Long-latency reflexes of hand muscles in idiopathic focal dystonia and their modification by botulinum toxin. *Brain* 1997; **120**: 409–16.

25 Gelb DJ, Yoshimura DM, Olney RK, Lowenstein DH, Aminoff MJ. Change in pattern of muscle activity following botulinum toxin injections for torticollis. *Ann Neurol* 1991; **29**: 370–6.

26 Priori A, Berardelli A, Mercuri B, Manfredi M. Physiological effects produced by botulinum toxin treatment of upper limb dystonia. Changes in reciprocal inhibition between forearm muscles. *Brain* 1995; **118**: 801–7.

27 Gilio F, Currà A, Lorenzano C *et al.* Effects of botulinum toxin A on intracortical inhibition in patients with dystonia. *Ann Neurol* 2000; **48**: 20–7.

28 Byrnes M, Thickbroom G, Wilson S *et al*. The corticomotor representation of upper limb muscles in writer's cramp and changes following botulinum toxin injection. *Brain* 1998; **121**: 977–88.

29 Brown P. Pathophysiology of spasticity. *J Neurol Neurosurg Psychiatry* 1994; **57**: 773–7.

30 Cosgrove APGH. Botulinum toxin A prevents the development of contractures in the hereditary spastic mouse. *Dev Med Child Neurol* 1994; **36**: 379–85.

31 Simpson LL. Clinically relevant aspects of the mechanism of action of botulinum neurotoxin. *J Voice* 1992; **6**: 358–64.

32 Gomez S, Queiros LZ. The effects of Black Widow spider venom on the innervation of muscles paralysed by botulinum toxin. *Q J Exp Physio* 1982; **67**: 495–506.

33 Duchen LW, Strich SJ. The effects of botulinum toxin on the pattern of innervation of skeletal muscle in the mouse. *Q J Exp Physio* 1968; **53**: 84–9.

34 Duchen LW. An electron microscopic study of the changes induced by botulinum toxin in the motor end plates of slow and fast skeletal muscles fibres of the mouse. *J Neurol Sci* 1971; **14**: 47–60.

35 Holland RL, Brown MC. Nerve growth in botulinum toxin poisoned muscles. *Neuroscience* 1981; **6**: 1167–79.

36 Simpson LL. Peripheral actions of the botulinum neurotoxins. *Botulinum Neurotoxin and Tetanus Toxin*. San Diego, CA: Academic Press, 1989: 153–78.

37 Pamphlett R. Early terminal and nodal sprouting of motor axons after botulinum toxin. *J Neurol Sci* 1989; **92**: 181–92.

38 Duchen LW, Strich T. The effects of botulinum toxin on the pattern of innervation of skeletal muscle in the mouse. *Q J Exp Physio* 1968; **53**: 84–9.

39 De Paiva A, Meunier F, Molgo J, Aoki K, Dolly J. Functional repair of motor endplates after botulinum toxin type A poisoning: biphasic switch of synaptic activity between nerve sprouts and their parent terminals. *Proc Natl Acad Sci U S A* 1999; **96**: 3200–5.

40 Alderson K, Holds JB, Anderson RL. Botulinum-induced alteration of nerve–muscle interactions in the human orbicularis oculi following treatment for blepharospasm. *Neurology* 1991; **41**: 1800–5.

41 Harris CP, Alderson K, Nebeker J, Holds JB, Anderson RL. Histologic features of human orbicularis oculi treated with botulinum A toxin. *Arch Ophthalmol* 1991; **109**: 393–5.

42 Ansved T, Odergren T, Borg K. Muscle fiber atrophy in leg muscles after botulinum toxin type A treatment of cervical dystonia. *Neurology* 1997; **48**: 1440–6.

43 Stahl JS, Averbuch-Heller L, Remler BF, Leigh RJ. Clinical evidence of extraocular muscle fiber-type specificity of botulinum toxin. *Neurology* 1998; **51**: 1093–9.

44 Kessler K, Skutta M, Benecke R. Long-term treatment of cervical dystonia with botulinum toxin A. Efficacy, safety, and antibody frequency. *J Neurol* 1999; **246**: 265–74.

45 Aoki K. A comparison of the safety margins of botulinum neurotoxin serotypes A, B and F in mice. *Toxicon* 2001; **39**: 1815–20.

46 Guyer B. Some unresolved issues with botulinum toxin. *J Neurol* 2001; **248**: 1–11–1/13.

47 Peng K, Merlino G, Foster SA, Spanoyannis A, Aoki KR. BOTOX® (botulinum toxin type A purified neurotoxin complex) is six-fold more potent than Dysport® in the mouse digit abduction scoring (DAS) assay. *Mov Disord* 1998; **13** (Suppl. 2): 110.

48 Dressler D, Rothwell J, Marsden C. Comparing biological potencies of Botox® and Dysport® with a mouse model may mislead. *J Neurol* 1998; **245**: 332.

49 Sampaio C, Ferreira JJ, Simoes F *et al*. DYSBOT. A single blind, randomized parallel study to determine whether any differences can be detected in the efficacy and tolerability of two formulations of botulinum toxin type A—Dysport® and Botox®—assuming a ratio of 4 : 1. *Mov Disord* 1997; **12**: 1013–8.

50 Marion MH, Sheehy MP, Sangla S, Soulayrol S. A study to compare the clinical efficacy of two different preparations of botulinum toxin in a group of patients with either hemifacial spasm or blepharospasm. *Mov Disord* 1994; **9** (Suppl. 1): 51.

51 Odergren T, Hjaltason H, Kaakkola S *et al*. A double blind, randomized, parallel group study to investigate the dose equivalence of Dysport® and Botox® in the treatment of cervical dystonia. *J Neurol Neurosurg Psychiatry* 1998; **64**: 6–12.

52 Ranoux D, Gury C, Khalf Y, Mas J, Zuber M. A randomized, double blind, crossover study to compare the clinical effects of BOTOX® and two different ratios of Dysport® in cervical dystonia. *Mov Disord* 2000; **15**: 141.

53 Wohlfarth K, Göschel H, Frevert J, Dengler R, Bigalke H. Botulinum toxin A toxins: units versus units. *Naunyn-Schmiedebergs Arch Pharmacol* 1997; **335**: 335–40.

54 Elston J. In: *Current therapy in neurologic disease*. Mosby Year Book, 1993: 276–81.

55 Tidswell P, King M. Comparison of two botulinum toxin preparations in the treatment of dystonias. *J Neurol Sci* 2001; **187**: S421.

56 Nussgens Z, Roggenkamper P. Comparison of two botulinum-toxin preparations in the treatment of essential blepharospasm. *Graefes Arch Clin Exp Ophthalmol* 1997; **235**: 197–9.

57 Van den Bergh P, Lison D. Dose standardization of botulinum toxin. In: Fahn S, Marsden C, DeLong M, eds. *Dystonia 3: Advances in Neurology*, Vol. 78. Philadelphia: Lippincott–Raven Publishers, 1998: 231–5.

58 Durif F. Clinical bioequivalence of the current commercial preparations of botulinum toxin. *Eur J Neurol* 1996; **2**: 17–18.

59 Dengler R, Neyer U, Wohlfarth K, Bettig U, Janzik HH. Local botulinum toxin in the treatment of spastic drop foot. *J Neurol* 1992; **239**: 375–8.

60 Schantz EJ, Johnson EA. Preparation and characterization of botulinum toxin type A for human treatment. In: Jankovic J, ed. *Therapy with Botulinum Toxin*. New York: Marcel Dekker Inc., 1994: 41–9.

61 Meyer K, Caputo F, Gasper C, Shopp G. Botulinum toxin type B, NeuroBloc®. Comparable systemic toxicities in adult and juvenile cynomolgus monkeys. *Mov Disord* 2000; **15** (Suppl. 3): 158–9.

62 Meyer KF, Eddie B. Perspectives concerning botulism. *Z Hyg Infektionskrankh* 1951; **133**: 255–63.

63 Schantz EJ, Sugiyama H. Toxic proteins produced by *Clostridium botulinum*. *J Agr Food Chem* 1974; **22**: 26–30.

64 Gill DM. Bacterial toxins. A table of lethal amounts. *Microbiol Rev* 1982; **46**: 86–94.

65 Tsui JKC, O'Brien CF. Clinical trials for spasticity. In: Jankovic J, ed. *Therapy with Botulinum Toxin*. New York: Marcel Dekker Inc., 1994: 523–33.

66 Konstanzer A, Ceballos-Baumann AO, Dressnandt J, Conrad B. Botulinum toxin A treatment in spasticity of arm and leg. *Mov Disord* 1992; **7**: 137.

67 Cullis P, Moore A, Chen R *et al*. An open label, forced dose-escalation safety study of botulinum toxin type B (Myobloc® injectable solution) in patients with cervical dystonia. Personal communication.

68 Scott AB. Botulinum toxin injection of eye muscles to correct strabismus. *Trans Am Ophthalmol Soc* 1981; **129**: 734–69.

69 Gartlan MG, Hoffman HT. Crystalline preparation of botulinum toxin type A (Botox®): degradation in potency with storage. *Otolaryngol Head Neck Surg* 1993; **108**: 135–40.

70 Greene P. *Clinical Trials for Cervical Dystonia 2*. Bethesda, MD: National Institute of Health, 1990: 53–6.

71 Greene P. Potency of frozen/thawed botulinum toxin type A in the treatment of torsion dystonia. *Otolaryngol Head Neck Surg* 1993; **109**: 968–9.

72 Setler P. The biochemistry of botulinum toxin type B. *Neurology* 2000; **55**: S22–8.

73 Borodic GE, Ferrante R, Pearce BL, Smith K. Histologic assessment of dose-related diffusion and muscle fiber response after therapeutic botulinum A toxin injections. *Mov Disord* 1994; **9**: 31–9.

74 Jankovic J, Brin MF. Therapeutic uses of botulinum toxin. *N Engl J Med* 1991; **324**: 1186–94.

75 Shaari CM, George E, Wu BL, Biller HF, Sanders I. Quantifying the spread of botulinum toxin through muscle fascia. *Laryngoscope* 1991; **101**: 960–4.

76 Borodic GE, Pearce LB, Smith K, Joseph M. Botulinum. A toxin for spasmodic torticollis: multiple vs. single injection points per muscle. *Head Neck* 1992; **14**: 33–7.

77 Walker FO, Scott GE, Butterworth J. Sustained focal effects of low-dose intramuscular succinyl-choline. *Muscle Nerve* 1993; **16**: 181–7.

78 Anonymous. Trauma and dystonia. *The Lancet* 1989; 759–60.

79 Comella CL. Electromyography-assisted botulinum toxin injections for cervical dystonia. In: Jankovic J, ed. *Therapy with Botulinum Toxin*. New York: Marcel Dekker Inc., 1994: 289–98.

80 Comella CL, Buchman AS, Tanner CM, Brown-Toms NC, Goetz CG. Botulinum toxin injection for spasmodic torticollis. Increased magnitude of benefit with electromyographic assistance. *Neurology* 1992; **42**: 878–82.

81 Buchman AS, Comella CL, Stebbins GT, Tanner CM, Goetz CG. Quantitative electromyographic analysis of changes in muscle activity following botulinum toxin therapy for cervical dystonia. *Clin Neuropharmacol* 1993; **16**: 205–10.

82 Ostergaard L, Fuglsang-Frederiksen A, Werdelin L, Sjo O, Winkel H. Quantitative EMG in botulinum toxin treatment of cervical dystonia. A double blind, placebo-controlled study. *Electroencephalogr Clin Neurophysiol* 1994; **93**: 434–9.

83 Cosgrove AP, Graham HK. Cerebral Palsy. In: Moore P. ed. *Handbook of Botulinum Toxin Treatment*. Oxford: Blackwell Scientific, 1995: 222–47.

84 Duane D, Stuart S, Case J, LaPointe L. Successful and safe use of botulinum toxin A in a patient with subclinical myasthenia gravis and lingual/brachial/manual dystonia. *Mov Disord* 2000; **15**: 149.

85 Erbguth F, Claus D, Engelhardt A, Dressler D. Systemic effect of local botulinum injections unmasks subclinical Lambert–Eaton syndrome. *J Neurol Neurosurg Psychiatry* 1993; **56**: 1235–6.

86 Metzer S, Jenkins T, McClellan VA. Effect of prior denervation surgery on outcome of botulinum toxin injection for torticollis. *Mov Disord* 1992; **7**: 131.

87 Sellin LC. The action of botulinum toxin at the neuromuscular junction. *Med Biol* 1981; **59**: 11–20.

88 Hughes R, Whaler BC. Influence of nerve-ending activity and of drugs on the rate of paralysis of rat diaphragm preparations by *Cl. botulinum* type A toxin. *J Physiol* 1962; **160**: 221–33.

89 Eleopra R, Tugnoli V, De Grandis D. The variability in the clinical effect induced by botulinum toxin type A. The role of muscle activity in humans. *Mov Disord* 1997; **12**: 89–94.

90 Hesse S, Jahnke MT, Luecke D, Mauritz KH. Short-term electrical stimulation enhances the effectiveness of botulinum toxin in the treatment of lower limb spasticity in hemiparetic patients. *Neurosci Lett* 1995; **201**: 37–40.

91 Hesse S, Reiter F, Konrad M, Jahnke MT. Botulinum toxin type A and short-term electrical stimulation in the treatment of upper limb flexor spasticity after stroke: a randomized, double blind, placebo-controlled trial. *Clin Rehabil* 1998; **12**: 381–8.

92 Arezzo J, Litwak M, Caputo F *et al*. Spread of paralytic activity in juvenile and adult monkeys for NeuroBloc® (botulinum toxin type B) and Botox® (botulinum toxin type A). *J Neurol Sci* 2001; **187**: S312.

93 Hott JS, Dalakas MC, Sung C, Hallett M, Youle RJ. Skeletal muscle-specific immunotoxin for the treatment of focal muscle spasm. *Neurology* 1998; **50**: 485–91.

94 World Health Organization (WHO). *ICIDH-2. International Classification of Functioning and Disability. Beta-2 Draft, Full Version*. Geneva: WHO, 1999.

95 World Health Organization (WHO). *The International Classification of Impairments, Disabilities and Handicaps*. Geneva: WHO, 1980.

96 Wade DT. *Neurological Rehabilitation*. London: Churchill Livingstone, 1990: 133–56.

97 Brin MF, Blitzer A, Herman S, Stewart C. Oro–facio–mandibular and lingual dystonia. In: Moore P, ed. *Handbook of Botulinum Toxin Treatment*. Oxford: Blackwell Scientific, 1995: 151–163.

98 Stebbins GT, Comella CL, Buchman A, Penn K. Changes in quality-of-life following Botox® injections for spasmodic torticollis. *Mov Disord* 1992; **7**: 135.

99 Knoll T, Gasser T, Arnold G *et al*. Psychopathology in patients with idiopathic dystonia improves under botulinum toxin treatment. *Mov Disord* 1992; **7**: 137.

100 Consky E, Basinski A, Belle L, Ranawaya R, Lang AE. The Toronto Western Spasmodic Torticollis Rating Scale (TWSTRS). Assessment of validity and inter-rater reliability. *Neurology* 1990; **40**: 445.

101 Tsui JK, Eisen A, Stoessel AJ, Calne S, Calne DB. Double blind study of botulinum toxin in spasmodic torticollis. *Lancet North Am Ed* 1986; **ii**: 245–7.

102 Greene P, Fahn S. Development of antibodies to botulinum toxin type A in torticollis patients treated with botulinum toxin injections. *Mov Disord* 1992; **7**: 134.

103 Hanna P, Jankovic J. Mouse bioassay versus Western blot assay for botulinum toxin antibodies. *Neurology* 1998; **50**: 1624–9.

104 Kessler KR, Benecke R. The EDB test—a clinical test for the detection of antibodies to botulinum toxin type A. *Mov Disord* 1997; **12**: 95–9.

105 Birklein F, Erbguth M. Sudomotor or sweating test for Bt antibodies. *Mov Disord* 2000; **15**: 146–7.

106 Hanna PA, Jankovic J, Vincent A. Comparison of mouse bioassay and immunoprecipitation assay for botulinum toxin antibodies. *J Neurol Neurosurg Psychiatry* 1999; **66**: 612–6.

107 Goschel H, Wohlfarth K, Frevert J, Dengler R, Bigalke H. Botulinum A toxin therapy: neutralising and nonneutralising antibodies—therapeutic consequences. *Exp Neurol* 1997; **147** (1): 96–102.

108 Dressler D, Dirnberger G, Bhatia K *et al*. Botulinum toxin antibody testing. Comparison of the mouse diaphragm bioassay and the mouse lethality bioassay *Mov Disord* 2000; **15**: 973.

109 Zuber M, Sebald M, Bathien N, de-Recondo J, Rondot P. Botulinum antibodies in dystonic patients treated with type A botulinum toxin. frequency and significance. *Neurology* 1993; **43**: 1715–8.

110 Jankovic J, Schwartz K. Response and immunoresistance to botulinum toxin injections. *Neurology* 1995; **45**: 1743–6.

111 Duane C, Clark M, LaPointe L, Case JLMD. Botulinum toxin A antibodies in initial and delayed resistance to botulinum toxin A therapy in cervical dystonia. *Mov Disord* 1995; **10**: 394.

112 Gonnering R. Negative antibody response to long-term treatment of facial spasm with botulinum toxin. *Am J Ophthalmol* 1988; **105**: 313–5.

113 Greene P, Fahn S, Diamond B. Development of resistance to botulinum toxin type A in patients with torticollis. *Mov Disord* 1994; **9**: 213–7.

114 Naumann M, Toyka K, Taleghani B, Reiners K, Bigalke H. Depletion of neutralizing antibodies re-sensitizes a secondary non-responder to botulinum A neurotoxin. *J Neurol Neurosurg Psychiatry* 1998; **65**: 924–7.

115 Dressler D, Zettl U, Benecke R. Can intravenous immunoglobulin improve antibody-mediated botulinum toxin therapy failure? *Mov Disord* 2000; **15**: 1279–81.

116 Lew MF, Adornato BT, Duane DD *et al*. Botulinum toxin type B. A double blind, placebo-controlled, safety and efficacy study in cervical dystonia. *Neurology* 1997; **49**: 701–7.

117 Jankovic J, Schwartz KS. Clinical correlates of response to botulinum toxin injections. *Arch Neurol* 1991; **48**: 1253–6.

118 Huygen P, Verhagen W, Van Hoof J. Vestibular hyperreactivity in patients with idiopathic spasmodic torticollis. *J Neurol Neurosurg Psychiatry* 1989; **52**: 782–5.

119 Riski J, Horner J, Nashold B. Swallowing function on patients with spasmodic torticollis. *Neurology* 1990; **40**: 1443–5.

120 Greene P, Kang U, Fahn S *et al*. Double blind, placebo-controlled trial of botulinum toxin injections for the treatment of spasmodic torticollis. *Neurology* 1990; **40**: 1213–8.

121 Blackie JD, Lees AJ. Botulinum toxin treatment in spasmodic torticollis. *J Neurol Neurosurg Psychiatry* 1990; **53**: 640–3.

122 Jankovic J, Schwartz K. Botulinum toxin injections for cervical dystonia. *Neurology* 1990; **40**: 277–80.

123 Committee on Safety of Medicines. Reminder: botulinum type A toxin (Dysport®)—severe dysphagia with unlicensed route of administration. *Curr Probl Pharmacovigil* 1993; **19**: 11.

124 Emmerson J. Botulinum toxin for spasmodic torticollis in a patient with myasthenia gravis. *Mov Disord* 1994; **9**: 367–79.

125 Schnider P, Brichta A, Schmied M, Auff E. Gallbladder dysfunction induced by botulinum A toxin. *Lancet North Am Ed* 1993; **342**: 811–2.

126 Critchley EM, Mitchell JD. Human botulism. *Br J Hosp Med* 1990; **43**: 290–2.

127 Girlanda P, Vita G, Nicolosi C, Milone S, Messina C. Botulinum toxin therapy: distant effects on neuromuscular transmission and autonomic nervous system. *J Neurol Neurosurg Psychiatry* 1992; **55**: 844–5.

128 Anonymous. Clinical use of botulinum toxin. National Institutes of Health Consensus development conference statement, November 12–14, 1990. *Arch Neurol* 1991; **48**: 1294–8.

129 LeWitt P, Trosch RM. Idiosyncratic adverse reactions to intramuscular botulinum toxin type A injection. *Mov Disord* 1997; **12**: 1064–7.

130 Glanzman RL, Gelb DJ, Drury I, Bromberg MB, Truong DD. Brachial plexopathy after botulinum toxin injections. *Neurology* 1990; **40**: 1143.

131 Sampaio C, Castro-Caldas A, Sales-Luis MI *et al.* Brachial plexopathy after botulinum toxin administration for cervical dystonia [letter]. *J Neurol Neurosurg Psychiatry* 1993; **56**: 220.

132 Anonymous. Botulinum toxin [editorial]. *Lancet North Am Ed* 1992; **340**: 1508–9.

133 Botox® data sheet 1999–2000. Allergan Inc.

134 Scott AB. Clostridial toxins as therapeutic agents. In: Simpson LL, ed. *Botulinum Neurotoxin and Tetanus Toxin*. San Diego, CA: Academic Press, Inc., 1989: 399–412.

135 Calne S. Local treatment of dystonia and spasticity with injections of botulinum A toxin. *Axone* 1993; **14**: 85–8.

136 Moser E, Ligon KM, Singer C, Sethi KD. Botulinum toxin A (Botox®) therapy during pregnancy. *Neurology* 1997; Suppl. 1: A399.

137 Thesleff S. Pharmacologic antagonism of clostridial toxins. In: Simpson LL, ed. *Botulinum Neurotoxin and Tetanus Toxin*. San Diego, CA: Academic Press, Inc., 1989.

138 McEvoy KM, Windebank AJ, Daube JR, Low PA. 3,4-Diaminopyridine in the treatment of Lambert–Eaton myasthenic syndrome. *N Eng J Med* 1989; **321**: 1567–71.

139 Molgio J, Lemeignan M, Thesleff S. Aminoglycosides and 3,4-Diaminopyridine on neuromuscular block caused by botulinum type A toxin. *Muscle Nerve* 1987; **10**: 464–70.

140 Simpson LL. A preclinical evaluation of aminopyridines as putative therapeutic agents in the treatment of botulism. *Infect Immun*, 1986; **52**: 858–62.

141 Davis LE, Johnson JK, Bicknell JM, Levy H, McEvoy KM. Human type A botulism and treatment with 3,4-diaminopyridine. *Electromyogr Clin Neurophysiol* 1992; **32**: 379–83.

142 Moore A. 2,4-Diaminopyridine for side-effects of therapeutic botulinum toxin A. *Mov Disord* 1994; **9**: 843.

143 Thesleff S, Zelena J, Hoffman WW. Restoration of function in botulinum paralysis by experimental nerve regeneration. *Proc Soc Exp Biol Med* 1964; **116**: 19–20.

144 Report of the Therapeutics and Technology Assessment Subcommittee of the American Academy of Neurology. Training. Guidelines for the use of botulinum toxin for the treatment of neurological disorders. *Neurology* 1994; **44**: 2401–3.

145 Whitaker J, Butler A, Semlyen J, Barnes M. Botulinum toxin for people with dystonia treated by an outreach nurse practitioner—a comparative study between a home and a clinic treatment service. *Arch Phys Med Rehab* 2001; **82**: 480–4.

146 Moore A, Rog D. Open label randomized controlled trial comparing botulinum toxin injections given by doctors and by specialist nurses. Submitted for publication 2002. In press.

EMG for identification of dystonic, tremulous and spastic muscles and techniques for guidance of injections

JÖRG WISSEL, JÖRG MÜLLER & WERNER POEWE

Introduction

Botulinum toxin (Bt) induces a focal, selective, graded, temporary paresis of the injected muscles. Beside the blockade of the neuromuscular junction, Bt has also a temporary inhibiting effect on the activity of gamma fusimotor fibres at the level of the muscle spindle [1], on the spinal interneurone excitability [2], on reciprocal muscle activation during gait [3], on cortical representation of injected muscles [4] and on cortical excitability in sensorimotor areas [5].

Correct selection and identification of affected muscles is crucial to the success of Bt injections and is mainly based on clinical features. However, this is not always possible on clinical grounds alone, and sometimes clinicians need other tools such as electromyography (EMG) and imaging techniques to find target muscles.

This chapter will discuss the general criteria for muscle selection for Bt treatment in patients with dystonia, tremor and spasticity. By way of example it covers patterns of activity in dystonic, tremulous and spastic muscles, and Bt injection guidance using EMG, electrical stimulation and imaging techniques.

General criteria for muscle selection and the role of EMG

The basis of successful Bt treatment is correct identification of muscles involved in the involuntary movement and associated pain. We recommend five sets of criteria to identify muscles for injection:

1 Bio-mechanical analysis of involuntary posture and movements during rest and voluntary activation.

2 Analysis of muscle tone and clonus activity during passive stretch of the affected muscles.

3 Visible and palpable muscle activity, stiffening and hypertrophy.

4 Location of uncomfortable stiffness or pain during rest, passive stretch or voluntary movement.

5 Poly EMG (simultaneous multichannel EMG) criteria.

In most cases of focal dystonias (e.g. rotational cervical dystonia [CD], jaw closure dystonia and flexor type writer's cramp), classical tremor syndromes (e.g. rest tremor in Parkinson's disease) and in typical syndromes with localized spasticity (e.g. clawed hand and flexed wrist or equinovarus foot position) clinical criteria alone are usually sufficient to select and identify muscles for Bt injections. However, even in the apparently straightforward situation of blepharospasm, the clinical picture may fail to reveal crucial elements of dystonic muscle activity, as was shown for patients with 'levator inhibition' with cocontraction of the pretarsal orbicularis oculi and levator palpebrae [6]. In CD, neck muscle activation patterns can change spontaneously despite constant dystonic head position [7].

We recommend poly EMG recordings to select muscles for injection or reinjection in all patients with complex involuntary posture or movements in dystonia or spasticity, and in patients with an inadequate response to previous Bt treatment. In patients with postural or action tremor of the arms poly EMG from antagonistic muscle groups before the first Bt injection is also useful to select the relevant muscles for injection. Remember that once muscles have been injected with Bt it may be many months before their EMG signal returns to normal, and the abnormal signal can hinder poly EMG interpretation during this time.

EMG patterns of dystonia, tremor and spasticity

EMG patterns of dystonia

The exact pathophysiological mechanisms underlying dystonia are still unclear. In idiopathic dystonia, conventional needle EMG and nerve conduction studies indicate that the peripheral motor nerves and large diameter corticospinal tract function normally [8]. Dystonic movements are probably based on a dysfunction of basal ganglia output to the motor cortex and to the brainstem, including the preparation of voluntary movements [9–14]. Poly EMG features of dystonia (Table 4.1 & Fig. 4.1) match the clinical impression of cocontraction of antagonistic muscles [15], with mainly tonic, non-reciprocal, EMG patterns during rest or voluntary movement [10,16–21]. In addition, there may be spontaneous and grouped slow rhythmical or irregular discharges [22,23].

Dystonic movements can be slow and sustained ('tonic'), resulting in abnormal postures, or rapid and/or jerky ('phasic') resulting in fast movements. Phasic movements in dystonia may be irregular or rhythmic (Fig. 4.2). Four EMG patterns can be distinguished [23], as shown in Table 4.2. These dystonic EMG patterns may occur alone (e.g. pure tonic or pure irregular-phasic pattern) or in various combinations. Tremor

Table 4.1 Poly EMG pattern of dystonia.

1	Spontaneous involuntary muscle activity at rest or during postural stress
2	Enhanced cocontraction of antagonistic muscles during voluntary movements
3	'Overflow' of muscle activity into muscles normally not involved in the movement

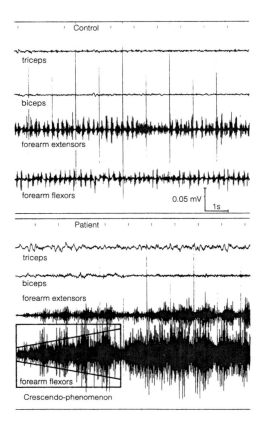

Fig. 4.1 Normal and dystonic EMG patterns during writing. Surface EMG recordings from elbow and forearm muscles during a standardized writing task. *Upper recording*: Normal control with reciprocal burst generation in forearm flexors and extensors. *Lower recording*: Patient with simple writer's cramp (task-specific flexion of wrist and all fingers) with increased tonic activation, disordered reciprocal innervation and cocontractions. Crescendo phenomenon during build-up of tonic contraction is a characteristic sign of dystonic activity in writer's cramp.

frequencies vary between 4 and 12 Hz [18,23]. Dystonic tremor usually has a frequency of 4–6 Hz [23–25], and has to be separated from a 10–12 Hz tremor of muscles activated to overcome dystonic posture [25]. Myoclonic patterns are usually superimposed on long-lasting tonic activation [26]. These dystonic jerks in idiopathic dystonia are clinically similar to those of primary myoclonus but back-averaging of cortical activity fails to reveal any preceding time-locked electroencephalogram (EEG) event [10].

At rest, mildly affected patients with dystonia sometimes have no involuntary muscle activity, whereas moderately and severely affected patients may show continuous dystonic EMG activity. Any attempt at voluntary movement, especially more delicate and precise manoeuvres such as writing (Fig. 4.1), may exacerbate involuntary muscle spasms with prolonged cocontracting activity in antagonists [10,22].

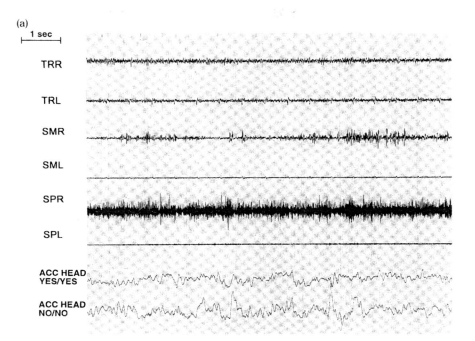

Fig. 4.2 Poly-EMG recordings were made of three symmetrical muscle pairs, with simultaneous accelerometric signals of head movement along two axes. Patients were sitting relaxed. (a) *Tonic EMG pattern:* Rotational torticollis and slight laterocollis to the right. The patient showed tonic EMG activity in the right splenius capitis (SPR) during spontaneous dystonic head posture. (b) *Irregular-phasic EMG pattern:* Retrocollis and rotational torticollis to the left. There is irregular phasic EMG activity in the right trapezius (TPR) and sternomastoid (SMR) and both splenii capitis (SPR, SPL) with additional interpolated, short-tremor episodes in both splenii during spontaneous dystonic head movements. (c) *Tremulous EMG pattern:* Tremulous rotational torticollis to the left. There is tremulous EMG activity in the right trapezius (TRR), both sternomastoids (SMR, SML) and both splenii capitis (SPR, SPL) with tremor oscillations in the accelerometer trace during spontaneous dystonic head movements. ACC, accelerometer recording; 'No/No', horizontal plane; TRL, left trapezius; 'Yes/Yes', vertical plane. (Figure 4.2 *continued on p. 80.*)

Types of EMG activity in cervical dystonia

Involuntary EMG activity

Patients with CD typically generate lengthy agonist bursts (tonic EMG pattern) and cocontraction in antagonistic muscles [16,23], sometimes with a prominent low-frequency tremor [23,25]. Irregular jerking of the head is associated with arrhythmic phasic or myoclonic EMG activity. In our own series, we analysed 145 poly EMGs of patients with CD before botulinum toxin type A (BtA) treatment. In every patient the EMG activity of three paired neck muscles (surface electrodes: sternomastoid and trapezius muscles; concentric needle electrodes: splenius capitis muscle) were recorded

(b)

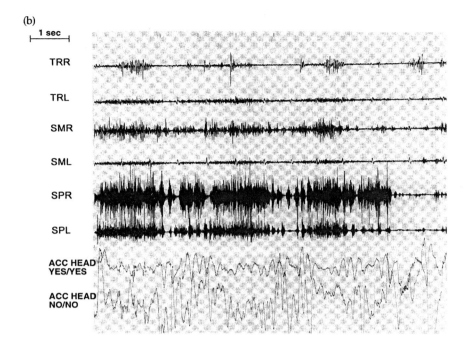

(c)

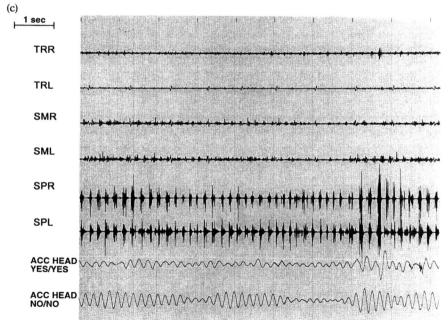

Fig. 4.2 *Continued*

Table 4.2 Classification of dystonic EMG activity.

Tonic	Several seconds of electromyographic interference pattern with only slight variations of amplitude and density (Fig. 4.2a)
Irregular-phasic	Bursts of variable amplitude, rhythmicity and duration (300 ms to several seconds, Fig. 4.2b)
Tremulous	Rhythmic bursts lasting mostly between 50 and 300 ms (Fig. 4.2c)
Myoclonic	Irregular bursts lasting less than 300 ms mostly superimposed on tonic activity

simultaneously under defined standardized conditions. In patients with phasic head movements a two-dimensional accelerometric system placed on the glabella was added to evaluate involuntary head movements. We made poly EMG recordings with patients sat upright and relaxed in a comfortable chair, during spontaneous head posturing or movement ('involuntary EMG activity'), with the patients performing a *geste antagonistique* ('effect of *geste* manoeuvre') and while turning the head from side to side ('voluntary head rotation').

Involuntary EMG activity in CD

The commonest pattern (31%) was purely tonic EMG activation of one to three neck muscles, depending on the type of postural abnormality. Combinations of different types of EMG activation were also common (Fig. 4.2 a,b & 4.3), and compound patterns with all four major types of activation were present in about 7% of tracings. We found short head tremor episodes in 75 polygrams (52%). The tremor frequencies ranged from 2 to 15 Hz and were clustered around a peak at 5 Hz (Figs 4.2c & 4.4). In patients with predominant low to middle frequency tremor (2–9 Hz), the tremor amplitude increased with voluntary movements directed away from the dystonic posture. The tremor frequencies were higher (9–15 Hz) in patients who tried to correct the dystonic posture (frequencies in the same range as isometric tremor) suggesting a different pathophysiological mechanism.

Effect of geste *manoeuvres*

Antagonistic gestures, such as touching the chin with a finger, are well known clinical features to reduce or abolish dystonic posturing in CD [27]. During such sensory tricks, the poly EMG usually shows a reduction or transformation of dystonic activity in the involved muscles (Fig. 4.5). Such a change in EMG activity helps to distinguish between genuinely dystonic muscle activity and compensatory activation to correct the dystonic posture.

Deuschl and colleagues [23] found a reduction or complete cessation of dystonic EMG activity during the *geste* in 72% of patients with CD. The *geste* effect was not related

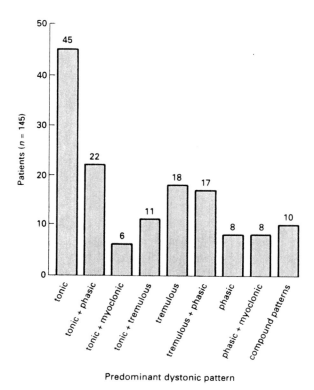

Fig. 4.3 Predominant dystonic patterns in cervical dystonia. Distribution of EMG patterns found in 145 polygrams of cervical muscles in patients with cervical dystonia.

to severity or duration of the disease and was not dependent on the type of dystonic EMG activity. However, a recent study [28] reported an inverse relation between disease duration and the duration of an effective *geste* manoeuvre.

In another study on the time course of *geste* effects in patients with CD [29] 52% of the patients with an effective *geste* manoeuvre showed marked reductions of dystonic EMG during arm movement, clearly beginning *before* the fingers touched the face. The remaining 48% showed *geste*-related EMG-effects only during finger contact in the facial target area. These results indicate different physiological mechanisms in clinically indistinguishable antagonistic gestures.

In a series of 60 patients with head tremor of different aetiology (dystonic and essential tremor) Masuhr and colleagues [30] were able to show that a significant decrease in tremor amplitude during the performance of a *geste* manoeuvre is a criterion that distinguishes dystonic from essential head tremor. Patients with tremulous CD showed a significant reduction in tremor amplitude during the *geste*, while patients with essential head tremor did not.

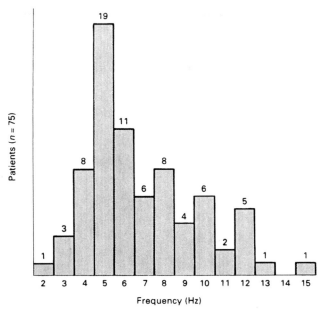

75 polygrams with significant tremor activity (>10%) in at least one investigated muscle

Fig. 4.4 Distribution of head tremor frequencies in cervical dystonia. Tremor episodes during relaxed sitting in a chair occurred in polygrams of 75 patients with cervical dystonia. Frequency analysis of the EMG recordings and accelerometric measurements revealed tremor frequencies between 2 and 15 Hz with a peak around 5 Hz.

EMG during voluntary head rotation

In most patients with CD the EMG activity during voluntary head rotation does not follow the normal synergistic pattern of muscle activation [23]. EMG of voluntary head rotation can therefore help to distinguish dystonic from physiological activation. Normal subjects rotate the head around a vertical axis mainly by activating the splenius capitis ipsilateral to the direction of rotation and the contralateral sternomastoid muscle. They simultaneously relax the antagonist pair. In dystonia there is asymmetric activation of the agonist pair and pathological cocontraction of the antagonist [23]. Muscles moving the head in the direction of dystonic posturing often show higher amplitude and denser recruitment than do the paired muscles that performing opposite rotations (Fig. 4.6a). Furthermore, when patients attempt to move the head in the direction opposite to the dystonic posture there is a failure of reciprocal inhibition (Fig. 4.6b).

Involvement of clinically unsuspected muscles

EMG studies showed that clinically unsuspected muscles may be actively contributing to dystonic posture or movement. In CD, the main types of head deviation are rotational

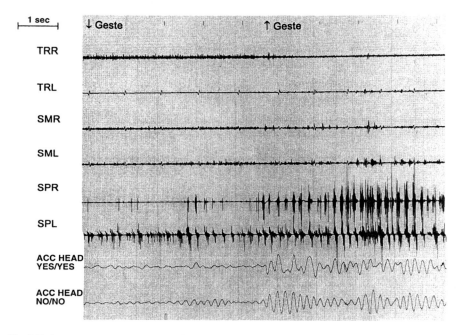

Fig. 4.5 Antagonistic gesture in cervical dystonia. The same patient as in Fig. 4.2(c) shows the positive effect of the antagonistic gesture of touching the chin with the right hand. The first 4 s represent recording during the gesture (↓*Geste*) whilst the last 4 s represent recording without the gesture (↑*Geste*). Tremulous EMG activity in the right splenius capitis (SPR) and both sternomastoids (SMR, SML) was reduced during this sensory trick, and reappeared when the gesture ended. For other abbreviations see Fig. 4.2.

Fig. 4.6 EMG polygrams, as recorded in Fig. 4.2, with the patient performing voluntary head rotation whilst sitting in a chair. (a) *Dystonic disturbances during head rotation:* Rotational torticollis to the right and head tremor when attempting to turn the head the other way. The beginning of the recording shows voluntary rotation to the right, in the direction of the dystonic posture, with enhanced EMG activation in the dystonic left sternomastoid (SML). Compare this with the unaffected right sternomastoid (SMR) during rotation to the left 3 s later. There is high-frequency tremor in both the left and the right splenius capitis (SPL, SPR) during rotation to the left, that is, away from the dystonic posture (antidystonic activation). (b) *Dystonic disturbances of reciprocal inhibition during head rotation:* Tremulous rotational torticollis to the left, laterocollis to the right and elevation of the right shoulder. At the beginning of the recording there is voluntary rotation to the left, in the direction of the dystonic posture, with enhanced EMG activation in the dystonic right sternomastoid (SMR). Compare this with the contralateral left sternomastoid (SML) during rotation to the right 3 s later. There is persistent tremulous EMG activity in the left splenius capitis (SPL) during rotation to the right, and persistent tremulous activity in the right trapezius (TRR) during rotation in both directions. Time marker, 1 s. ACC, accelerometer recording; 'No/No', horizontal plane; TRL, left trapezius; 'Yes/Yes', vertical plane.

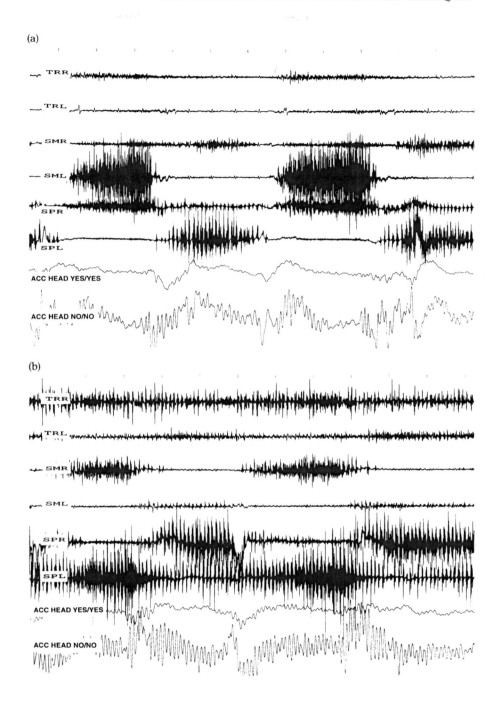

Table 4.3 EMG criteria for muscle selection in cervical dystonia.

1	Spontaneous tonic or phasic EMG bursts of variable duration at rest
2	Spontaneous tremor episodes with characteristic low to middle (4–9 Hz) frequencies
3	Disturbance of antagonistic muscle activation during voluntary head rotation
4	Reduction of dystonic EMG activity during sensory tricks

Table 4.4 Criteria for muscle selection in writer's cramp.

1	Clinically identified dystonic finger, wrist and elbow deviation or movements as assessed by the Writer's Cramp Rating Scale [35] and mirror movements or posture in the affected arm while writing with the other hand
2	Poly EMG during writing: build-up of tonic EMG activity ('crescendo phenomenon') and transformation of normal antagonistic burst pattern to a sustained tonic or tremulous EMG activity

torticollis, laterocollis, retrocollis and anterocollis. In 100 patients, Deuschl and colleagues [23] found rotational torticollis in 72, laterocollis in 11, retrocollis in nine and a complex multidimensional head deviation in eight patients. If Bt is given purely according to the direction of dystonic head movement, patients with rotational torticollis should receive Bt injections into the splenius capitis muscle ipsilateral and the sternomastoid muscle contralateral to the side of chin deviation. However, poly EMG in rotational torticollis showed that this pattern of activation accounted for only 39 of 72 cases. There was underlying activity of either the ipsilateral splenius capitis or contralateral sternomastoid muscles in eight cases, and of the contralateral sternomastoid and both splenius capitis muscles in 25 patients [23].

In our own series of patients with rotational CD, more detailed needle EMG examinations detected further muscles involved, especially the contralateral trapezius, the ipsilateral semispinalis capitis and cervicis muscles and the ipsilateral levator scapulae muscle. Thus, it may be worth using surface and/or needle EMG to identify dystonic muscles in patients with complex multidimensional head deviation, or if patients with simple torticollis, laterocollis or retrocollis fail to respond adequately to clinically directed Bt injections. The major criteria for EMG identification of relevant dystonic muscles for Bt injection in CD are summarized in Table 4.3.

Writer's cramp

Writer's cramp (WC) is the most prevalent task specific dystonia. Table 4.4 [35] summarizes the criteria for muscle selection in Bt treatment of WC. The forearm muscles most often involved in WC are the flexor carpi ulnaris and radialis, flexor digitorum superficialis, flexor pollicis longus and extensor digitorum communis muscles [31–35].

In most cases there is no involuntary dystonic EMG activation during rest or postural stress in patients with WC, and poly EMG must therefore be performed during the specific task. Wire electrodes introduced into forearm muscles reveal loss of normal alternating agonist–antagonist bursts, and show cocontracting phasic spasms, tonic cocontracting and tremor episodes [36]. Although such invasive recordings can identify dystonic muscle activity, it is hardly possible to use wire electrodes in the setting of a dystonia clinic.

We assessed the value of surface EMG of elbow and forearm flexors and extensors using poly EMG while the subject was writing, and compared surface poly EMG findings from 24 patients with WC with those from 25 healthy volunteers during a standardized writing task [18,37]. Most patients showed pathologically enhanced cocontractions of forearm flexors and extensors. In all but two recordings from patients with WC, sustained tonic activity contaminated phasic burst generation in forearm muscles regardless of the direction of the writing movement. The tonic EMG activation showed a typical crescendo-type build-up in 16 cases (Figs 4.1), and 50% of the patients had tremor episodes with frequencies between 6 and 16 Hz [25]. Compared to controls 10 patients showed enhanced tonic EMG activity in the triceps muscle.

Nevertheless it is usually possible to plan Bt injections on the basis of the clinically apparent finger, wrist and elbow deviations alone (semiquantitative evaluation with the Writer's Cramp Rating Scale [35]), and invasive or surface EMG is not necessary unless the clinical situation is uncertain.

Poly EMG features in tremor

Tremor is defined as an involuntary rhythmic movement of one or multiple body parts [38]. The majority of tremors can be classified according to clinical criteria (see Table 4.5 [39]). Surface EMG, or in special circumstances needle or fine wire electrodes, can give a measure of the frequency and rhythmicity and typically shows rhythmic EMG bursts lasting between 50 and 300 ms in tremulous muscles. We use at least two channels and record EMG simultaneously from an antagonist pair of muscles to see whether the EMG is synchronous or alternating and whether Bt injections should be placed only in one or in both antagonistic muscles. Therefore, we recommend recordings of antagonistic muscles before Bt treatment of postural and kinetic hand tremor, and in tremor syndromes where the clinical identification of tremulous muscle activation is uncertain.

Table 4.5 Clinical criteria for tremor classification [39].

1	Activation condition (rest, posture, action, intention)
2	Frequency range (low, <4 Hz; medium, 4–7 Hz; high >7 Hz)
3	Presence or absence of additional neurological symptoms (e.g. akinesia, dystonia, polyneuropathy, etc.) or signs of systemic diseases (e.g. endocrinopathies)
4	Clinical course of the condition
5	Sensitivity to specific medication or alcohol

The mechanical motion of tremor can be evaluated using a device to measure the acceleration (accelerometer) of the tremulous body part [40]. Acceleration as the second time derivative of motion accentuates the movement, making the tremor easier to see [40]. Computers can analyse the output of uni-, bi- or triaxial accelerometer systems to generate a spectral analysis which represents the power at different frequencies in the signal [30,41]. We recommend sequential measurements of the acceleration of the tremulous body part to evaluate treatment-related changes in tremor amplitude [40].

An excellent way to study the physiology of postural hand tremor is to use a uniaxial accelerometer system placed on the dorsum of the hand and surface EMG of forearm extensor and flexor muscles combined with a fast Fourier analysis and load of 500 g [40]. This method allows separation of tremor from mechanical reflexes or central oscillators [39,40]. In contrast to a central oscillator, tremor from mechanical reflexes shows a decreased frequency peak in the fast Fourier analysis with weight load compared with frequency peak without weight load [39,40].

EMG recordings in combination with EEG are only helpful in specific conditions [39]: identification of dystonic tremor (see Table 4.2 and paragraph 'Effect of *geste* manoeuvres' in above Section), primary orthostatic tremor, and the differential diagnosis of myoclonus, asterixis ('negative myoclonus') and clonus (see following Section). Orthostatic tremor shows a synchronous 13–18 Hz EMG activity in antagonistic leg muscles (e.g. rectus femoris muscle and knee flexors) only during stance. Asterixis shows synchronous arrhythmic pauses of EMG activity in antagonistic muscles during voluntary contraction, while myoclonus of spinal origin mostly shows a pseudo-rhythmic EMG patterns without a relation to cortical spikes in EEG. *Epilepsia partialis continua* or cortical myoclonus may be diagnosed by simultaneous EEG and EMG recordings to establish a relation between cortical spikes and rhythmic EMG activation in the monitored muscles [39].

Poly EMG features in spasticity

Spasticity has been defined as a motor disorder characterized by a velocity-dependent increase in tonic stretch reflexes, and with exaggerated tendon jerks, resulting from hyperexcitability of the stretch reflex [42] as one component of the upper motorneurone syndrome (UMNS).

Young [43] includes other 'positive symptoms' such as exaggerated cutaneous reflexes (painful flexor or adductor spasms), mass reflexes, abnormal postures, and 'negative symptoms' such as paresis, lack of dexterity and fatigability in the syndrome of spastic paresis, which is the common clinical pattern in patients following lesions of the central motor system in adulthood.

Spastic dystonia is used to describe abnormal postures present in patients with UMNS [43]. These abnormal postures of the arm or leg may be produced by a combination of soft-tissue changes and continuous muscle activity dependent upon continuous

Table 4.6 Poly EMG features and typical EMG pattern in spasticity.

1	Velocity dependent increase in EMG activity during passive stretch of the affected muscle (see Fig. 4.7)
2	Clonus activity (grouped low frequency rhythmic EMG bursts) following passive stretch of the affected muscle, with a modulating effect on clonus by increasing or decreasing the stretch to the monitored muscle (see Figs 4.8 & 4.9)
3	Spontaneous or stimuli related spasms (rapid phasic, non-rhythmic EMG activation)
4	Persistent tonic EMG activity during movement in muscles involved in spastic dystonia (see Fig. 4.10)
5	Loss of phasic EMG activity in agonist muscles as a result of the central paresis
6	Cocontracting EMG pattern of antagonist muscles but no correlation with severity of exaggerated reflexes and movement disorder resulting from spasticity

supraspinal drive to the α-motorneurone pool [44]. Peripheral secondary structural changes may also be relevant, including alterations in tendon compliance, changes in muscle fibres and connective tissue viscosity [45–47]. However, extensive investigation of voluntary movements and EMG activity of arm and leg muscles has not revealed any consistent relationship between exaggerated reflexes and clinical spasticity with its associated disabling movement disorder [48].

Poly EMG features of spasticity match the clinical impression of an increased muscle tone with a velocity dependent increase in EMG activity in stretched muscles and cocontraction of antagonistic muscles during voluntary movement. In addition, in many patients clonus may generate slow rhythmical discharges following passive stretch [49]. The poly EMG features and typical EMG pattern of spasticity are summarized in Table 4.6.

Types of poly EMG pattern in spasticity

Use a standardized programme of surface poly EMG, simultaneously recording agonists and antagonists [48]. Record during rest (e.g. supine position with spontaneous joint position), during passive slow and fast stretch of the muscle, and during voluntary movement (single or multijoint movements such as simple alternating extension and flexion of the joint, or dynamic EMG during instrumented gait analysis or fine arm motor tasks such as writing a standard text).

Poly EMG recordings during rest

The majority of patients with spasticity due to supratentorial lesions generate no involuntary muscle activity during rest. In some patients with spastic dystonia poly EMG may show continuous tonic EMG activity in muscles responsible for the spastic-dystonic

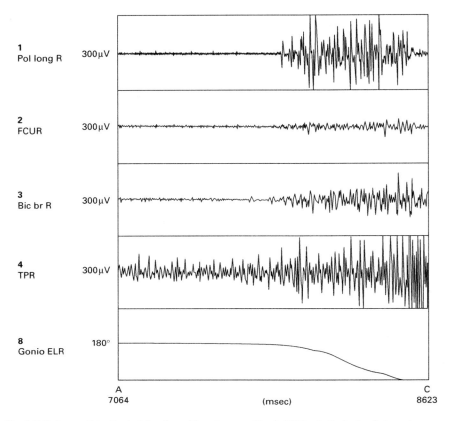

Fig. 4.7 Enhanced kinetic stretch reflex with an increased tonic EMG activity during fast passive extension of the elbow (stretch to the monitored flexor muscles of the upper limb) in a patient with a Wernicke–Mann type spasticity in the upper right limb. Pol long R, right pollicis longus; FCUR, right flexor carpi ulnaris; Bic br R, right biceps brachii; TPR, right trapezius; Gonio ELR, goniometer placed at the right elbow.

posture during rest [44]. However patients with lesions of the spinal cord often suffer from spontaneous or triggered painful flexor or extensor spasms with brisk, phasic, short duration EMG bursts.

Poly EMG recordings during passive stretch

As a characteristic feature, patients with spasticity show a velocity dependent increase in tonic EMG activity during passive stretch of the monitored muscle (Fig. 4.7). A certain velocity of movement is needed to elicit such stretch reflexes (critical angular velocity >40°/s [49]). This emphasizes that spasticity is due to an enhanced kinetic stretch reflex [49]. This phenomenon results in an increased tonic EMG activity which is an enhanced tonic stretch reflex (Fig. 4.7). Furthermore, tonic stretch reflexes demonstrate a linear

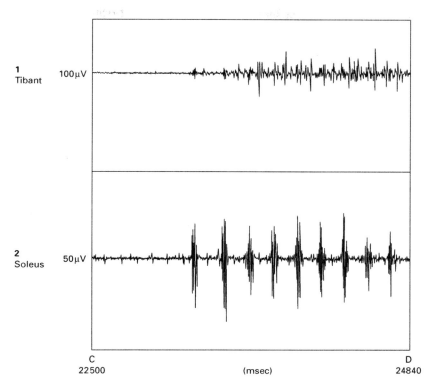

Fig. 4.8 Rhythmic EMG (clonus) activity following fast passive stretch of the triceps surae muscle in a patient following stroke. Tib ant, tibial anterior muscle; Soleus, soleus muscle.

velocity dependence; that is, the faster the movement, the greater the muscle contraction or EMG activity provoked [46].

Clonus activity may follow a fast passive stretch of the affected muscle, and produces low frequency rhythmic EMG activity (Fig. 4.8), with modulation in EMG amplitude by increasing or decreasing the stretch to the monitored muscle [49].

Poly EMG recordings during voluntary movement

In patients with spastic paresis, dynamic EMG of fine voluntary arm movements such as writing a standard text shows a loss of selective phasic EMG activity of agonists, and co-contracting antagonists. There is increased tonic background EMG activity in muscles normally not involved (non-selected synergistic EMG activity) in the fine motor task.

In patients with spastic-dystonic posture, recordings of voluntary movements show a persistent tonic EMG activity in the muscle responsible for the abnormal dystonic posture (Fig. 4.9).

In the leg there are typical changes in kinematic and kinetic parameters in instrumented gait analysis in adult patients with cerebral lesions as well as in children with

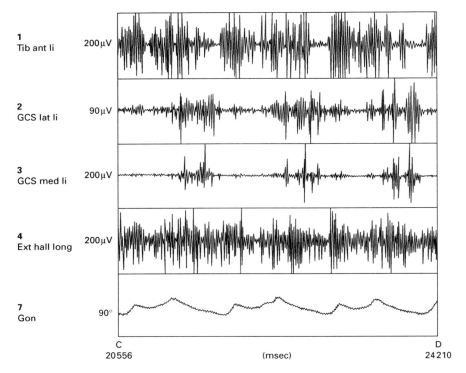

Fig. 4.9 Persistent tonic EMG activity in the extensor hallucis longus muscle (trace 4) in a patient with the clinical picture of a painful striatal toe (spastic dystonia) following stroke. Dynamic EMG (instrumented gait analysis) showing three gait cycles; beginning and end of the recording with initial foot contact. Tib ant li, left tibial anterior muscle; GCS lat li, left gastrocnemius muscle (lateral head); GCS med li, left gastrocnemius muscle (medial head); Ext hall long, left extensor hallucis longus muscle; Gon, goniometer at the left ankle.

cerebral palsy. Dynamic EMG shows a pattern of cocontraction of anterior tibial and gastrocnemius muscles during the gait cycle only in children with cerebral palsy [50]. Instrumented gait analysis in adults with supratentorial lesions did not show this cocontracting pattern of antagonists. Adults with spastic gait disorders often display a disabling clonus like EMG activity in the triceps surae muscle during the early stance phase (Fig. 4.10) of gait cycle, the so called premature activity [51].

Guiding botulinum toxin injections

Once muscles for Bt injection have been selected, the next crucial step is the correct targeting of the Bt injections. Superficially localized and palpable muscles can be injected using anatomical landmarks without other specific guidance techniques. We recommend guided injections if muscles are small or deep. There are three principal options for muscle identification and targeting of Bt injections:

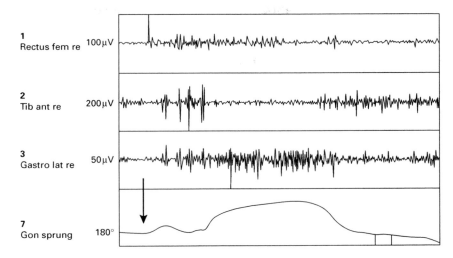

Fig. 4.10 Instrumented gait analysis of a patient with right hemiparesis following stroke showing premature activity (clonus activity: phasic rhythmic activity) in the gastrocnemius and tibial anterior muscles during early stance phase. Recording of one gait cycle, rhythmic EMG activity in gastrocnemius and tibial anterior muscles directly following passive stretch related to initial foot contact (arrow). Rectus fem re, right rectus femoris muscle; Tib ant re, right tibial anterior muscle; Gastro lat re, right gastrocnemius muscle (lateral head); Gon sprung, goniometer at the right ankle.

- Record EMG activity.
- Stimulate selected muscles electrically using a (at the tip) non-isolated hollow Teflon-coated needle.
- Use imaging techniques such as CT or sonography to plan the injection and to identify the tip of the needle in the muscle.

EMG and electrical stimulation for targeting botulinum toxin injections

Using a Teflon-coated monopolar EMG needle, EMG and electrical stimulation can help to guide Bt injections into previously selected muscles. Also, in patients with CD, EMG can identify dystonic muscle activity in deep neck muscles, especially in levator scapulae, semispinalis cervicis and the scalenes. In a blinded study in CD, outcomes were significantly better with supplementary EMG for both muscle selection and injections than with BtA injections directed on clinical grounds alone [52]. The percentage of improved patients was the same in both groups, but those who responded showed greater benefit with EMG guidance, especially in retrocollis, head tilt and shoulder elevation.

EMG guidance for injection is indispensable in spasmodic dysphonia and jaw opening dystonia [53,54]. Similarly, we recommend EMG guidance or electrical stimulation for Bt injections in writer's cramp and limb spasticity when small or thin hand/forearm or foot/crural muscles are targeted. There are no relevant prospective studies comparing guided and non-guided Bt injections, but most specialists agree that reliable, accurate injections to these muscles are impossible without EMG guidance.

In practice, insert a monopolar Teflon-coated EMG needle into the expected anatomical position with the indifferent electrode and earth placed nearby. Monitor EMG activity during spontaneous dystonic or tremulous movements, passive stretch and active movements, or deliver repetitive electrical stimuli given with increasing current, and monitor the corresponding movements. If the needle position is correct the EMG monitor or sound should confirm motor unit potentials during the movements, and electrical stimulation should produce a corresponding movement of the muscle or joint. If the needle is out of position, move it until clear and crisp motor unit action potentials appear, or stimuli elicit movement of the targeted muscle. Another way to identify the target muscle is to move the relevant joint passively to induce a corresponding movement of the properly placed needle.

Imaging techniques for guiding botulinum toxin injections

When selecting deep muscles, imaging techniques such as computed tomography (CT) or ultrasound may help to verify the position of the needle tip before Bt injection.

Radiological procedures using CT to calculate and guide the depth and direction of the needle path are well established and part of most software programs of CT units. A good example is directing Bt injections into the psoas muscle in adult patients with uni- or bilateral hip flexor spasticity. We recommend the so called 'posterior' approach with insertion of the needle into the paraspinal region at lumbar segments 2–4 under CT guidance (Fig. 4.11). Alternatively, ultrasound can verify needle position in the psoas muscle (Fig. 4.12). Ultrasound is helpful in both the 'posterior' or 'ventral' approach

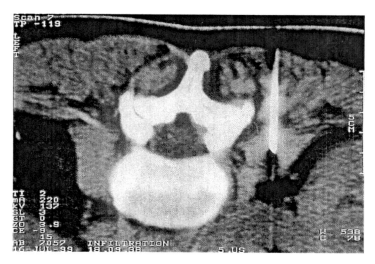

Fig. 4.11 Guidance of Bt-injection into the psoas muscle: Computed tomography scan showing the injection needle within the right psoas muscle at segments L3/L4.

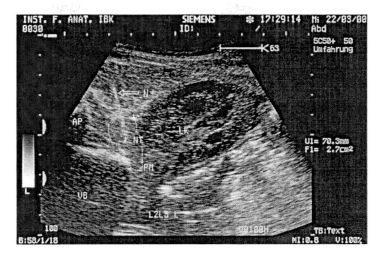

Fig. 4.12 Guidance of Bt injection into the psoas muscle: ultrasound scan showing the injection needle within the psoas muscle. N, needle; *tip of the needle; LK, left kidney; VB, body of the vertebra; AP, anterior portion of the intervertebral joint; L2L3L, segments L2/L3.

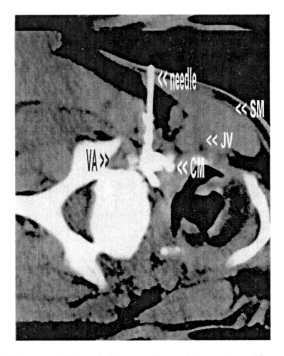

Fig. 4.13 CT-guided injection of Bt into the longus colli muscle in a patient with severe anterocollis (with permission of the Department of Neurology [M. Naumann] and the Institute of Neuroradiology [M. Bendszus], University of Würzburg, Germany). CM, contrast medium; JV, jugular vein; SM, sternomastoid muscle; VA, vertebral artery.

(ventral approach: needle insertion medially from the anterior superior iliac spine) of ilio-psoas muscle injections. CT guided injections may also be very helpful in identifying and injecting the longus colli muscle in patients with CD and severe anterocollis (Fig. 4.13).

Ultrasound may usefully guide injections into small muscles in children with CP (see Chapter 11), into salivary glands for siallorhea (see Chapter 14), and into sphincter muscles (see Chapter 15).

Conclusion

In most focal dystonias with obvious dystonic posturing, in typical tremor syndromes or in syndromes with localized spasticity, clinical criteria are usually sufficient to select and identify muscles for Bt injections. Poly EMG recordings may be of great value in identifying active muscles in complex CD, postural and kinetic hand tremor or spastic dystonia, and may be the only way to identify the muscles involved in task specific dystonias or focal limb spasticity. Guidance is essential when injecting Bt into muscles in delicate places, such as in laryngeal and jaw opening dystonia, or in small hand and foot muscles as well as muscles in deeper layers such as the psoas muscle. In complex CD EMG guidance is recommended to detect dystonic EMG activity while injecting Bt. To confirm the exact needle position in task specific dystonia, hand tremor or spastic paretic forearm or small hand or foot muscles we recommend electrical stimulation as well as EMG guidance. When injecting Bt into deeper muscles such as psoas, verify the needle position using imaging techniques such as CT or ultrasound.

References

1 Rosales R, Arimura K, Takenaga S, Osame M. Extrafusal and intrafusal muscle effects in experimental botulinum toxin A injection. *Muscle Nerve* 1996; **19**: 488–96.

2 Priori A, Berardelli A, Mercuri B, Manfredi M. Physiological effects produced by the botulinum toxin treatment of upper limb dystonia. Changes in reciprocal inhibition between forearm muscles. *Brain* 1995; **118**: 801–7.

3 Wissel J, Müller J, Baldauf A *et al.* Gait analysis to assess the effects of botulinum toxin type A treatment in cerebral palsy: an open-label study in 10 children with equinus gait pattern. *European J Neurol* 1999; **6** (Suppl. 4): S63–7.

4 Byrnes ML, Thickbroom GW, Wilson SA *et al.* The corticomotor representation of upper limb muscles in writer's cramp and changes following botulinum toxin injection. *Brain* 1998; **121**: 977–88.

5 Gilio F, Curra A, Lorenzano C *et al.* Effects of botulinum toxin type A on intracortical inhibition in patients with dystonia. *Ann Neurol* 2000; **48**: 20–6.

6 Aramideh M, Bour LJ, Koelman JH *et al.* Abnormal eye movements in blepharospasm and involuntary levator palpebrae inhibition. Clinical and pathophysiological considerations. *Brain* 1994; **117**: 1457–74.

7 Münchau A, Filipovic S, Oester-Barkey A *et al.* Spontaneously changing muscular activation pattern in patients with cervical dystonia. *Mov Disord* 2001; **16**: 1091–7.

8 Berardelli A, Rothwell JC, Hallett M *et al.* The pathophysiology of primary dystonia. *Brain* 1998; **121**: 1195–212.

9 Tolosa E, Montserrat L, Bayes A. Blink reflex studies in focal dystonias, enhanced excitability of brainstem interneurons in cranial dystonia and spasmodic torticollis. *Mov Disord* 1988; **3**: 61–9.

10 Rothwell JC, Obeso JA, Day BL, Marsden CD. Pathophysiology of dystonias. Motor control mechanisms in health and disease. In: Desmedt JE, ed. *Motor Control Mechanisms in Health and Disease*. New York: Raven Press, 1983: 851–72.

11 Ikoma K, Samii A, Mercuri B, Wassermann EM, Hallett M. Abnormal cortical motor excitability in dystonia. *Neurology* 1996; **46**: 1371–6.

12 Ridding MC, Sheean G, Rothwell JC, Inzelberg R, Kujirai T. Changes in the balance between motor cortical excitation and inhibition in focal, task specific dystonia. *J Neurol Neurosurg Psychiatry* 1995; **59**: 493–8.

13 Deuschl G, Toro C, Matsumoto J, Hallett M. Movement-related cortical potentials in writer's cramp. *Ann Neurol* 1995; **38**: 509–14.

14 Kaji R, Ikeda A, Ikeda T *et al.* Physiological study of cervical dystonia. Task specific abnormality in contingent negative variation. *Brain* 1995; **118**: 511–22.

15 Oppenheim H. Über eine eigenartige krampfkrankheit des kindlichen und jugendlichen alters (dystonica lordotica progressiva, dystonia musculorum deformans). *Neurol Zentralblatt* 1911; **30**: 1090–107.

16 Thompson PD, Stell R, Maccabe JJ *et al.* Electromyography of neck muscles and treatment in spasmodic torticollis. In: Berardelli A, Benecke R, Manfredi M, Marsden CD, eds. *Motor Disturbances II*. New York: Academic Press, 1990: 289–304.

17 Cohen LG, Hallett M. Hand cramps. Clinical features and electromyographic patterns in a focal dystonia. *Neurology* 1988; **38**: 1005–12.

18 Kleppek B, Wissel J, Kabus C, Schelosky L, Poewe W. Veränderungen in der oberflächenelektromyographie von ober und unterarmmuskeln bei 24 patienten mit graphospasmus. In: Huffmann G, Braune H-J, Henn K-H, eds. *Extrapyramidale Erkrankungen*. Reinbek: Einhorn Presse Verlag, 1994: 385–9.

19 Hoefer PFA, Putnam TJ. Action potentials of muscles in athetosis and Sydenham chorea. *Arch Neurol Psychiatr* 1940; **44**: 517–31.

20 Herz E. *Dystonia, Part I Arch Neurol Psychiatr* 1944; **51**: 305–18.

21 Cooper IS. *Involuntary Movement Disorders*. New York: Harper & Row, 1969.

22 Yanagisawa N, Goto A. Dystonia musculorum deformans: analysis with electromyography. *J Neurol Sci* 1971; **13**: 39–65.

23 Deuschl G, Heinen F, Kleedorfer B *et al.* Clinical and polymyographic investigation of spasmodic torticollis. *J Neurol* 1992; **1**: 9–16.

24 Jedynak CP, Bonnet AM, Agid Y. Tremor and idiopathic dystonia. *Mov Disord* 1991; **6**: 230–6.

25 Wissel J, Schelosky L, Ebersbach G, Poewe W. The concept of 'dystonic tremor'. *Mov Disord* 1992; **7** (Suppl. 1): 90.

26 Obeso JA, Rothwell JC, Day BL, Marsden CD. Myoclonic dystonia. *Neurology* 1983; **33**: 825–30.

27 Naumann M, Magyar S, Reiners K, Erbguth F, Leenders KL. Sensory tricks in cervical dystonia. Perceptual dysbalance of parietal cortex modulates frontal motor programming. *Ann Neurol* 2000; **47**: 322–8.

28 Müller J, Wissel J, Ebersbach G, Masuhr F, Poewe W. Clinical characteristics of the *geste antagoniste* in cervical dystonia. *J Neurol* 2001; **248**: 478.

29 Wissel J, Müller J, Ebersbach G, Poewe W. Trick manoeuvres in cervical dystonia. Investigation of movement- and touch-related changes in polymyographic activity. *Mov Disord* 1999; **14**: 994–9.

30 Masuhr F, Wissel J, Müller J, Scholz U, Poewe W. Quantification of sensory trick impact on tremor amplitude and frequency in 60 patients with head tremor. *Mov Disord* 2000; **15**: 960–4.

31 Cohen LG, Hallett M, Geller BD, Hochberg F. Treatment of focal dystonias of the hand with botulinum toxin injections. *J Neurol Neurosurg Psychiatry* 1989; **52**: 355–63.

32 Rivest J, Lees AJ, Marsden CD. Writer's cramp: treatment with botulinum toxin injections. *Mov Disord* 1991; **1**: 55–9.

33 Tsui JKC, Bhatt M, Calne S, Calne DB. Botulinum toxin in the treatment of writer's cramp: a double-blind study. *Neurology* 1993; **43**: 183–5.

34 Karp BI, Cole RA, Cohen LG *et al*. Long-term botulinum toxin treatment of focal hand dystonia. *Neurology* 1994; **44**: 70–6.

35 Wissel J, Kabus C, Wenzel R *et al*. Botulinum toxin in writer's cramp: objective response evaluation in 31 patients. *J Neurol, Neurosurgery Psychiatry* 1996; **61**: 172–5.

36 Cohen LG, Hallett M. Hand cramps. Clinical features and electromyographic patterns in a focal dystonia. *Neurology* 1988; **38**: 1005–12.

37 Wissel J, Belian R, Kleppek B *et al*. Clinical features and surface electromyographic patterns in 24 patients with writer's cramp and 25 healthy controls. *Mov Disord* 1992; **7** (Suppl. 1): 132.

38 Elble RJ, Koller WC. The definition and classification of tremor. In: Elble RJ, Koller WC, eds. *Tremor.* Baltimore: The Johns Hopkins University Press, 1990: 1–9.

39 Deuschl G, Krack P, Lauk M, Timmer J. Clinical neurophysiology of tremor. *J Clin Neurophysiol* 1996; **13**: 110–21.

40 Hallett M. Overview of human tremor physiology. *Mov Disord* 1998; **13** (Suppl. 3): 43–8.

41 Wissel J, Masuhr F, Schelosky L, Ebersbach G, Poewe W. Quantitative assessment of botulinum toxin treatment in 43 patients with head tremor. *Mov Disord* 1997; **12**: 722–6.

42 Lance JW. Symposium synopsis. In: Feldman RG, Qoung RR, Koella WP, eds. *Spasticity. Disordered Motor Control.* Chicago: Yearbook Medical, 1980: 485–94.

43 Young RR. Spasticity: a review. *Neurology* 1994; **44** (Suppl. 9): S12–20.

44 Burke D. Spasticity as an adaptation to pyramidal tract injury. In: Waxman SG, ed. *Advances in Neurology: Functional Recovery in Neurological Disease.* New York: Raven Press, 1987: 401–23.

45 Dietz V, Berger W. Normal and impaired regulation of muscle stiffness in gait: a new hypothesis about muscle hypertonia. *Exp Neurol* 1983; **79**: 680–78.

46 Thilmann AF, Fellows SJ, Garms E. The mechanism of spastic muscle hypertonus: variation in reflex gain over the time course of spasticity. *Brain* 1991; **114**: 233–44.

47 Dwyer NJ, Ada L, Neilson PD. Spasticity and muscle contracture following stroke. *Brain* 1996; **119**: 1737–49.

48 Dietz V. Neurophysiology of gait disorders: present and future applications. *Electroencephalogr Clin Neurophysiol* 1997; **103**: 333–55.

49 Sheean GL. Pathophysiology of spasticity. In: Sheean G, ed. *Spasticity Rehabilitation.* London: Churchill Communications Europe Limited, 1998: 17–38.

50 Berger W, Quintern J, Dietz V. Pathophysiological aspects of gait in children with cerebral palsy. *Electroencephalogr Clin Neurophysiol* 1982; **53**: 538–48.

51 Hesse S, Krajnik J, Luecke D *et al*. Ankle muscle activity before and after botulinum toxin therapy for lower limb extensor spasticity in chronic hemiparetic patients. *Stroke* 1996; **27**: 455–60.

52 Comella LC, Buchmann AS, Tanner CM, Brown-Toms NC, Goetz CG. Botulinum toxin injection for spasmodic torticollis, increased magnitude of benefit with electromyographic assistance. *Neurology* 1992; **42**: 878–82.

53 Brin MF, Blitzer A, Herman S, Stewart C. Oromandibular dystonia. Treatment of 96 patients with botulinum toxin type A. In: Jankovic J, Hallett M, eds. *Therapy with Botulinum Toxin.* New York: Marcel Dekker Inc., 1994: 429–35.

54 Ludlow CL, Rhew K, Nash EA. Botulinum toxin injection for adductor spasmodic dysphonia. In: Jankovic J, Hallett M, eds. *Therapy with Botulinum Toxin.* New York: Marcel Dekker Inc., 1994: 437–50.

PART TWO

Movement disorders

CHAPTER 5

Fundamentals of dystonia

MITCHELL F. BRIN

Introduction

Dystonia is a neurological syndrome dominated by involuntary muscle contractions that may be sustained (tonic), spasmodic (rapid or clonic), irregular or repetitive. The muscle activity frequently causes abnormal postures including twisting (e.g. torticollis), flexion or extension (e.g. anterocollis, retrocollis, writer's cramp), adduction or abduction (e.g. spasmodic dysphonia). Dystonia can involve any voluntary muscle. It is one of the more frequently misdiagnosed neurological conditions because the movements and resulting postures are often unusual, and dystonia is rare [1]. Many patients initially receive a psychiatric diagnosis, thought to be anxious or imagining symptoms, or to have real symptoms but not of physical origin. Some are labelled as malingerers or simply antisocial. Where the doctor accepts the illness as physical, other more common disorders may come to mind first. Some common errors appear in Table 5.1.

Prevalence of dystonia

The prevalence of dystonia is unclear, but we estimate there are at least 250 000 cases of idiopathic dystonia in the US (NIH Dystonia Workshop, February 1993 & [2]). About one in 3000 people receive a diagnosis of dystonia, but the true prevalence is probably much higher. Focal dystonia affects about 300 persons per million people, nine times the prevalence of generalized dystonia [2]. Writer's cramp may be the most common form of focal dystonia, although cervical dystonia is probably more commonly seen and diagnosed in clinics.

Classification of dystonia

Classification of dystonia by aetiology, clinical distribution and symptoms, and age at onset (Table 5.2 [3,4]) gives clues about prognosis and management. The history may reveal factors potentially leading to dystonia [5]. By definition, patients with idiopathic primary dystonia have no evidence by history, examination or laboratory studies of any identifiable cause. There must be a normal perinatal and early developmental history, no prior personal or family history of relevant neurological illness, and no exposure to drugs known to cause acquired dystonia (e.g. phenothiazines). There must also be

Table 5.1 Common misdiagnoses of dystonia.

All dystonia: psychogenic, stress, nervousness
Blepharospasm: dry eye syndrome, tics
Cervical dystonia: stiff neck, arthritis (degenerative joint disease)
Writer's cramp: carpal tunnel syndrome, tennis elbow, strain
Spasmodic dysphonia: sore throat, laryngitis, vocal abuse
Oromandibular dystonia: temporomandibular joint syndrome

normal intellectual, pyramidal, cerebellar and sensory examinations and diagnostic studies [6,7]. Any relevant abnormalities may point to a secondary or symptomatic dystonia.

The clinical features are often clues to aetiology. Primary dystonia is typically action-induced. Symptoms are enhanced with use of the affected body part and the region may appear normal at rest. Secondary dystonia frequently results in fixed dystonic postures. The presence of extensive dystonia limited to one side of the body (hemidystonia) suggests a secondary cause such as a structural brain lesion.

When classified by distribution, dystonia may be focal, segmental or generalized. Focal dystonia involves one small group of muscles in one body part, segmental disease involves a contiguous group of muscles, and generalized dystonia is widespread. Common examples of focal dystonia include blepharospasm (forced, involuntary eye-closure), oromandibular dystonia (face, jaw, or tongue), torticollis or cervical dystonia (neck), writer's cramp (action-induced dystonic contraction of hand muscles), and spasmodic dysphonia (vocal cords). Patients with dystonia limited to one region of the body (focal or segmental dystonia) are deemed to be the best candidates for treatment with botulinum toxin type A (BtA). However, patients with severe generalized dystonia may benefit when selected regions of the body are treated.

Various members of families with dystonia may have generalized, segmental, or focal dystonia, linking the milder to the more generalized syndromes. This gives rise to the concept that the less affected individuals have a *forme fruste*, or more limited manifestation of generalized dystonia. The presence of dystonic symptoms in other family members supports the concept that the focal involvement is dystonic and genetic in these cases.

Genetics

Idiopathic torsion dystonia (ITD) probably has many causes, and clinical and ethnic subtypes of ITD have been proposed (Table 5.3 [8–35]). Family and linkage studies indicate that several of these subtypes have different genetic bases. These subtypes include autosomal dominant dopa-responsive dystonia (DRD) [36–38], X-linked Filipino torsion dystonia (XLTD) [39–44], and autosomal dominant (non-dopa responsive) ITD

Table 5.2 Classification of dystonia.*

I Age at onset
  A Infantile (<2 years)
  B Childhood (2–26 years)
  C Adult (>26 years)
II Aetiology
  A Primary
    1 With hereditary pattern
      (a) Autosomal dominant
        Classical types
          Childhood-onset dystonia
          Focal dystonia
        Variant types
          Dopa-responsive dystonia
          Myoclonic dystonia
      (b) X-linked recessive
    2 Sporadic (without a documented hereditary pattern)
      Classical types
      Variant types
  B. Symptomatic
    1 Associated with hereditary neurological syndromes and with known enzyme defect
      (1) Wilson's disease
      (2) GM1 gangliosidosis
      (3) GM2 gangliosidosis
      (4) Hexosaminidase A and B deficiency
      (5) Metachromatic leukodystrophy
      (6) Lesch–Nyhan syndrome
      (7) Homocystinuria
      (8) Glutaric acidemia
      (9) Triosephosphate isomerase deficiency
      (10) Methylmalonic aciduria
    2 Associated with probable hereditary neurological syndromes, without known enzyme defect, but with a chemical marker
      (1) Leigh's disease
      (2) Familial basal ganglia calcifications
      (3) Hallervorden–Spatz disease
      (4) Dystonic lipidosis (sea-blue histiocytosis)
      (5) Juvenile neuronal ceroid-lipofuscinosis
      (6) Ataxia-telangiectasia
      (7) Neuroacanthocytosis
      (8) Hartnup's disease
      (9) Intraneuronal inclusion disease
      (10) Hereditary bilateral optic atrophy with dystonia (mitochondrial)
    3 Associated with hereditary neurological syndromes, without known enzyme defect or chemical marker
      (1) Huntington's disease
      (2) Hereditary juvenile dystonia-parkinsonism
      (3) Pelizaeus–Merzbacher disease
      (4) Progressive pallidal degeneration
      (5) Joseph's disease
      (6) Rett's syndrome
      (7) Spinocerebellar degenerations

Continued on p. 104

Table 5.2 *Continued*

    (8)   Olivopontocerebellar atrophies
    (9)   Hereditary spastic paraplegia with dystonia
  4 Due to known environmental cause
    (1)   Perinatal cerebral injury
        (a) Athetoid cerebral palsy
        (b) Delayed onset dystonia
    (2)   Encephalitis and postinfectious
          Reye's syndrome
          Subacute sclerosing leucoencephalopathy
          Wasp sting
          Creutzfeldt–Jakob disease
    (3)   Head trauma
    (4)   Thalamotomy
    (5)   Brainstem lesion, including pontine myelinolysis
    (6)   Focal cerebral vascular injury
    (7)   Arteriovenous malformation
    (8)   Brain tumour
    (9)   Multiple sclerosis
    (10) Cervical cord injury
    (11) Peripheral injury Drugs: D2-receptor antagonists, levodopa, ergotism, anticonvulsants
    (12) Toxins: Mn, CO, carbon disulphide, cyanide, methanol, disulfiram
    (13) Metabolic: hypoparathyroidism
  5 Dystonia associated with parkinsonism
  6 Psychogenic dystonia
  7 Pseudodystonia
    (14) Sandifer syndrome
    (15) Stiff-person syndrome
    (16) Rotational vertebral subluxation
    (17) Soft tissue mass causing postural abnormality
    (18) Bone disease
    (19) Ligamentous absence, laxity or damage
    (20) Congenital muscular torticollis
    (21) Congenital postural torticollis
    (22) Congenital Klippel–Feil syndrome
    (23) Posterior fossa tumour
    (24) Syringomyelia
    (25) Arnold Chiari malformation
    (26) Trochlear nerve palsy
    (27) Vestibular torticollis
III Distribution
  A Focal
    1 Blepharospasm (forced, involuntary eye-closure)
    2 Oromandibular dystonia (face, jaw, or tongue)
    3 Torticollis (neck)
    4 Writer's cramp (action-induced dystonic contraction of hand muscles)
    5 Spasmodic dysphonia (vocal cords)
  B Segmental (cranial/axial/crural)
  C Multisegmental
  D Generalized (ambulatory, non-ambulatory)

*This table is expanded from those presented by [3] and [4]. Consult these reviews for references.

Table 5.3 Dystonia: molecular classification (updated from [8]).

OMIM designation (OMIM #)	Location	Major citations	Classic/variant	Typical age onset	Primary phenotype/Comment
DYT1 (128100)	9q34	[9]	Classic	Child or adolescent: <28 years	AD childhood and adolescent limb onset. AJ: most due to single mutation (GAG deletion) in torsinA. NJ: some due to torsinA mutation, or mutations at other locations, incl. chrom 8 (DYT6)
DYT2 (224500)	Unknown	[10]	–		AR in Gypsies, presence as a distinct entity is disputed
DYT3 (314250)	Xq13.1	[11]	Variant	Adult	X-linked parkinsonism-dystonia ('Lubag'. Philippines)
DYT4 (128101)	Unknown	[12,13]	Variant	Adult	AD hereditary whispering dysphonia in Australian family
DYT5 (128230)	14q22.1–22.2	[14]	Variant	Child or adolescent	DRD. Due to mutation in GTP cyclohydrolase I gene. Sex influenced
DYT6 (602629)	8p21-q22	[15]	Classic	Child or adolescent	Mennonite/Amish families with mixed (cranial/cervical or limb onset) phenotype
DYT7 (602124)	18p	[16]	Classic	Adult	German. adult cervical. cranial or brachial-onset
DYT8 (118800)	2q33-q35	[17–19]	Variant	Child or adolescent	Paroxysmal dystonia; paroxysmal dystonic choreoathetosis. May be a channelopathy
DYT9 (601042)	1p	[20]	Variant	Child or adolescent	Paroxysmal choreoathetosis with episodic ataxia and spasticity
DYT10 (128200)	16p11.2-q12.1	Possible [21] Reported in [22–25]	Variant	Child or adolescent	PKC; overlaps with OMIM 602066
DYT11 (159900)	11q23	[26–29]	Variant	Child or adolescent	Myoclonic dystonia: hereditary alcohol-responsive myoclonus. Mutation in dopamine D2-receptor in one family. Gene identified as a gene encoding varepsilon-sarcoglycan [29]
	7q21		Variant		
DYT12 (128235)	19q13	[30–32]	Variant	Child or adolescent	RDP
DYT13 (not assigned)	1p36	[33]	Classic	–	Cranial-cervical-brachial in one Italian family with 11 members
LDYT1 (535000)	mtDNA	[34,35]	Variant	Child or adolescent	Leber's hereditary optic neuropathy

AD. autosomal dominant: AJ. Ashkenazi Jewish.: AR. autosomal recessive: CSE. choreoathetosis/spasticity. episodic: DRD. dopa-responsive dystonia: NJ, non-Jewish: OMIM. online Mendelian inheritance in man (http://www3.ncbi.nlm.nih.gov/Omim/): PKC. paroxysmal kinesigenic choreoathetosis: RDP. rapid-onset dystonia-parkinsonism: XR. X-linked recessive.
The torsinA protein is the gene product of the DYT1 gene mutation on chromosome 9.

due to the *DYT1* gene mapped to chromosome 9q34 [45–47]. Both DRD and XLTD are rare 'variant' forms of ITD in which parkinsonism as well as dystonia are common expressions of the disease gene. In contrast, studies of families in which dystonia is due to the *DYT1* gene describe dystonia as the only clinical abnormality.

Idiopathic dystonia linked to the *DYT1* gene, also known as primary generalized torsion dystonia (PTD), dystonia musculorum deformans, or Oppenheim's dystonia, is one of the most severe forms of the inherited dystonias [45]. It is inherited as an autosomal dominant disease with 30–40% penetrance [45]. The symptoms usually start in an arm or leg in childhood, and generalize by adulthood. Occasionally onset is in later life, with the symptoms typically presenting in the cranial structures (e.g. neck, larynx and upper face), and tending to remain localized [48]. The cause for this variation in distribution with different age of onset is not known, but presumably reflects the underlying neurobiology [49]. Although the deletion mutation is most prevalent in Ashkenazi Jews due to a founder mutation [45], it can appear in most ethnic populations, including African-American and Asian. In some cases the deletion is a spontaneous mutation [47,50].

A decade of work on *DYT1* dystonia led to the identification of torsinA, the protein product of the *DYT1* gene, and its localization to chromosome 9q34.1 [51–54]. Recently a mutation of the dopamine D2-receptor in one family with the distinct but related hereditary disorder of myoclonus-dystonia was reported [27] in addition to linkage of myoclonic dystonia to chromosome 7 [29,55] where the gene product is varepsilon-sarcoglycan.

The role of torsinA in cellular function is not known. In most pedigrees with the clinical syndrome of childhood onset PTD, there is a single amino acid (glutamic acid) deletion at residue 303 [54]. This alteration in the amino acid sequence of the protein is necessary to produce clinical symptoms, but is not sufficient as not all gene carriers develop dystonia. The reason for the lack of complete penetrance is unknown, but it may be attributable to some property of the abnormal torsinA in dystonia, for example, the precipitation of neuronal dysfunction by an environmental factor(s) or by other modifier genes resulting in alterations of gene–gene/protein–protein interactions.

Laboratory and autopsy studies

Laboratory investigations are typically normal in patients with idiopathic dystonia. Patients with secondary dystonia will have laboratory findings consistent with the underlying disorder.

There are no consistent brain pathological findings in patients with idiopathic dystonia. Among the various reviews [56–60] of primarily idiopathic dystonia, the most frequently cited lesions are in the basal ganglia, including the putamen, head of caudate, and upper brainstem. The putamen and the striatopallidal–thalamo–cortical circuit appear to be the most likely sites in which to search for the unknown defect in primary dystonia [61].

Neuroimaging in dystonia

Brain lesions causing symptomatic dystonia point towards the basal ganglia as one probable generator of dystonic movements. In symptomatic dystonia, most abnormalities involve the lentiform nuclei and the thalamus [57], with the putamen and globus pallidus being the most frequent sites of pathology. In line with these observations functional neuroimaging studies demonstrate altered neuronal activity of the basal ganglia nuclei and their projection areas. Several positron emission tomography (PET) and functional magnetic resonance imaging (fMRI) studies identified a relative overactivity of the prefrontal motor planning areas, premotor area, supplementary motor area, anterior cingulate cortex and the thalamus during movements [62–64]. At rest and during movements there are increases in glucose metabolism and regional cerebral blood flow (PET) mainly at the lateral portions of the lentiform nuclei, again emphasizing increased activity of putaminal neurones. Radiotracer studies of the striatal dopaminergic system using single photon emission computed tomography (SPECT) reveal a decrease of the postsynaptic dopamine D2-receptor binding at the putamen with no change in presynaptic tracer accumulation at the striatal dopaminergic neurones [65].

Neurophysiology

According to a highly simplified but practical model [66], basal ganglia nuclei are organized into major motor loops: the direct circuit evolves a stimulating net effect on the frontal motor cortex while the indirect, D2-receptor mediated, circuit yields an inhibitory net effect. A reduced D2-receptor level may therefore lead to a reduced inhibitory effect on the frontal motor areas. In addition, increased activity of putaminal neurones via the direct motor loop would increase motor cortex activation due to a disinhibition of the thalamus.

Changes in neuronal activity of basal ganglia circuits greatly affect cortical motor activity. Transcranial magnetic stimulation (TMS) studies demonstrated a shorter silent period indicating a reduced cortical inhibition in primary dystonia [67]. Thus dysbalance in this cortical inhibitory network may lead to cortical overflow and uncontrolled, overshooting and dystonic movements. The lack of selectivity in attempts to perform specific movements and the slowness of voluntary and involuntary movements reflect pathological coactivation of antagonist muscles [68]. Dystonic cocontraction of antagonistic muscle groups is also linked to reduced reciprocal inhibition [69].

Contributions of the sensory systems to the pathophysiology of dystonia

The sensory trick

Sensory tricks often ameliorate dystonic movements and postures and can be effective in many different parts of the body. These sensory tricks are also known as '*gestes antagonistiques*' or incorrectly described as the 'counterpressor' phenomenon. Patients with cervical dystonia often find that gently touching the chin, back of head, or top of head will relieve symptoms. Force is not needed. In one series 88.9% of patients reported using sensory tricks to keep the head in the midline position [70]. The physiology of sensory tricks remains unclear, but there is evidence that they initiate a sensorimotor servomechanism that switches off the dystonic drive during the trick. In one study, 13 of 25 patients performing sensory tricks to dampen their idiopathic cervical dystonia had markedly reduced (50% or more) dystonic EMG activity even before the hand touched the face [71]. Some patients have reduced dystonia while merely thinking about their sensory trick [72]. PET studies show that sensory tricks in cervical dystonia lead to a significant decrease in the activity of the supplemental motor area and the primary motor cortex at the same time as the markedly reduced EMG activity [73].

The role of botulinum toxin

BtA may also modify the sensory feedback loop to the central nervous system and this mechanism may be partially responsible for its beneficial effect in dystonia. Ludlow *et al.* [74] and Zwirner *et al.* [75] proposed that reduced muscle activity and therefore feedback to laryngeal motoneurone pools may be a primary mechanism of action of BtA. We suggested that BtA might directly affect sensory afferents by blocking intrafusal fibres, decreasing activation of muscle spindles [76]. This would change activity in the sensory afferent system by reducing the Ia motorneurone traffic. Filippi *et al.* [77] supported this hypothesis by establishing that local injections of BtA directly reduce afferent Ia fibre traffic, and therefore modulate sensory feedback. This may account for the clinical observation that injections of BtA may have an effect on regional non-injected muscles, most striking in spastic limbs [78].

Further support for this mechanism derives from the cumulative work of Ryuji Kaji and colleagues [79–84]. He showed that the increase in severity of dystonic writer's cramp associated with enhancing Ia muscle spindle activity with the tonic vibration manoeuvre can be decreased by intramuscular injections of dilute lidocaine (lignocaine) which preferentially affects the afferent innervation of the muscle spindle. Both ethanol and lidocaine block sodium channels, although ethanol blocks the channels for longer than the anaesthetic. Kaji has coined the treatment of lidocaine plus ethanol as the 'muscle afferent block' or 'MAB', and has shown an effect in neck, jaw [83] and limb dystonia [79,80], and in spasticity [82,84]. The benefit for each treatment only lasts a few weeks and so muscle afferent block is of limited use in most dystonic and spastic situations. However, this model of Ia afferent blockade supports the proposed mechanism of action of BtA in conditions associated with excessive muscle contraction, as well as the importance of the afferent system in the clinical manifestations of dystonia [85].

Trauma and dystonia

Trauma is generally accepted as a factor in the pathogenesis of dystonia [86–89], although not everyone agrees [90]. Head/neck trauma precedes 5–21% of cases of cervical dystonia [91–95]. Patients with spasmodic dysphonia may report the onset of symptoms immediately after a laryngeal/pharyngeal trauma, most often following a viral infection. Whereas approximately 20% of our patients have a clear family history of dystonia, and therefore a genetic predisposition to the development of symptoms, some of the 'sporadic' cases may also be genetically susceptible or 'primed', and develop symptoms after exposure to the appropriate environmental factors ('trigger factors') such as exposure to infections or trauma. Limb dystonia [96–98] and jaw dystonia [99,100] may occur after peripheral traumas. Similar models have been proposed for other movement disorders [101]. There is a growing body of experimental evidence that appropriately predisposed people may develop dystonia with overactivity [102,103].

In our practice, we accept trauma as a trigger for dystonia when the onset of the dystonia is within 6–12 months of the identified trauma. In many cases, the peripheral injury which preceded the dystonia was acute, brief and well defined. In some of our patients the injury was relatively mild or chronic, or repetitive, as had been noted by Schott [104]. The dystonia typically occurs in the traumatized body part or region and in many cases is associated with pain. Sometimes the dystonic posture evolves as the pain improves.

Therapy of dystonia

There are several options for patients with dystonia. Apart from the rare instances when there is specific treatment for the underlying cause, all provide symptomatic relief only. Some patients choose no treatment. Apart from levodopa in DRD [38,105], no drug or surgical approach has emerged as uniformly effective and risk-free. Clinicians must choose treatment strategies that minimize risk, so reversible treatments should precede surgery and any drugs that may cause irreversible complications. There have been very few systematic drug trials in dystonia [106], and much of what we know about pharmacotherapy derives from empirical observations [107].

As genetic research advances there is growing concern about the use of destructive central nervous system surgery. The goal of this research is to clarify the causes of dystonia and develop specific treatments, as one does not want to ablate regions of the brain that may hold receptors or other structures important to future drug or restorative surgery.

Specific treatment for an underlying identified biochemical defect is available for only a limited number of symptomatic dystonias [108]. The most notable is Wilson's disease. For tardive dystonia, the best treatment is discontinuation of offending medications when possible, and providing the patient with a list of these medications to avoid.

DRD usually starts in childhood with gait disturbance and is often familial. Most patients respond dramatically to less than 500 mg/day levodopa (with carbidopa). For this reason, levodopa is first typically tried.

Patients with focal dystonia

Most focal dystonias are now treated effectively with local injections of BtA, which has been in use since the early 1980s. The response is often dramatic and BtA has replaced pharmacotherapy or surgery for many indications. Although BtA is licensed in many countries for only a limited palette of blepharospasm and related facial dystonia, hemi-facial spasm, and cervical dystonia (BtA and botulinum toxin type B [BtB]), it is also accepted as safe, effective and appropriate therapy for spasmodic dysphonia, and for many cases of oromandibular dystonia, writer's cramp and other focal dystonias [76,109–115].

Patients with more than focal dystonia

Patients with more than focal dystonia (segmental, multifocal, generalized) usually receive other drugs. However, many benefit from BtA directed towards one or several discrete regions of particularly troublesome dystonia. Initial drug treatment is usually with either an anticholinergic, benzodiazepine or baclofen. The choice usually depends on the patient's age, prior treatment attempts, and other concurrent medications or medical problems. The general strategy is to start with a low dose, gradually increasing it as tolerated and required. If it does not help at a dose causing adverse effects, then it is gradually tapered and discontinued before the next drug is tested. If it does help it can be continued and additional medication tried if necessary. In difficult cases, dopamine depleting and receptor-blocking agents may be worthwhile.

Intrathecal baclofen, used for patients with spasticity of spinal origin, has been tested in a limited number of studies and shows promise for patients with dystonia [116]. In our report [117], we reviewed our results in screening 25 dystonia patients and implanting pumps in 13. Intrathecal baclofen continued to work in six individuals (55%), but five had severe complications. Nevertheless, some patients derive significant benefit from intrathecal baclofen and so it is worth further study.

Consider central nervous system or peripheral surgery in only the most refractory cases that are unresponsive to BtA or BtB and/or extensive trials with other drugs. Peripheral surgery may be worthwhile in patients with cervical dystonia who fail with botulinum toxin (Bt). On a background of experience from other techniques, and from anatomical and electrophysiological studies, Claude Bertrand has popularized selective peripheral denervation [118,119]. Following the lead of Cooper [120] in 1964 and then Hassler and Dieckman [121], he attempted to avoid the sequelae of bilateral cervical rhizotomy by performing thalamotomy for rotatory torticollis [122,123]. After studying the cervical muscles using EMG and nerve blocks, Bertrand then combined thalamotomy with selective peripheral denervation [124–126]. His early experience demonstrated that peripheral denervation on its own could provide symptomatic relief in rotatory torticollis. Although championed by Bertrand at Notre-Dame Hospital (Montreal, Canada) since 1978 [125,127], the procedure is also currently performed in other centres within the US and Europe [128–132]. The major concerns are dysphagia and limitation of range of movement after surgery [133].

Central nervous system surgery is also reserved for patients with intractable disease, unresponsive to traditional drug and/or Bt therapy. Most practitioners have abandoned thalamotomy [134,135] because of the significant potential for serious side-effects. Most patients required bilateral operations which increase the risk of speech disturbance and dysphagia. Early stereotactic neurosurgeons, including Gros [136], Caracalos [137] and Cooper [138], tried pallidal lesions as well and reported these results alongside the thalamotomy studies. Pallidal ablation seemed encouraging, and Cooper's three reported patients derived substantial benefit [138].

With advances in surgical technique, movement disorder teams have re-explored neurosurgery for dystonia (for review, see [139]). Vitek *et al.* [140] and independently Iacono *et al.* [141], and others [140–155] have recently reported benefit from pallidotomy in patients with medically intractable dystonia.

Deep brain stimulation (DBS) is a new surgical technique that simulates the effects of a lesion and is now used for essential tremor and the motor features of Parkinson's disease. In comparison to pallidotomy, DBS has the advantages that: (a) it is not necessary to make a lesion other than that produced by the placement of the stimulation electrodes and, accordingly, it is associated with a decreased risk of adverse effects; (b) stimulation settings and the response to stimulation can be modified at any time postoperatively to maximize symptomatic relief; (c) if there are complications of stimulation, such as paresthesias, dysarthria or dysphagia, stimulation parameters can be modified or stimulation discontinued; (d) bilateral stimulation does not carry many of the risks associated with bilateral lesions. DBS of the thalamus was explored in a few patients with dystonia [156–159]. The authors reported moderate improvement in contralateral signs and symptoms. Encouraged, investigators are exploring DBS of thalamus and other nuclei, especially the internal segment of the globus pallidum (GPi), with fair to excellent results [139,154,160–163].

Acknowledgements

This work was supported, in part, by the Bachmann–Strauss Dystonia and Parkinson Foundation, and the US Public Health Grant FD-R-001452.

References

1 Fahn S. The varied clinical expressions of dystonia. *Neurol Clin* 1984; **2**: 541–54.

2 Nutt JG, Muenter MD, Aronson A, Kurland LT, Melton LJ III. Epidemiology of focal and generalized dystonia in Rochester. *Minnesota Mov Disord* 1988; **3**: 188–94.

3 Fahn S, Marsden CD, Calne DB. Classification and investigation of dystonia. In: Marsden CD, Fahn S, eds. *Movement Disorders 2*. London: Butterworths, 1987: 332–58.

4 Calne DB, Lang AE. Secondary dystonia. *Adv Neurol* 1988; **50**: 9–33.

5 Jankovic J. Post-traumatic movement disorders: central and peripheral mechanisms. *Neurology* 1994; **44**: 2006–14.

6 Marsden CD, Harrison MJG. Idiopathic torsion dystonia (dystonia musculorum deformans). A review of forty-two patients. *Brain* 1974; **97**: 793–810.

7 Burke RE, Brin MF, Fahn S, Bressman SB, Moskowitz C. Analysis of the clinical course of non-Jewish, autosomal dominant torsion dystonia. *Mov Disord* 1986; **1**: 163–78.

8 Brin MF. Dystonia: genetics and treatment with botulinum toxin. In: Smith B, Adelman G, eds. *Neuroscience Year (Encyclopedia of Neuroscience)*. Amsterdam: Elsevier 1997: 56–8.

9 Ozelius LJ, Hewett JW, Page CE *et al*. The early-onset torsion dystonia gene (*DYT1*) encodes an ATP binding protein. *Nat General* 1997; **17**: 40–8.

10 Gimenez-Roldan S, Lopez-Fraile IP, Esteban A. Dystonia in Spain: study of a Gypsy family and general survey. *Adv Neurol* 1976; **14**: 125–36.

11 Haberhausen G, Schmitt I, Köhler A *et al*. Assignment of the dystonia–parkinsonism syndrome locus, *DYT3*, to a small region within a 1.8-Mb YAC Contig Xq13 1. *Am J Hum Genet* 1995; **57**: 644–50.

12 Parker N. Hereditary whispering dysphonia. *J Neurol Neurosurg Psychiatry* 1985; **48**: 218–24.

13 Kandil MR, Tohamy SA, Fattah MA, Ahmed HN, Farwiez HM. Prevalence of chorea, dystonia and athetosis in Assiut, Egypt: a clinical and epidemiological study. *Neuroepidemiology* 1994; **13**: 202–10.

14 Ichinose H, Ohye T, Takahashi E *et al*. Hereditary progressive dystonia with marked diurnal fluctuation caused by mutations in the *GTP cyclohydolase I* gene. *Nat Genet* 1994; **8**: 236–42.

15 Almasy L, Bressman SB, Raymond D *et al*. Idiopathic torsion dystonia linked to chromosome 8 in two Mennonite families. *Ann Neurol* 1997; **42**: 670–3.

16 Leube B, Rudnicki D, Ratzlaff T *et al*. Idiopathic torsion dystonia: assignment of a gene to chromosome 18p in a German family with adult onset, autosomal dominant inheritance and purely focal distribution. *Hum Mol Genet* 1996; **5**: 1673–7.

17 Fink JK, Rainer S, Wilkowski J *et al*. Paroxysmal dystonic choreoathetosis: tight linkage to chromosome 2q. *Am J Hum Genet* 1996; **59**: 140–5.

18 Fouad GT, Servidei S, Durcan S, Bertini E, Ptacek LJ. A gene for familial paroxysmal dyskinesia (FPD1) maps to chromosome 2q. *Am J Hum Genet* 1996; **59**: 135–9.

19 Raskind WH, Bolin T, Wolff J *et al*. Further localization of a gene for paroxysmal dystonic choreoathetosis to a 5 cM region on chromosome 2q34. *Hum Genet* 1998; **102**: 93–7.

20 Auburger G, Ratzlaff T, Lunkes A *et al*. A gene for autosomal dominant paroxysmal choreoathetosis/spasticity (CSE) maps to the vicinity of a potassium channel gene cluster on chromosome 1p, probably within 2 cM between D1S443 and D1S197. *Genomics* 1996; **31**: 90–4.

21 Smith LA, Heersema PH. Periodic dystonia. *Mayo Clin Proc* 1941; **16**: 842–6.

22 Lance JW. Sporadic and familial varieties of tonic seizures. *J Neurol Neurosurg Psychiatry* 1963; **26**: 51–9.

23 Kertesz A. Paroxysmal kinesigenic choreoathetosis. An entity within the paroxysmal choreoathetosis syndrome. Description of 10 cases, including one autopsied. *Neurology* 1967; **17**: 680–90.

24 Walker ES. Familial paroxysmal dystonic choreoathetosis: a neurologic disorder simulating psychiatric illness. *Johns Hopkins Med J* 1981; **148**: 108–13.

25 Tomita H, Nagamitsu S, Wakui K *et al*. Paroxysmal kinesigenic choreoathetosis locus maps to chromosome 16p11.2-q12.1. *Am J Hum Genet* 1999; **65**: 1688–97.

26 Gasser T, Bereznai B, Muller B *et al*. Linkage studies in alcohol-responsive myoclonic dystonia. *Mov Disord* 1996; **11**: 363–70.

27 Klein C, Brin MF, Kramer P *et al*. Association of a missense change in the D2-dopamine receptor with myoclonus dystonia. *Proc Natl Acad Sci U S A* 1999; **96**: 5173–6.

28 Nygaard TG, Raymond D, Chen C *et al*. Localization of a gene for myoclonus-dystonia to chromosome 7q21-q31. *Ann Neurol* 1999; **46**: 794–8.

29 Zimprich A, Grabowski M, Asmus F *et al*. Mutations in the gene encoding varepsilon-sarcoglycan cause myoclonus-dystonia syndrome. *Nat Genet* 2001; **29**: 66–9.

30 Dobyns WB, Ozelius LJ, Kramer PL *et al*. Rapid-onset dystonia-parkinsonism. *Neurology* 1993; **43**: 2596–602.

31 Ishikawa A, Miyatake T. A family with hereditary juvenile dystonia-parkinsonism. *Mov Disord* 1995; **10**: 482–8.

32 Brashear A, deLeon D, Bressman SB *et al*. Rapid-onset dystonia-parkinsonism in a second family. *Neurology* 1997; **48**: 1066–9.

33 Valente EM, Bentivoglio AR, Cassetta E *et al*. DYT13, a novel primary torsion dystonia locus, maps to chromosome 1p36.13–36.32 in an Italian family with cranial-cervical or upper-limb onset. *Ann Neurol* 2001; **49**: 362–6.

34 Novotny EJ Jr, Singh G, Wallace DC *et al*. Leber's disease and dystonia: a mitochondrial disease. *Neurology*. 1986; 36: 1053–60.

35 Jun AS, Brown MD, Wallace DC. A mitochondrial DNA mutation at np 14459 of the ND6 gene associated with maternally inherited Leber's hereditary optic neuropathy and dystonia. *Proc Natl Acad Sci U S A* 1994; **91**: 6206–10.

36 Kwiatkowski DJ, Nygaard TG, Schuback DE *et al*. Identification of a highly polymorphic microsatellite VNTR within the argininosuccinate synthetase locus: exclusion of the dystonia gene on 9q32–34 as the cause of dopa-responsive dystonia in a large kindred. *Am J Hum Genet* 1991; **48**: 121–8.

37 Nygaard TG, Marsden CD, Fahn S. Dopa-responsive dystonia: long-term treatment response and prognosis. *Neurology* 1991; **41**: 174–81.

38 Nygaard TG, Trugman JM, de Yebenes JG, Fahn S. Dopa-responsive dystonia: the spectrum of clinical manifestations in a large North American family. *Neurology* 1990; **40**: 66–9.

39 Takahashi H, Snow B, Waters C *et al*. Evidence for nigrostriatal lesions in Lubag (X-linked dystonia-parkinsonism in the Philippines). *Neurology* 1992; **42**: 441.

40 Lee LV, Kupke KG, Caballar Gonzaga F, Hebron Ortiz M, Muller U. The phenotype of the X-linked dystonia–parkinsonism syndrome. An assessment of 42 cases in the Philippines. *Medicine (Balt)* 1991; **70**: 179–87.

41 Wilhelmsen KC, Weeks DE, Nygaard TG *et al*. Genetic mapping of the 'Lubag' (X-linked dystonia-parkinsonism) in a Filipino kindred to the pericentromeric region of the X chromosome. *Ann Neurol* 1991; **29**: 124–31.

42 Fahn S, Moskowitz CX. X-linked recessive dystonia and parkinsonism in Filipino males. *Annals of Neurology* 1988; **24**: 179.

43 Kupke KG, Lee LV, Muller U. Assignment of the X-linked torsion dystonia gene to Xq21 by linkage analysis. *Neurology* 1990; **40**: 1438–42.

44 Kupke KG, Lee LV, Viterbo GH *et al*. X-linked recessive torsion dystonia in the Philippines. *Am J Med Genet* 1990; **36**: 237–42.

45 Ozelius L, Kramer PL, Moskowitz CB *et al*. Human gene for torsion dystonia located on chromosome 9q32-q34. *Neuron* 1989; **2**: 1427–34.

46 Kramer PL, de Leon D, Ozelius L *et al*. Dystonia gene in Ashkenazi Jewish population is located on chromosome 9q32–34. *Ann Neurol* 1990; **27**: 114–20.

47 Risch NJ, Bressman SB, deLeon D *et al*. Segregation analysis of idiopathic torsion dystonia in Ashkenazi Jews suggests autosomal dominant inheritance. *Am J Hum Genet* 1990; **46**: 533–8.

48 Bressman SB, de Leon D, Kramer PL *et al*. Dystonia in Ashkenazi Jews: clinical characterization of a founder mutation. *Ann Neurol* 1994; **36**: 771–7.

49 Ozelius LJ, Hewett JW, Page CE *et al*. The gene (*DYT1*) for early-onset torsion dystonia encodes a novel protein related to the Clp protease/heat shock family. *Adv Neurol* 1998; **78**: 93–105.

50 Klein C, Brin MF, de Leon D *et al*. Novo mutations (GAG deletion) in the *DYT1* gene in two non-Jewish patients with early-onset dystonia. *Hum Mol Genet* 1998; **7**: 1133–6.

51 Kramer PL, de Leon D, Ozelius L *et al*. Dystonia gene in Ashkenazi Jewish population is located on chromosome 9q32–34 [see comments]. *Ann Neurol* 1990; **27**: 114–20.

52 Ozelius LJ, Kramer PL, de Leon D *et al*. Strong allelic association between the torsion dystonia gene (*DYT1*) and loci on chromosome 9q34 in Ashkenazi Jews. *Am J Hum Genet* 1992; **50**: 619–28.

53 Ozelius LJ, Hewett J, Kramer P *et al*. Fine localization of the torsion dystonia gene (*DYT1*) on human chromosome 9q34: YAC map and linkage disequilibrium. *Genome Res* 1997; **7**: 483–94.

54 Ozelius LJ, Hewett JW, Page CE *et al*. The early-onset torsion dystonia gene (*DYT1*) encodes an ATP-binding protein. *Nat Genet* 1997; **17**: 40–8.

55 Nygaard TG, Raymond D, Chen C *et al*. Localization of a gene for myoclonus-dystonia to chromosome 7q21-q31 [see comments]. *Ann Neurol* 1999; **46**: 794–8.

56 Obeso JA, Gimenez Roldan S. Clinicopathological correlation in symptomatic dystonia. *Adv Neurol* 1988; **50**: 113–22.

57 Marsden CD, Obeso JA, Zarranz JJ, Lang AE. The anatomical basis of symptomatic hemidystonia. *Brain* 1985; **108**: 463–83.

58 Narbona J, Obeso JA, Tunon T, Martinez Lage JM, Marsden CD. Hemidystonia secondary to localized basal ganglia tumour. *J Neurol Neurosurg Psychiatry* 1984; **47**: 704–9.

59 Jankovic J, Patel SC. Blepharospasm associated with brainstem lesions. *Neurology* 1983; **33**: 1237–40.

60 Zweig RM, Hedreen JC, Jankel WR *et al*. Pathology in brainstem regions of individuals with primary dystonia. *Neurology* 1988; **38**: 702–6.

61 Hedreen JC, Zweig RM, DeLong MR, Whitehouse PJ, Price DL. Primary dystonias: a review of the pathology and suggestions for new directions of study. *Adv Neurol* 1988; **50**: 123–32.

62 Playford ED, Passingham RE, Marsden CD, Brooks DJ. Increased activation of frontal areas during arm movement in idiopathic torsion dystonia. *Mov Disord* 1998; **13**: 309–18.

63 Ceballos-Baumann AO, Passingham RE, Warner T *et al*. Overactive prefrontal and underactive motor cortical areas in idiopathic dystonia. *Ann Neurol* 1995; **37**: 363–72.

64 Preibisch C, Berg D, Hofmann E, Solymosi L, Naumann M. Cerebral activation patterns in patients with writer's cramp: a functional magnetic resonance imaging study. *J Neurol* 2001; **248**: 10–7.

65 Naumann M, Pirker W, Reiners K *et al*. Imaging the pre- and postsynaptic side of striatal dopaminergic synapses in idiopathic cervical dystonia: a SPECT study using [123I]epidepride and [123I]beta-CIT. *Mov Disord* 1998; **13**: 319–23.

66 Alexander GE, Crutcher MD, DeLong MR. Basal ganglia-thalamocortical circuits: parallel substrates for motor, oculomotor, 'prefrontal' and 'limbic' functions. *Prog Brain Res* 1990; **85**: 119–46.

67 Ikoma K, Samii A, Mercuri B, Wassermann EM, Hallett M. Abnormal cortical motor excitability in dystonia. *Neurology* 1996; **46**: 1371–6.

68 Berardelli A, Rothwell JC, Hallett M *et al*. The pathophysiology of primary dystonia. *Brain* 1998; **121**: 1195–212.

69 Panizza M, Lelli S, Nilsson J, Hallett M. H-reflex recovery curve and reciprocal inhibition of H-reflex in different kinds of dystonia. *Neurology* 1990; **40**: 824–8.

70 Jahanshahi M. Factors that ameliorate or aggravate spasmodic torticollis. *J Neurol Neurosurg Psychiatry* 2000; **68**: 227–9.

71 Wissel J, Muller J, Ebersbach G, Poewe W. Trick manoeuvres in cervical dystonia: investigation of movement- and touch-related changes in polymyographic activity. *Mov Disord* 1999; **14**: 994–9.

72 Greene PE, Bressman S. Exteroceptive and interoceptive stimuli in dystonia. *Mov Disord* 1998; **13**: 549–51.

73 Naumann M, Magyar S, Reiners K, Erbguth F, Leenders KL. Sensory tricks in cervical dystonia: perceptual dysbalance of parietal cortex modulates frontal motor programming. *Annals of Neurology* 2000; **47**: 322–8.

74 Ludlow CL, Hallett M, Sedory SE, Fujita M, Naunton RF. The pathophysiology of spasmodic dysphonia and its modification by botulinum toxin. In: Berardelli A, Benecke R, Manfredi M, Marsden CM, eds. *Motor Disturbances II*. New York: Academic Press, 1990; 273–88.

75 Zwirner P, Murry T, Swenson M, Woodson G. Effects of botulinum toxin therapy in patients with adductor spasmodic dysphonia: acoustic, aerodynamic, and videoendoscopic findings. *Laryngoscope* 1992; **102**: 400–6.

76 Brin MF, Blitzer A, Stewart C, Fahn S. Treatment of spasmodic dysphonia (laryngeal dystonia) with local injections of botulinum toxin: review and technical aspects. In: Blitzer A, Brin MF, Sasaki CT, Fahn S, Harris KS, eds. *Neurological Disorders of the Larynx*. New York: Thieme, 1992: 214–28.

77 Filippi GM, Errico P, Santarelli R, Bagolini B, Manni E. Botulinum toxin A effects on rat jaw muscle spindles. *Acta Oto-Laryngol* 1993; **113**: 400–4.

78 Borg-Stein J, Pine ZM, Miller JR, Brin MF. Botulinum toxin for the treatment of spasticity in multiple sclerosis. New observations. *Am J Phys Med Rehabil* 1993; **72**: 364–8.

79 Kaji R, Rothwell JC, Katayama M *et al*. Tonic vibration reflex and muscle afferent block in writer's cramp. *Ann Neurol* 1995; **38**: 155–62.

80 Kaji R, Kohara N, Katayama M *et al*. Muscle afferent block by intramuscular injection of lidocaine for the treatment of writer's cramp. *Muscle Nerve* 1995; **18**: 234–5.

81 Kaji R, Shibasaki H, Kimura J. Writer's cramp: a disorder of motor subroutine? [Editorial; comment.] *Ann Neurol* 1995; **38**: 837–8.

82 Kaji R, Mezaki T, Kubori T, Murase N, Kimura J. Treatment of spasticity with botulinum toxin and muscle afferent block. *Rinsho Shinkeigaku* 1996; **36**: 1334–5.

83 Yoshida K, Kaji R, Kubori T, Kohara N, Iizuka T, Kimura J. Muscle afferent block for the treatment of oromandibular dystonia. *Mov Disord* 1998; **13**: 699–705.

84 Mezaki T, Kaji R, Hirota N, Kohara N, Kimura J. Treatment of spasticity with muscle afferent block. *Neurology* 1999; **53**: 1156–7.

85 Hallett M. Physiology of dystonia. *Adv Neurol* 1998; **78**: 11–8.

86 Brin MF, Fahn S, Bressman SB, Burke RE. Dystonia precipitated by peripheral trauma. *Neurology* 1986; **36** (Suppl. 1): 119.

87 Jankovic J, Van der Linden C. Dystonia and tremor induced by peripheral trauma: predisposing factors. *J Neurol Neurosurg Psychiatry* 1988; **51**: 1512–9.

88 Gordon M, Brin MF, Giladi N, Hunt A, Fahn S. Dystonia precipitated by peripheral trauma. *Mov Disord* 1990; **5** (Suppl. 1): 236.

89 Jankovic J. Can peripheral trauma induce dystonia and other movement disorders? Yes! *Mov Disord* 2001; **16**: 7–12.

90 Weiner WJ. Can peripheral trauma induce dystonia? No! *Mov Disord* 2001; **16**: 13–22.

91 Chan J, Brin M, Fahn S. Idiopathic cervical dystonia: clinical characteristics. *Mov Disord* 1991; **6**: 119–26.

92 Jankovic J, Leder S, Warner D, Schwartz K. Cervical dystonia: clinical findings and associated movement disorders. *Neurology* 1991; **41**: 1088–91.

93 Rondot P, Marchand MP, Dellatolas G. Spasmodic torticollis—review of 220 patients. *Can J Neurol Sci* 1991; **18**: 143–51.

94 Lowenstein DH, Aminoff MJ. The clinical course of spasmodic torticollis. *Neurology* 1988; **38**: 530–2.

95 Samii A, Pal PK, Schulzer M, Mak E, Tsui JKC. Post-traumatic cervical dystonia: a distinct entity? *Canadian Journal of Neurological Sciences* 2000; **27**: 55–9.

96 Frucht S, Fahn S, Ford B. Focal task-specific dystonia induced by peripheral trauma. *Mov Disord* 2000; **15**: 348–50.

97 Hollinger P, Burgunder J. Post-traumatic focal dystonia of the shoulder. *Eur Neurol* 2000; **44**: 153–5.

98 Thyagarajan D, Kompoliti K, Ford B. Post-traumatic shoulder 'dystonia': persistent abnormal postures of the shoulder after minor trauma. *Neurology* 1998; **51**: 1205–7.

99 Schrag A, Bhatia KP, Quinn NP, Marsden CD. Atypical and typical cranial dystonia following dental procedures. *Movement Disord* 1999; **14**: 492–6.

100 Sankhla C, Lai EC, Jankovic J. Peripherally induced oromandibular dystonia. *J Neurol Neurosurg Psychiatry* 1998; **65**: 722–8.

101 Barbeau A. Aetiology of Parkinson's disease: a research strategy. *Can J Neurol Sci* 1984; **11**: 24–8.

102 Byl N, Wilson F, Merzenich M *et al.* Sensory dysfunction associated with repetitive strain injuries of tendinitis and focal hand dystonia: a comparative study. *J Orthop Sports Phys Ther* 1996; **23**: 234–44.

103 Byl NN, Merzenich MM, Jenkins WM. A primate genesis model of focal dystonia and repetitive strain injury: (i) learning-induced dedifferentiation of the representation of the hand in the primary somatosensory cortex in adult monkeys. *Neurology* 1996; **47**: 508–20.

104 Schott GD. The relationship of peripheral trauma and pain to dystonia. *J Neurol Neurosurg Psychiatry* 1985; **48**: 698–701.

105 Fletcher NA, Holt IJ, Harding AE *et al.* Tyrosine hydroxylase and levodopa responsive dystonia. *J Neurol Neurosurg Psychiatry* 1989; **52**: 112–4.

106 Burke RE, Fahn S, Marsden CD. Torsion dystonia: a double-blind, prospective trial of high-dosage trihexyphenidyl. *Neurology* 1986; **36**: 160–4.

107 Greene P, Shale H, Fahn S. Analysis of open-label trials in torsion dystonia using high dosages of anticholinergics and other drugs. *Mov Disord* 1988; **3**: 46–60.

108 Bressman SB, Greene PE. Treatment of hyperkinetic movement disorders. *Neurol Clin* 1990; **8**: 51–75.

109 American Academy of Neurology. Assessment: the clinical usefulness of botulinum toxin A in treating neurologic disorders. *Report of the Therapeutics and Technology Assessment Subcommittee of the American Academy of Neurology. Neurology* 1990; **40**: 1332–6.

110 American Academy of Ophthalmology (AAO). Statement. Botulinum A toxin for ocular muscle disorders. *Lancet* 1986; **1**: 76–7.

111 American Academy of Ophthalmology (AAO). Statement. Botulinum toxin therapy of eye muscle disorders. Safety and effectiveness. *Ophthalmology* 1989; **2**: 37–41.

112 American Academy of Otolaryngology—Head and Neck (AAO—HNS). American Academy of Otolaryngology-Head and Neck Surgery policy statement: Botox® for spasmodic dysphonia. *AAO-HNS Bull* 1990; **9**: 8.

113 National Institutes of Health Concensus Development Conference. Clinical use of botulinum toxin. National Institutes of Health Consensus Development Statement. *Arch Neurol* 1990; **48**: 1294–8.

114 Jankovic J, Brin M. Therapeutic uses of botulinum toxin. *N Engl J Med* 1991; **324**: 1186–94.

115 Brin MF. Interventional neurology: treatment of neurological conditions with local injection of botulinum toxin. *Arch Neurobiol* 1991; **54**: 173–89.

116 Narayan RK, Loubser PG, Jankovic J, Donovan WH, Bontke CF. Intrathecal baclofen for intractable axial dystonia [see comments]. *Neurology* 1991; **41**: 1141–2.

117 Ford B, Greene P, Louis ED *et al*. Use of intrathecal baclofen in the treatment of patients with dystonia. *Arch Neurol* 1996; **53**: 1241–6.

118 Bertrand C, Molina Negro P, Bouvier G, Gorczyca W. Observations and analysis of results in 131 cases of spasmodic torticollis after selective denervation. *Appl Neurophysiol* 1987; **50**: 319–23.

119 Bertrand CM. Selective peripheral denervation for spasmodic torticollis: surgical technique, results and observations in 260 cases. *Surg Neurol* 1993; **40**: 96–103.

120 Cooper IS. Effects of thalamic lesions on torticollis. *N Engl J Med* 1964; **270**: 967–72.

121 Hassler R, Dieckmann G. Stereotactic treatment of different kinds of spasmodic torticollis. *Confin Neurol* 1970; **32**: 135–43.

122 Bertrand CM. The treatment of spasmodic torticollis with particular reference to thalamotomy. In: Mortley T, ed. *Current Controversies in Neurosurgery*. Philadelphia: WB Saunders, 1976: 455–9.

123 Bertrand CM, Molina-Negro P, Martinez SN. Stereotactic targets for dystonias and dyskinesias: relationship to corticobulbar fibers and other adjoining structures. *Adv Neurol* 1979; **24**: 395–9.

124 Bertrand C, Molina-Negro P, Martinez SN. Combined stereotactic and peripheral surgical approach for spasmodic torticollis. *Appl Neurophysiol* 1978; **41**: 122–33.

125 Bertrand C, Molina NP, Martinez SN. Technical aspects of selective peripheral denervation for spasmodic torticollis. *Appl Neurophysiol* 1982; **45**: 326–30.

126 Bertrand CM. Stereotactic and peripheral surgery for the control of movement disorders. In: Barbeau A, ed. *Disorders of Movements: Current Status of Modern Therapy*. Lancaster: MTP Press, 1981: 191–208.

127 Bertrand CM, Molina Negro P. Selective peripheral denervation in 111 cases of spasmodic torticollis: rationale and results. *Adv Neurol* 1988; **50**: 637–43.

128 Arce C, Russo L. Selective peripheral denervation: a surgical alternative in the treatment of spasmodic torticollis. Review of fifty-five patients. *Mov Disord* 1992; **7**: 128.

129 Davis DH, Ahlskog JE, Litchy WJ, Root LM. Selective peripheral denervation for torticollis: preliminary results. *Mayo Clin Proc* 1991; **66**: 365–71.

130 Munchau A, Palmer JD, Dressler D *et al*. Prospective study of selective peripheral denervation for botulinum-toxin resistant patients with cervical dystonia. *Brain* 2001; **124**: 769–83.

131 Bertrand CM, Benabou R. Surgical treatment of spasmodic torticollis: selective peripheral denervation revisited. In: Germano I, ed. *Neurosurgical Treatment of Movement Disorders*. Park Ridge: American Association of Neurological Surgeons, 1998: 239–54.

132 Krauss JK, Toups EG, Jankovic J, Grossman RG. Symptomatic and functional outcome of surgical treatment of cervical dystonia. *J Neurol Neurosurg Psychiatry* 1997; **63**: 642–8.

133 Munchau A, Good CD, McGowan S *et al*. Prospective study of swallowing function in patients with cervical dystonia undergoing selective peripheral denervation. *J Neurol Neurosurg Psychiatry* 2001; **71**: 67–72.

134 Tasker RR. Outcome after stereotactic thalamotomy for dystonia and hemiballismus. Comment. *Neurosurgery* 1995; **36**: 507–8.

135 Tasker RR, Doorly T, Yamashiro K. Thalamotomy in generalized dystonia. *Adv Neurol* 1988; **50**: 615–32.

136 Gros C, Frerebeau P, Perez-Dominguez E, Bazin M, Privat JM. Long-term results of stereotaxic surgery for infantile dystonia and dyskinesia. *Neurochirurgia (Stuttg)* 1976; **19**: 171–8.

137 Caracalos A. Results of 103 cryosurgical procedures in involuntary movement disorders. *Confin Neurol* 1972; **34**: 74–83.

138 Cooper IM, Bravo GM. Alleviation of dystonia musculorum deformans and other involuntary movement disorders of childhood by chemopallidectomy and chemopallido-thalamectomy. *Clin Neurosurg* 1958; **5**: 127–49.

139 Brin MF, Germano I, Danisi F, Weisz D, Olanow CW. Deep brain stimulation in the treatment of dystonia. In: Krauss JK, Jankovic J, Grossman RG, eds. *Surgery for Parkinson's Disease and Movement Disorders*. Philadelphia: Lippincott, Williams & Wilkins, 2001: 307–15.

140 Vitek JL, Zhang J, Evatt M *et al*. Pallidotomy for dystonia: clinical outcome and neuronal activity. *Adv Neurol* 1998; **78**: 211–9.

141 Iacono RP, Kuniyoshi SM, Lonser RR *et al*. Simultaneous bilateral pallidoansotomy for idiopathic dystonia musculorum deformans. *Pediatr Neurol* 1996; **14**: 145–8.

142 Vitek JL, Evatt M, Zhang J *et al*. Pallidotomy as a treatment for medically intractable dystonia. *Annals of Neurology* 1997; **42**: 409.

143 Shima F, Sakata S, Sun S-J *et al*. The role of the descending pallido-reticular pathway in movement disorders. In: Segawa M, Nomura Y, eds. *Age-Related Dopamine-Dependent Disorders*. New York: Karger, 1995: 197–207.

144 Gibson GJ, Douglas NJ, Stradling JR, London DR, Semple SJ. Sleep apnoea: clinical importance and facilities for investigation and treatment in the UK. Addendum to the 1993 Royal College of Physicians Sleep Apnoea report [see comments]. *J R Coll Physicians Lond* 1998; **32**: 540–4.

145 Lozano AM, Kumar R, Gross RE *et al*. Globus pallidus internus pallidotomy for generalized dystonia. *Mov Disord* 1997; **12**: 865–70.

146 Ondo WG, Desaloms JM, Jankovic J, Grossman RG. Pallidotomy for generalized dystonia. *Mov Disord* 1998; **13**: 693–8.

147 Teive H, Sa D, Grande CV *et al*. Bilateral simultaneous globus pallidus internus pallidotomy for generalized post-traumatic dystonia. *Mov Disord* 1998; **13**: 33.

148 Lin JJ, Lin GY. Bilateral posteroventral pallidotomy in treatment of generalized dystonia. *Mov Disord* 1998; **13**: 68.

149 Rezak M, Vergenz SM, Eller TW, Bernstein LP, Nenonene EK. Successful treatment of segmental idiopathic dystonia with internal segment pallidotomy. *Mov Disord* 1998; **13**: 98.

150 Sterio D, Beric A, Alterman R, Kelly P. Pallidotomy treatment for torsion dystonia. *Mov Disord* 1998; **13**: 198.

151 Teive HA, Sa DS, Grande CV, Antoniuk A, Werneck LC. Bilateral pallidotomy for generalized dystonia. *Arq Neuropsiquiatr* 2001; **59**: 353–7.

152 Yoshor D, Hamilton WJ, Ondo W, Jankovic J, Grossman RG. Comparison of thalamotomy and pallidotomy for the treatment of dystonia. *Neurosurgery* 2001; **48**: 818–24.

153 Adler CH, Kumar R. Pharmacological and surgical options for the treatment of cervical dystonia. *Neurology* 2000; **55**: S9–14.

154 Tronnier VM, Fogel W. Pallidal stimulation for generalized dystonia. Report of three cases. *J Neurosurg* 2000; **92**: 453–6.

155 Lin JJ, Lin GY, Shih C *et al*. Benefit of bilateral pallidotomy in the treatment of generalized dystonia. Case report. *J Neurosurg* 1999; **90**: 974–6.

156 Benabid AL, Pollack P, Limousin P, Hoffman D. Chronic stimulation of the ventrolateral thalamic nucleus in dystonia. Focus on dystonia: A satellite meeting of the 11th Parkinson's Disease Symposium, Rome (25 March 1994), p. 26.

157 Blond S, Siegfried J. Thalamic stimulation for the treatment of tremor and other movement disorders. *Acta Neurochir (Suppl)(Wien)* 1991; **52**: 109–11.

158 Sellal F, Hirsch E, Barth P, Blond S, Marescaux C. A case of symptomatic hemidystonia improved by ventroposterolateral thalamic electrostimulation. *Mov Disord* 1993; **8**: 515–8.

159 Benabid AL, Pollak P, Gao D *et al*. Chronic electrical stimulation of the ventralis intermedius nucleus of the thalamus as a treatment of movement disorders. *J Neurosurg* 1996; **84**: 203–14.

160 Islekel S, Zileli M, Zileli B. Unilateral pallidal stimulation in cervical dystonia. *Stereotact Funct Neurosurg* 1999; **72**: 248–52.

161 Andaluz N, Taha JM, Dalvi A. Bilateral pallidal deep brain stimulation for cervical and truncal dystonia. *Neurology* 2001; **57**: 557–8.

162 Ghika J, Vingerhoets F, Temperli P, Pollo C, Villemure J-G. Ventrooralis nucleus thalamic deep brain stimulation (Voa-DBS), but not pallidal DBS (GPi-DBS), is effective in generalized postanoxic dystonia with necrosis of bilateral pallida. *Neurology* 2000 **54** (Suppl. 3): A220.

163 Kumar R, Dagher A, Hutchison WD, Lang AE, Lozano AM. Globus pallidus deep brain stimulation for generalized dystonia: clinical and PET investigation. *Neurology* 1999; **53**: 871–4.

CHAPTER 6

Blepharospasm, oromandibular dystonia, Meige's syndrome and hemifacial spasm

MITCHELL F. BRIN, FABIO DANISI & ANDREW BLITZER

Introduction

Botulinum toxin type A (BtA) therapy is now established treatment for patients with blepharospasm, hemifacial spasm and oromandibular dystonia, including bruxism. In most situations it is accepted as a first-line therapy for the spasms, associated discomfort and pain. Table 6.1 summarizes the literature on treating these disorders with BtA (p. 127). We do not discuss botulinum toxin type B because there is no published experience using it for these conditions.

Blepharospasm

Clinical presentation and epidemiology

Blepharospasm is characterized by involuntary, inappropriate, forceful eye closure [1]. It typically affects both eyes symmetrically, although sometimes there is marked asymmetry. The most common presentation is essential blepharospasm (referred to below as 'blepharospasm'), which is a form of adult-onset focal dystonia. When it is associated with oromandibular dystonia, laryngeal or cervical dystonia, the complex is called segmental cranial dystonia, or Meige's syndrome.

Blepharospasm, like other presentations of focal, adult-onset idiopathic dystonia, typically begins insidiously in the 5th to 7th decade of life. Estimates of the prevalence of blepharospasm range from 16 to 133 per million people[2], and it is more common in women. Disease progression is generally very slow and although it usually remains focal, over decades the dystonic features may spread to nearby facial muscles or, less commonly, to other parts of the body. There may be a family history of blepharospasm, other focal dystonias, movement disorder or tics.

There may be a long prodrome of sensory symptoms such as photophobia and ocular discomfort. Initially, the dystonic muscle contractions are intermittent. If the disease progresses, the blepharospasm can increase in both frequency and intensity, leading to functional blindness in some patients. Typically, most symptoms stabilize after 2–3 years but with fluctuations in intensity. However, in the absence of therapy, some patients can have a protracted progression of symptoms. Blepharospasm may be task specific and occur mainly with certain activities, and not with others. It may be worse in bright light, and when the patient is tired, anxious or particularly needs to see. Many patients complain of worsening symptoms as the day wears on.

As with other focal dystonias, blepharospasm can be a prominent component of generalized primary (idiopathic torsion dystonia) and symptomatic dystonias [3]. Blepharospasm is seen in about a quarter of patients with progressive supranuclear palsy. In patients with Parkinson's disease, an exaggerated blink reflex is thought to be the basis of the Meyerson's sign, also known at the glabellar tap sign. Sustained eye closure can be triggered by visual stimuli brought into close range. Infrequently, patients with Parkinson's disease have significant blepharospasm superimposed on their hypomimia. Dystonic facial grimacing is also seen as a dystonic hyperkinesia associated with levodopa therapy. Blepharospasm sometimes occurs in tardive dystonia. Evaluation of any patient with dystonia requires an accurate and detailed drug history. Psychogenic blepharospasm is rare.

Differential diagnosis

The diagnosis is made on a typical history, even in the absence of physical signs. Patients may present to ophthalmologists with sore eyes. Even if slit lamp examination of the eyelids reveals chronic ocular surface disorders such as blepharitis, meibomian gland dysfunction or dry eyes, appropriate local treatment usually has no effect on the primary symptoms. It is possible that these disorders trigger blepharospasm in individuals who are genetically or otherwise susceptible. By contrast, in secondary blepharospasm the ophthalmological cause is usually acute and obvious (e.g. corneal abrasions). Also, the characteristic fluctuations experienced by patients in idiopathic blepharospasm are not evident.

Apraxia of eyelid opening This is sometimes described as 'atypical blepharospasm' or 'akinetic blepharospasm' or 'involuntary levator palpebrae inhibition'. It is characterized by excessive eyelid closure, but is primarily due to failure to activate the levator palpebrae muscle. It is encountered in basal ganglia disorders. Careful examination may be required to differentiate apraxia from flaccid ptosis and from subtle blepharospasm where there is inappropriate contraction of the fine muscles on the eyelids. A useful clue is that even in mild blepharospasm the lower lid is usually slightly raised.

Motor tics These can frequently present as increased blink rate, or forceful blinking, and even persistent disabling blepharospasm. They can usually be distinguished from blepharospasm by the earlier age at onset, the sense of inner tension relieved by the movement, and the presence of other tics and comorbid conditions, such as obsessive-compulsive disorder and attention deficit/hyperactivity disorder.

Psychogenic Functional or psychogenic (previously called 'hysterical') blepharospasm is unusual. Note that some patients with idiopathic blepharospasm may become secondarily depressed or anxious, and unhelpful suggestions from poorly informed laymen or doctors may exacerbate this.

Oromandibular dystonia, lower facial dystonia and Meige's syndrome

Clinical presentation

Oromandibular dystonia This is dystonia involving the masticatory, the *lower* facial and the tongue muscles, producing spasms and jaw deviation. In the early 16th century Brueghel often painted faces with open mouths and contracted facial muscles, since postulated to have had oromandibular dystonia [4]. In 1899, Gowers described many conditions producing tonic or clonic jaw contractions [5]. The differential diagnosis of *tonic* spasms nowadays includes tetanus, trauma, hysteria, brainstem lesions, tardive levodopa induced, and hypothermia. Causes of *clonic* spasms include convulsions, rigors, paralysis agitans, facial pain and chorea.

Meige's syndrome Just after the turn of the century, Meige reported a syndrome of spasms of the eyelids and contractions of the pharyngeal, jaw and tongue muscles [6]. Characteristic of dystonia, these spasms were often provoked by voluntary action (talking, eating), or lessened by humming, singing, yawning, or voluntarily opening the mouth. Some of the patients with Meige's syndrome developed other signs of dystonia including torticollis or writer's cramp. In 1976, Marsden concluded that blepharospasm and oromandibular dystonia were within the spectrum of adult-onset segmental torsion dystonia [7], and this is now generally accepted [8].

Differential diagnosis

The aetiology and differential diagnosis of oromandibular dystonia is similar to that of other focal or segmental dystonias [9]. Oromandibular dystonia is particularly common in patients with chromosome-8 linked dystonia in the Amish/Mennonite population [10]. Misdiagnosis is widespread because the condition is uncommon. Most patients are initially diagnosed as having *temporomandibular joint disorder*, and treated with a variety of appliances [8,11] but, for many patients, these treatments are inadequate. Nevertheless, dental appliances may be useful for treating some cases of orofacial dyskinesias, and some of these patients may have oromandibular dystonia [12]. The true incidence of benefit from physical treatments is not known; most patients present to a referral centre only after failing conservative therapies in the community.

Bruxism is a diurnal or nocturnal jaw-associated malady in which patients clench, grind, brace and gnash their teeth. Sustained or repetitive muscle contractions associated with bruxism typically occur in sleep [13], a time when most classical movement disorders such as oromandibular dystonia are not present. However, bruxism may also occur during the day and simulate the symptoms of oromandibular dystonia. Symptoms of bruxism (for review, see [14]) may be caused by drugs, idiopathic or post-traumatic oromandibular dystonia, hemifacial spasm, postanoxic brain damage, coma, cerebellar damage, Rett's syndrome, Whipple's disease and be present in patients with mental retardation. Because of the similarities in aetiologies and phenomenology, some have proposed that bruxism represents a variant of dystonia [14].

Classification

The classification of patients with oromandibular dystonia is based on the clinical features. Patients may have oromandibular dystonia that is predominantly jaw closing, jaw opening, or jaw deviation dystonia. Many patients with jaw deviation also have jaw opening, and are classified as primarily jaw opening dystonia in the following discussion. There may be associated involuntary tongue movements.

General considerations

During the neurological evaluation, the physician evaluates the patient in an attempt to diagnose an underlying cause or contributing factors. For patients with dystonia, we obtain a careful medication history, caeruloplasmin levels, liver and thyroid function tests, erythrocyte sedimentation rate (ESR), antinuclear antibody, serum protein electrophoresis and immunoprotein electrophoresis to screen for inherited metabolic or inflammatory disorders that may result in symptomatic dystonia. We recommend more extensive testing when there is a strong clinical suspicion of secondary dystonia. We do not obtain magnetic resonance imaging (MRI) of the brain unless we suspect a symptomatic dystonia. If an underlying biochemical basis is identified, then specific therapy is instituted.

Treatment for craniofacial dystonias

We counsel patients about the treatments available. These include no therapy (the disorder is not life threatening per se), supportive therapies, physical therapies, pharmacotherapy, BtA injections and surgery (Fig. 6.1).

Support systems

The most extensive support system is the network of concerned patients who participate in support groups and national and international foundations that promote education and research on dystonia. This is supplemented by increasingly easy access to patient support materials on the World-wide Web (see www.wemove.org). The importance of this type of support can not be underestimated. Some countries have a developing

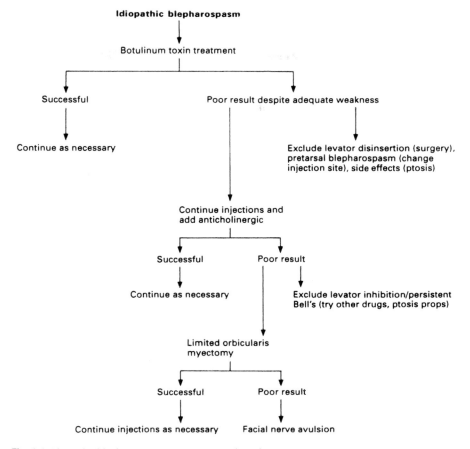

Fig. 6.1 Idiopathic blepharospasm: management algorithm.

network of dystonia nurses, who become experts in counselling, help to run support groups, and deal with welfare agencies as an advocate for the patient and to raise public awareness. Professional emotional support may also be helpful. Reactive or primary depression often aggravates disability [15–22] and can be helped by supportive psychotherapy.

Physical measures

Physical measures include physical therapy, biofeedback [23], and braces that mimic the simple *geste antagonistique* using minimal force. Some devices physically obstruct the involuntary posturing, such as neck collars for cervical dystonia [24] and dental braces for oromandibular dystonia [25]. Prescribe these with care as the force of dystonic posturing may bend or break them, and can lead to skin abrasions and pressure sores. Eyelid crutches alone rarely work for blepharospasm, but can be useful to override the flaccid ptosis that may follow BtA treatment. Manipulation-based therapists (physical therapists, chiropractors) should not use force in therapy, but should use treatments that assist patients to use their own resources to compensate for postural abnormalities. None of these therapies have been subjected to double blind evaluation.

Pharmacotherapy

Nearly every neuropharmacological agent has been tried in primary dystonia and no single agent has emerged as a cure. Pharmacotherapy typically is associated with more systemic side-effects than BtA. Monotherapy with oral agents is not as useful as BtA in patients with focal or segmental cranial dystonia. However, oral medications are frequently used as an adjunct to BtA, and may help 'take the edge off' the dystonic symptoms. The medications used for focal and segmental cranial dystonia are the same as those for other forms of dystonia. These include anticholinergic agents such as trihexyphenidyl, oral baclofen, benzodiazepines and tetrabenazine. We start at a low dose and slowly increase the dose until there is benefit or intolerable side-effects appear. Combinations may be useful. Oral medications typically play a greater role in patients with more generalized dystonia.

Hemifacial spasm

Epidemiology and clinical presentation

Hemifacial spasm is peripherally induced. *It is not generally considered a form of focal dystonia.* It is characterized by recurrent involuntary twitches of the muscles innervated by the facial nerve, and is typically unilateral. There are rare cases of bilateral hemifacial spasm reported in the literature in which there is asymmetrical onset and an asynchronous discharge pattern [26]. The twitches can be tonic, clonic or mixed. The prevalence of hemifacial spasm in women is 14.5/100 000 population, in men 7.4/100 000. Most patients are between 20 and 80 years old.

Typically it starts in the orbicularis oculi and spreads slowly to other muscles over months or years. Eye closure spasms and mouth retraction/elevation are the most commonly encountered movements, but any other posture induced by a facial nerve innervated muscle can occur. Stapedius contraction can sometimes cause a clicking sound in the ear. The spasms can continue during sleep. They may be worsened by stress, chewing, speaking, light, and cold. Hemifacial spasm may be partly posture dependent. Mild facial weakness develops in proportion to the duration of the illness. In between the obvious spasms, facial asymmetry may be present and may be due to the weakness or to synkinesis, contracture, or mild persistent spasm. The combination of a mild lower motor neuron facial weakness with a slightly closed palpebral fissure is characteristic and nearly always diagnostic. There are no other associated cranial nerve signs in the classical disorder.

Most causes of hemifacial spasm are extra-axial and intracranial. The most common cause is vascular compression of the nerve by an aberrant arterial loop (typically a branch of the posterior inferior cerebellar artery) or vein. Additional causes include tumours, vascular malformations, and localized infectious processes [27].

In addition to a comprehensive history, examination, and relevant blood studies [28], we perform a brain MRI, and rarely a MR angiogram to rule out a structural lesion at the level of the brainstem. MR angiographic tomography (MRAT) is a useful technique which combines vascular imaging with an image of the brainstem parenchyma and the facial nerve origin, and usually demonstrates the vascular compression directly. Investigation may be unnecessary in long-standing and typical adult-onset cases unless neurosurgical treatment is being considered.

Differential diagnosis

The differential diagnosis of hemifacial spasm includes essential blepharospasm, which is typically bilateral. Focal seizures are less frequent, although *epilepsia partialis continua* may localize to the face. *Facial myokymia* is characterized by subtle, continuous, ripple-like quivering, usually over small areas of the face. *Facial tics* usually are not limited to one side of the face. A Bell's palsy or other peripheral damage to the facial nerve may result in aberrant regeneration and *synkinesia*, and there is a clear history that the lower motorneurone facial weakness came before the facial twitching.

Management of hemifacial spasm

Explain to patients that the facial nerve is probably being irritated by a blood vessel and that although the condition is unpleasant, it is not dangerous and the movements should not spread elsewhere. Unfortunately, they are likely to persist indefinitely. Systemic drugs include oral anticonvulsants, baclofen and benzodiazepines, but unfortunately often have little effect on hemifacial spasm. The choice of treatment lies between BtA injections and base of the brain microvascular decompression surgery. Relatively young fit patients often choose neurosurgery whereas older patients prefer injections. Doxorubicin (Adriamycin) intramuscular injections have been used [29], but we do not recommend this approach because of its toxicity.

Pharmacotherapy

Pharmacotherapy with anticonvulsants such as carbamazepine or valproic acid is sometimes helpful. However, patients are rarely well controlled on oral medications alone. Our oral agent of choice is carbamazepine. Start at lower doses and increase more slowly than in epilepsy. We use a similar approach for valproic acid, clonazepam, gabapentin and baclofen.

Surgery

Surgery is indicated as primary therapy for the rare patients with symptomatic hemi-facial spasm due to mass lesions at the base of the brain [30,31]. Selected patients with typical hemifacial spasm may also benefit. The facial nerve root entry zone (REZ) is visualized via a retro-mastoid craniectomy using a microsurgical technique. If vascular compression of the facial nerve is identified, the artery and nerve are either separated by an Ivalon sponge or larger arteries are retracted using a dural based sling. Patients usually stay in hospital for about a week.

Based on the surgical literature, in experienced hands more than 90% of patients with hemifacial spasm achieve either partial or excellent control of their hemifacial spasm, and the relief appears to be long lasting. Complications are usually transient, but permanent neurological deficits are encountered, especially ipsilateral hearing loss and facial weakness; rarely, brainstem stroke and death occur. Because of the potentially serious surgical complications, we typically refer patients for surgery only if they fail more than one medication and several trials of botulinum toxin (Bt) (Fig. 6.2).

Treating with botulinum toxin (Table. 6.1 [32–38])

General considerations

BtA is dramatically effective and is currently the treatment of choice for most cases of hemifacial spasm, and for many focal dystonias including blepharospasm, Meige's syndrome and jaw dystonia. The list of areas treated has expanded to include dystonic

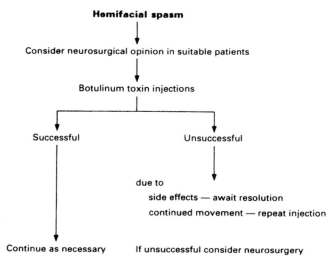

Fig. 6.2 Hemifacial spasm: management algorithm.

Table 6.1 Selection of larger BtA studies on blepharospasm, hemifacial spasm and oromandibular dystonia.

Authors	Type	Design	n	Dose	Rating	Results
Jankovic & Orman [32]	BS	Randomized, double blind, placebo-controlled, crossover	11	25 mu Botox® per side	Pt self-assessment Fahn scale Videotapes	60.7% improvement (self-assessment) 71.6% improvement (Fahn scale) Mean duration 12.5 weeks
Brin et al. [33]	BS	Open label	49	Total of 47.3 mu (mean) Botox® per session	Pt self-assessment	Moderate to marked improvement in 69% of patients. Mean duration 12.9 weeks
Taylor et al. [34]	BS	Open label	235	2.5–5.0 mu Botox® in each of 4–6 sites per side	Spasms relief on severity scale	98% responders Mean duration 14.4 weeks
Nüssgens & Roggenkämper [35]	BS	Randomized, double blind, active-controlled, crossover	212	Total of 45.4 mu (mean) Botox®: 182.1 mu (mean) Dysport®	Subjective assessment	Mean duration Botox® 7.98 weeks Dysport® 8.03 weeks Less ptosis in the Botox® group
Chen et al. [36]	HFS	Open label	137	12–15 mu Botox® on one side	Subjective assessment of spasm relief and intensity	Improvement of spasms in 88% of treatments Mean duration 20 weeks
Jitpimolard et al. [37]	HFS	Open label	175	92 mu Dysport® at 3 sites on one side	Subjective improvement on 0–100 scale	Mean improvement of 77.2% Mean 3.4 months
Blitzer et al. [11]	OMD	Open label	20	Individually 10–40 mu Botox® per muscle (EMG)	Physician and pt self-assessment	Overall 47% improvement of symptoms
Jankovic et al. [38]	OMD	Open label	45	Individually 25–50 mu Botox® per muscle	Subjective assessment (severity, overall response 0–4)	Moderate improvement in 73% of patients. Mean duration 7.7 weeks

BS, blepharospasm; EMG, electromyography; HFS, hemifacial spasm; mu, mouse unit; OMD, oromandibular dystonia.

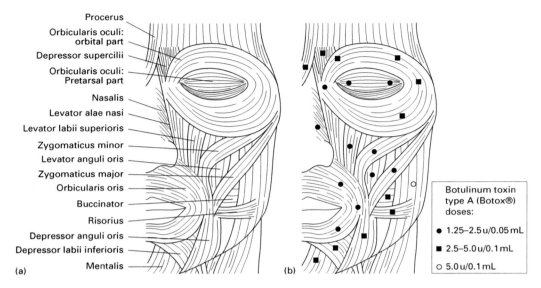

Procerus
Orbicularis oculi: orbital part
Depressor supercilii
Orbicularis oculi: Pretarsal part
Nasalis
Levator alae nasi
Levator labii superioris
Zygomaticus minor
Levator anguli oris
Zygomaticus major
Orbicularis oris
Buccinator
Risorius
Depressor anguli oris
Depressor labii inferioris
Mentalis
(a)
(b)

Botulinum toxin type A (Botox®) doses:
● 1.25–2.5 u/0.05 mL
■ 2.5–5.0 u/0.1 mL
○ 5.0 u/0.1 mL

Fig. 6.3 (a) The facial musculature. The treating physician must observe the abnormal facial movements closely to identify which muscle(s) to inject with botulinum toxin. EMG guidance is useful when there is a need to identify some of the deeper-set muscles of the lower face. (b) Samples of sites and maximum initial doses of BtA as Botox® injections for facial dystonia and hemifacial spasm. Dysport® doses given in Table 6.2.

and non-dystonic involuntary movements in different parts of the body and with a variety of causes. The American Academy of Ophthalmology [39,40], American Academy of Neurology [41], American Academy of Otolaryngology [42] and the National Institutes of Health [43] have released statements on the therapeutic efficacy of Bt in well-studied human conditions. There are books devoted to the topic [44,45], and courses held at most neurological academies.

When using BtA, there is considerable variation among clinicians in terms of injection techniques, number of injections per muscle, doses, combinations of muscles injected, and the use of electromyography (EMG). We typically start with small doses for the first treatment, since it is difficult to predict the degree of initial response in individual patients. We explain this approach to our patients, to prevent inappropriate expectations and to encourage them to appreciate that the overall treatment strategy is to gradually improve symptoms while minimizing side-effects. Dosing and targeting become more precise over the course of a few treatment sessions as the individual patient profile and requirements become more evident. It is much easier to achieve a good outcome if there are good records, and it is important to record the drug used, and the dose and site of injections given, not least because the next treatment may be given elsewhere or by a different clinician. For facial muscles use a diagram such as Fig. 6.3.

We obtain informed consent before starting BtA injections [46]. We discuss the alternative treatments, and explain the procedures and the potential benefits and risks associated with BtA injections.

Blepharospasm and other eyelid contractions

In 1973, Dr Alan Scott, an American ophthalmologist, was searching for a medical treatment for strabismus and showed that Bt can be injected into the lateral rectus of monkeys to produce selective relaxation of the muscle without significant systemic or local reactions [47]. When tested in patients the relaxation lasted for several months and was clinically useful. His success in strabismus marked the beginning of clinical use of BtA, and it was soon extended to blepharospasm. BtA injections have been convincingly shown to be effective and substantially relieve blepharospasm (Table 6.1).

After Scott's pioneer work many open-label and several double blind, placebo-controlled studies were performed in essential blepharospasm with success rates of usually 90%. Controlled studies show a good to excellent improvement of symptoms in 66–98% of patients treated, and BtA is clearly superior to placebo. The benefit lasts between 2.0 and 3.5 months.

Dose and dilution for the first injection

DOSES: A HEALTH WARNING

Please read the warning on p. 35 about doses of Bt. There are three preparations available. *Dysport®* and *Botox®* are type A toxins (BtA), *NeuroBloc®/MYOBLOC™* is type B (BtB). Even though the doses for each are quoted in mouse units (mu), the three preparations have different dose schedules: one mu of *Dysport®* is **not** the same as one mu of *Botox®*, and neither is equivalent to one mu of *NeuroBloc®/MYOBLOC™*.

Tailor the dose and injection sites to the patient. We generally start with a concentration of 5 mu Botox® in 0.1 mL (50 mu/mL) for the orbicularis oculi muscles, and give a total dose of around 20 mu Botox® per side. For Dysport®, use 100–200 mu/mL with total dose of 80 mu per side. This initial dose may be inadequate, and some centres start with larger doses. The range of doses used for initial therapy is outlined in Table 6.2 with dose modifier guidelines in Table 6.3 [48]. Figure 6.3 is provided for anatomical reference. Inject subcutaneously, using a 30–32 gauge needle without EMG guidance. Larger needles are more likely to lead to bruising.

Typically, we inject three or four sites in the orbital part of orbicularis oculi. As shown in Fig. 6.3, the initial sites are the medial and lateral superior palpebral part of the orbicularis oculi, the lateral canthus and the inferolateral portion of the orbicularis oculi. For the initial treatment, each injection includes 2.5–5.0 mu Botox® in 0.05–0.1 mL, or 20–40 mu Dysport®. Avoid injecting directly over the meridian of the eye, to prevent spread to the levator palpebrae and development of ptosis. We do not at first inject the pretarsal part of the orbicularis, leaving that to subsequent injection sessions if a different pattern is required. We usually avoid injecting the inferomedial portion of the

Table 6.2 Patterns of spasm, muscles, initial botulinum toxin type A (BtA) dosing in adults.

Clinical pattern	Potential muscles involved	Dose* (mu) Botox® (starting dose total per muscle; range)	Dose* (mu) Dysport® (starting dose total per muscle; range)	Starting dose is divided into the following number of injection sites per muscle
Forced eye closure for blepharospasm	Orbicularis oculi (including lateral canthus)	20 (10–30)	80 (40–140)	4
Forced eye closure for hemifacial spasm	Orbicularis oculi (including lateral canthus)	7.5 (7.5–20.0)	60 (30–120)	3
Jaw closing	Masseter, temporalis	25 (15–50)	100 (60–200)	4
Jaw closing	Internal pterygoid	15 (5–40)	60 (20–160)	2
Jaw opening	External pterygoid	15 (10–40)	60 (40–160)	3
	Digastric	5 (2.5–20.0)	20 (10–80)	2
Facial muscle spasm	Zygomaticus minor, zygomaticus major, levator anguli oris, levator labii superioris, risorius, depressor anguli oris, depressor labii inferioris	2.5 (2.5–7.5)	10 (10–30)	1–2
	Mentalis, buccinator	5 (2.5–10.0)	20 (10–40)	2
Lip pursing	Orbicularis oris	5 (2.5–5.0)	10 (5–15)	2–4 per lip
Neck band spasm	Platysma	5 (2.5–10.0) per strand	20 (10–30) per strand	1–3 per strand

*See dose modifiers (Table 6.3) and general guidelines.

pretarsal, as it is fairly vascular, and BtA may spread to the inferior oblique and inferior rectus, or it may interfere with function of the lacrimal duct (Fig. 6.3b).

Patients with *lid opening apraxia* receive small doses of BtA to the pretarsal, or preseptal and orbital region of the orbicularis oculi.

Ask patients to keep a diary to track their response using a visual analogue scale [49,50]. They should return to the office after about 1 month for an assessment of their response to therapy. This visit is particularly important to assess their requirements for future injections.

Table 6.3 Dose modifiers (adapted from [48]).

Modifiers	Dose per muscle	
	Decrease dose if	Increase dose if
Patient weight	Very low and muscles small	N/a
Likely duration of therapy	Chronic	Acute
Muscle bulk	Very small	Very large
Number of body regions treated simultaneously	Many	Few
Spasms	Mild	Severe
Concern for excessive weakness	High	Low
Previous results of therapy	Too much weakness	Inadequate muscle relaxation
Sternocleidomastoid, digastric or perilingual/pharyngeal injections	Bilateral injection	—
Prior denervation or nerve injury (hemifacial spasm, peripheral denervation surgery, Bell's palsy)	Present	—

Treatment effects

BtA begins to work between 1 day and 10 days after injection, usually reaching peak effect within 2–4 weeks. The typical duration of action is 3–4 months, with considerable variation in individual responses, but 85–90% of patients respond satisfactorily. Avoid injecting more than every 3 months because of the potential risk of developing immunoresistance to BtA due to blocking antibodies. We have not seen resistance develop in our blepharospasm patients despite over a decade of therapy in some. This is likely to be due to the lower dose of BtA used (usually <100 mu Botox®) compared to other presentations of dystonia (e.g. cervical dystonia).

Repeat injections

Refine doses and targeting at each subsequent visit. Increase the dose if the patient reports inadequate reduction of the dystonic contractions and there is no ptosis or other adverse event. Consider injections to the pretarsal part of orbicularis oculi. This may produce an excessive response with side-effects and the patient should be warned accordingly. However, adjusting the dose and site of injection is the primary way to establish the most favourable response to BtA. If there are signs of unwanted spread to other muscles, most notably the levator palpebrae and the extraocular muscles, either concentrate the solution of BtA and/or reduce the dose and adjust the site of injection.

If the patient remains visually disabled despite adequate orbicularis oculi weakness, it is worth adding a systemic anticholinergic, such as benzhexol, or a benzodiazepine, such as lorazepam or diazepam, starting at a low dose and gradually increasing until

Blepharospasm severity

	OD	OS	
None	☐	☐	0
Minimal, increased blinking present only with external stimuli (e.g. bright light, wind, reading, driving, etc.).	☐	☐	1
Mild, but spontaneous eyelid fluttering (without actual spasm), definitely noticeable, possibly embarrassing, but not functionally disabling.	☐	☐	2
Moderate, very noticeable spasm of eyelids only, mildly incapacitating	☐	☐	3
Severe, incapacitating spasm of eyelids and possibly other facial muscles.	☐	☐	4

Blepharospasm frequency

	OD	SO	
None	☐	☐	0
Slightly increased frequency of blinking	☐	☐	1
Eyelid fluttering lasting less than 1 second in duration	☐	☐	2
Eyelid spasm lasting more than 1 second, but eyes open more than 50% of waking time	☐	☐	3
Functionally blind due to persistent eye closure (blepharospasm) more than 50% of the waking time	☐	☐	4

Disability rating scale
0, Normal; 1, slight disability, no functional impairment; 2, moderate disability, no functional impairment; 3, moderate disability, functional impairment; 4, incapacitated.

Assessment of peak effect
0, No effect; 1, mild effect, no functional improvement; 2, moderate improvement, no change in functional disability; 3, moderate improvement in both severity and function; 4, marked improvement in both severity and function.

To determine the global peak effect, subtract 1 point for non-disabling complication and 2 points for a disabling complication.

Fig. 6.4 Blepharospasm rating scales.

either there is a response or side-effects supervene. In spite of this, a very few patients remain visually disabled.

Side-effects

Side-effects are relatively common early in therapy during the period of dose optimization, but are usually mild, and they are invariably self-limiting. Discuss them with the patient before treatment. The most common side-effects are dry eye (7%) and a partial ptosis (3–10%) due to a spread of the toxin to the levator palpebrae muscle. Also, abolishing the spasm may lead to changes in local fluid dynamics and tissue fluid accumulation with eyelid edema. It usually resolves within 1–2 weeks. If there is profound weakness of levator palpebrae, ptosis props may allow the patient to see. They are also helpful in patients who have lid-opening apraxia. Ptosis props will not prevent normal or pathological *active* blinking and eye closure, and we warn patients that as BtA wears off their spasms will again be troublesome. Some patients may have Bell's phenomenon [51–53] so that even when lids are open, repeated or tonic vertical displacement of the eye prevents useful vision.

Occasionally patient cannot close an eye properly and should be warned to protect it, perhaps taping it shut at night to help avoid exposure keratopathy. Other side-effects of BtA injected around the eyes include blurring of vision and diplopia. Frank diplopia is quite rare (<1%). Rarely, patients develop a somatic rash and/or report a flu-like syndrome. If a rash occurs consistently after BtA, it sometimes responds to pretreatment with diphenhydramine.

Treatment alternatives after botulinum toxin therapy failure

Surgery may help the few patients with blepharospasm who fail BtA therapy and pharmacotherapy. The most common operation is myectomy of the orbicularis oculi [54]. It may be combined with a blepharoplasty to treat dermatochalasis of the upper lid region for those patients whose excessive skin folds above the upper lid create a virtual blepharoptosis, in the absence of a true lid droop. Surgical myectomy is irreversible, and patients should be referred only to surgeons experienced in this procedure. The major complication is excessive weakness of orbicularis oculi. The lid will not close fully and keratopathy may ensue. Refinement of the procedure, and the combined use of surgery and BtA therapy improve the outcome [55,56]. Brow ptosis may need to be managed surgically by brow fixation to the underlying periosteum. Lower lid entropion can occur and responds to taping of the lid.

Oromandibular dystonia

Treatment of jaw dystonia requires a detailed knowledge of the local anatomy (Fig. 6.5) and management of potential complications of therapy. Most patients should be evaluated by a neurologist, otolaryngologist, and speech and language pathologist. In selected cases where there are signs or symptoms of temporomandibular joint dysfunction (TMD), including joint pain or click or restricted jaw mobility, an evaluation by a TMD specialist may be appropriate. We have seen cases where oromandibular dystonia and TMD coexist and these require a coordinated treatment approach. Injections are performed in outpatients, except for patients who have severe oromandibular dystonia and require nasogastric or parenteral feeding until treatment permits resumption of oral feeding. Patients with bruxism have also been treated with BtA with good results [57–60].

Muscle selection

Table 6.4 lists the muscles controlling jaw movements.

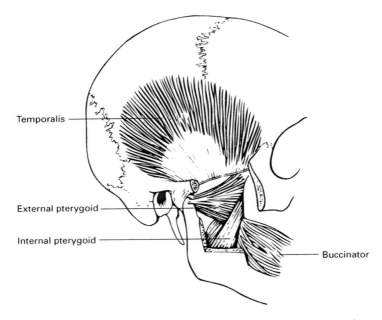

Fig. 6.5 Jaw muscles. The zygomatic arch with the masseter muscle, which inserts into the mandible, have been removed to reveal the underlying musculature.

Table 6.4 Muscles affecting jaw and tongue movement.

Muscle	Primary functions
Masseter	Jaw closing
Temporalis	Jaw closing; anterior fibres assist in jaw opening, deviation and protrusion
Internal pterygoid	Jaw closing
Digastric (anterior and posterior)	Jaw opening
External pterygoid	Jaw opening, deviation to opposite side and protrusion
Genioglossus	Tongue protrusion, jaw opening
Hyoglossus	Tongue protrusion, jaw opening
Geniohyoid	Jaw opening
Myohyoid	Elevation of hyoid, jaw opening

JAW CLOSING

The best results are seen in patients with jaw closing and jaw deviation. For jaw-closing dystonia, at the first visit we typically treat the masseters and temporalis muscles bilaterally. If the results with repeated treatments are inadequate, then we also treat the internal pterygoid muscles. We avoid the internal pterygoid muscles at first because they are close to the lingual muscles and there is a risk of dysphagia.

JAW OPENING

Patients with jaw opening are more challenging to treat. Treatment is straightforward if external pterygoid involvement is prominent. However, the digastrics and base-of-tongue muscles may also be involved, and aggressive injection into these muscles can cause unwanted dysphagia. Use EMG guidance for injection into the digastrics, to ensure that the needle tip is in the target muscle and not the lingual muscles. If activation of the tongue muscles results in increased EMG activity with the needle in place, withdraw it from the lingual muscles. Except in very rare situations, we strictly avoid injecting the lingual muscles because of the increased risk of associated dysphagia.

Jaw deviation and protrusion Jaw deviation is caused by the contralateral external pterygoid muscle contracting more than the ipsilateral muscle. For relief of pure jaw deviation, inject the contralateral external pterygoid muscle. For jaw protrusion, inject both external pterygoid muscles. For mixed jaw protrusion and deviation, inject the contralateral external pterygoid with a larger dose than the ipsilateral.

First botulinum toxin injection and use of electromyography

All pterygoid muscle injections are performed with EMG guidance as the muscles are not easy to palpate. We use EMG for the other jaw muscles (digastrics, masseters, temporalis) to improve the precision and accuracy, and to help to inject regions of active contraction. This is particularly important when performing follow-up injections, when there can be islands of still-weakened or inactive muscle from previous injection cycles. The EMG responses to gestures and movements, such as opening the mouth, or side-to-side motion when injecting the lateral pterygoids, or opening the mouth forcefully when injecting the digastric muscles, all help to place the toxin injections precisely.

Dose and dilution

As noted above for blepharospasm, we begin with small to modest doses, and titrate subsequently according to the clinical response, selecting the muscles that on clinical examination have the greatest spasm, and drawing upon our previous experience. Table 6.2 outlines average doses of BtA [61]. After a careful examination, adjust the dose according to factors such as the force of contractions, characteristics of the condition, etc. (Table 6.3). The usual dilution of Botox® is 50 mu/mL, and of Dysport® 200 mu/mL. Distribute toxin between three and five sites in each muscle. Even when the initial treatment was inadequate, we discourage 'boosters' because of our concern about antibody development. We have observed resistance to therapy in patients with oromandibular dystonia. All of these patients were exposed to the original lot of Botox® (lot 79–11) [62]. With the current Botox®, which has a significantly lower protein exposure, we anticipate a lower rate of immunoresistance [63,64].

Injections of the external and internal pterygoid muscles

A special note should be made regarding injections of the external pterygoid muscles. Although a percutaneous approach can be used for the external pterygoid muscles, reaching the muscle through the coronoid notch, and impaling the muscle perpendicularly, we use an intraoral approach under EMG guidance. This approach permits injection along the full length of the muscle, whereas the percutaneous approach only permits injection through one point perpendicular to the muscle. The needle insertion is just lateral to the most posterior molar tooth, lateral to the palpable pterygoid plate and impaling the muscle parallel to the muscle fibres, aiming in the direction of the temporomandibular joint. If the needle is placed too far medially, rhinolalia, nasal regurgitation and Eustachian tube dysfunction may occur from toxin diffusing into the palatine muscles. Because the external pterygoid muscle area is highly vascular, always aspirate before injecting the toxin.

Approach the internal pterygoid from the angle of the mandible, but directing the EMG needle superiorly and anteriorly, hugging the inside of the mandible to avoid the lingual muscles and the resulting dysphagia.

Effects of treatment

The duration of benefit, as reported in our initial series [61] and that of others [65], is approximately 4 months, being longest in the jaw-closing patients and shortest in the jaw deviation group. Two-thirds of patients have a moderate to marked improvement [65]. Rare complications of treating oromandibular dystonia include weakness of jaw-closing and jaw-opening muscles. In our series, treating these patients for over 17 years, we have had only one case of clinically evident haematoma occurring, and that occurred in a patient after an external pterygoid injection. Within a few minutes of the injection, the patient experienced local pain and then mild swelling in the region of the upper mandible. The patient was treated with ice and there were no sensory symptoms or persistent complaints. Dry mouth has not occurred as a side-effect in our series. Diffusion of the toxin to tongue or pharyngeal muscles may lead to dysphagia. For treatment of Bt-induced dysphagia see Chapter 8. These injections should be performed by physicians skilled in the anatomy and the management of potential side-effects.

Lower facial muscles (Meige's syndrome)

The diagnostic and therapeutic approach used for blepharospasm also applies when there is dystonia of the lower face involving muscles innervated by the seventh nerve, such as in Meige's syndrome. The more diffuse the dystonia, the more we rely on adjunctive pharmacotherapy (see above). BtA is our usual first-line therapy if symptoms are mainly facial. There are no randomized controlled trials, and most authors report on the focal symptoms and not the global symptomatology. Unlike in blepharospasm, we tend to use EMG guidance for hyperkinetic lower facial muscles, particularly the deep muscles, such as zygomaticus major and minor, and buccinator. However, some physicians give injections free hand. Use as fine a needle as possible, usually 30–32 gauge. Typical *initial* doses for lower facial muscles are given in Table 6.2.

In general, muscles that elevate facial expression need lower doses and more caution than those depressing facial expression, such as those below the angle of the orbicularis oris. We often start with a lower dose and risk under-treating to minimize adverse events such as excessive facial flattening when injecting zygomaticus, or drooling when injecting orbicularis oris.

Hemifacial spasm

Bt injections can provide relatively long-lasting relief or substantial reduction in symptoms in the majority of patients. They have the advantage of being simple, safe and usually indefinitely repeatable. Several open and a few controlled studies have reported good to excellent improvement of spasms in 76–100% of patients injected, and are listed in Table 6.1. In these trials (and from subsequent world-wide experience), the mean duration of benefit ranged between 2.6 and 4.0 months, with some patients responding for much longer to a single treatment session. Unfortunately, there are some patients who do not respond well, or who regularly suffer from side-effects and cannot tolerate an efficacious dose. Neurosurgical referral can be offered at any stage.

When injecting BtA, the approach to hemifacial spasm is similar to that for blepharospasm. However, perhaps because there is usually neurogenic damage to the facial nerve, hemifacial spasm needs a smaller initial dose and fewer injections. Inject subcutaneously, using a 30–32 gauge needle without EMG guidance. Larger needles may lead to bruising. We usually start with no more than 2.5 mu Botox® at 25 mu/mL (10–20 mu Dysport® at 200 mu/mL) into each of the upper and lower lateral orbicularis oculi and the lateral canthus (Fig. 6.4). This initial dose is often inadequate, and some centres start with twice as much. However, there is a greater chance of unwanted facial muscle weakness because the facial nerve may be more susceptible to the effects of the toxin in hemifacial spasm than in blepharospasm. The smaller dose is mandatory in post-Bell's palsy synkinesis, where the facial muscles are often very sensitive to BtA. Injections into the pretarsal portion of orbicularis oculi are rarely needed. We do not treat the lower facial spasms until we have seen the response to the orbicularis oculi injections. Many patients are satisfied by relief of the periorbital spasms. If not, and the first injection does not suppress perioral or platysmal spasms, cautiously extend the injections and increase the dose. The site of injection can be varied as required. Multiple small doses are preferable, 'customised' to the individual patient. Injections can be extended into the mid and lower face and also to the platysma.

Side-effects

These are similar to side-effects after BtA for blepharospasm. Side-effects due to excessive focal facial weakening are very noticeable because of the asymmetry, and may be longer lasting in hemifacial spasm than in blepharospasm. Occasionally patients like to receive injections bilaterally to even up the face. Reassure patients that the iatrogenic component of the facial weakness will recover in most cases. It is worth warning patients about this side-effect, and telling them that if they receive regular BtA injections the iatrogenic palsy may disguise progression of the underlying weakness. Tell them in advance that there is no evidence that BtA contributes to that progression.

Acknowledgements

This work was supported by the Bachmann–Strauss Dystonia and Parkinson Foundation. The editors have provided the Dysport® doses in this chapter, as the authors have not used Dysport® for this indication.

References

1 Fahn S. Blepharospasm: a form of focal dystonia. *Adv Neurol* 1988; **49**: 125–33.

2 Defazio G, Livrea P. Epidemiology of primary blepharospasm. *Mov Disord* 2002; **17**: 7–12.

3 Jankovic J, Ford J. Blepharospasm and orofacial-cervical dystonia: clinical and pharmacological findings in 100 patients. *Ann Neurol* 1983; **13**: 402–11.

4 Parkes D, Schachter M. Meige, Brueghel or Blake. *Neurology* 1981; **31**: 498.

5 Gowers WR. *Manual of Diseases of the Nervous System*, 3rd edn. London: Churchill, 1899.

6 Meige H. Les convulsions de la face: une forme clinique de convulsions faciales, bilaterale et mediane. *Rev Neurol (Paris)* 1910; **21**: 437–43.

7 Marsden CD. Blepharospasm-oromandibular dystonia syndrome (Brueghel's syndrome). A variant of adult-onset torsion dystonia? *J Neurol Neurosurg Psychiatry* 1976; **39**: 1204–9.

8 Thompson PD, Obeso JA, Delgado G, Gallego J, Marsden CD. Focal dystonia of the jaw and the differential diagnosis of unilateral jaw and masticatory spasm. *J Neurol Neurosurg Psychiatry* 1986; **49**: 651–6.

9 Brin MF. Advances in dystonia: genetics and treatment with botulinum toxin. In: Smith B, Adelman G, eds. *Neuroscience Year, Supplement to the Encyclopedia of Neuroscience*. Boston: Birkhauser, 1992: 56–8.

10 Almasy L, Bressman SB, Raymond D *et al.* Idiopathic torsion dystonia linked to chromosome 8 in two Mennonite families. *Ann Neurol* 1997; **42**: 670–3.

11 Blitzer A, Brin MF, Greene PE, Fahn S. Botulinum toxin injection for the treatment of oromandibular dystonia. *Ann Otol Rhinol Laryngol* 1989; **98**: 93–7.

12 Sutcher HD, Underwood RB, Beatty RA, Sugar O. Orofacial dyskinesia: a dental dimension. *JAMA* 1971; **216**: 1459–63.

13 Dyken ME, Rodnitzky RL. Periodic, aperiodic and rhythmic motor disorders of sleep. *Neurology* 1992; **42** (Suppl. 6): 68–74.

14 Watts MW, Tan EK, Jankovic J. Bruxism and cranial-cervical dystonia: is there a relationship? *Cranio* 1999; **17**: 196–201.

15 Kraft IA. A psychiatric study of two patients with dystonia musculorum deformans. *South Med J* 1966; **59**: 284–8.

16 Tolosa ES. Clinical features of Meige's disease (idiopathic orofacial dystonia). A report of 17 cases. *Arch Neurol* 1981; **38**: 147–51.

17 Jahanshahi M, Marsden CD. Depression in torticollis: a controlled study. *Psychol Med* 1988; **18**: 925–33.

18 Jahanshahi M, Marsden CD. A longitudinal follow-up study of depression, disability, and body concept in torticollis. *Behav Neurol* 1990; **3**: 233–46.

19 Murry T, Cannito MP, Woodson GE. Spasmodic dysphonia—emotional status and botulinum toxin treatment. *Arch Otolaryngol Head Neck Surg* 1994; **120**: 310–6.

20 Lauterbach EC, Price ST, Spears TE, Jackson JG, Kirsh AD. Serotonin responsive and non-responsive diurnal depressive mood disorders and pathological affect in thalamic infarct associated with myoclonus and blepharospasm. *Biol Psychiatry* 1994; **35**: 488–90.

21 Tucha O, Naumann M, Berg D, Alders GL, Lange KW. Quality of life in patients with blepharospasm. *Acta Neurol Scand* 2001; **103**: 49–52.

22 Cairns SL, LeBow MD. Meige's disease misdiagnosed as anxiety disorder. *J Behav Ther Exp Psychiatry* 1991; **22**: 221–3.

23 Jankovic J, Leder S, Warner D, Schwartz K. Cervical dystonia: clinical findings and associated movement disorders. *Neurology* 1991; **41**: 1088–91.

24 Krack P, Schneider S, Deuschl G. *Geste* device in tardive dystonia with retrocollis and opisthotonic posturing. *Mov Disord* 1998; **13**: 155–7.

25 Frucht S, Fahn S, Ford B, Gelb M. A *geste antagoniste* device to treat jaw-closing dystonia. *Movement Disord* 1999; **14**: 883–6.

26 Tan EK, Jankovic J. Bilateral hemifacial spasm: a report of five cases and a literature review. *Movement Disord* 1999; **14**: 345–9.

27 Boghen DR, Lesser RL. Blepharospasm and hemifacial spasm. *Curr Treat Options Neurol* 2000; **2**: 393–400.

28 Sindou M, Keravel Y, Moller AR. *Hemifacial Spasm*. Vienna: Springer-Verlag, 1997.

29 Wirtschafter JD, McLoon LK. Long-term efficacy of local doxorubicin chemomyectomy in patients with blepharospasm and hemifacial spasm. *Ophthalmology* 1998; **105**: 342–6.

30 Chung SS, Chang JW, Kim SH *et al.* Microvascular decompression of the facial nerve for the treatment of hemifacial spasm: preoperative magnetic resonance imaging related to clinical outcomes. *Acta Neurochir (Wien)* 2000; **142**: 901–6.

31 Barker FG, Jannetta PJ, Bissonette DJ *et al.* Microvascular decompression for hemifacial spasm. *J Neurosurg* 1995; **82**: 201–10.

32 Jankovic J, Orman J. Botulinum A toxin for cranial-cervical dystonia: a double blind, placebo-controlled study. *Neurology* 1987; **37**: 616–23.

33 Brin MF, Fahn S, Moskowitz C *et al.* Localized injections of botulinum toxin for the treatment of focal dystonia and hemifacial spasm. *Mov Disord* 1987; **2**: 237–54.

34 Taylor JD, Kraft SP, Kazdan MS *et al.* Treatment of blepharospasm and hemifacial spasm with botulinum A toxin: a Canadian multicentre study. *Can J Ophthalmol* 1991; **26**: 133–8.

35 Nussgens Z, Roggenkamper P. Comparison of two botulinum-toxin presses in the treatment of essential blepharospasm. *Graefes Arch Clin Exp Ophthalmol* 1997; **235**: 197–9.

36 Chen RS, Lu CS, Tsai CH. Botulinum toxin a injection in the treatment of hemifacial spasm. *Acta Neurol Scand* 1996; **94**: 207–11.

37 Jitpimolmard S, Tiamkao S, Laopaiboon M. Long-term results of botulinum toxin type A (Dysport®) in the treatment of hemifacial spasm: a report of 175 cases. *J Neurol Neurosurg Psychiatry* 1998; **64**: 751–7.

38 Jankovic J, Schwartz K, Donovan DT. Botulinum toxin treatment of cranial-cervical dystonia, spasmodic dysphonia, other focal dystonias and hemifacial spasm. *J Neurol Neurosurg Psychiatry* 1990; **53**: 633–9.

39 American Academy of Ophthalmology (AAO). Statement. Botulinum-A toxin for ocular muscle disorders. *Lancet* 1986; **1**: 76–7.

40 American Academy of Ophthalmology (AAO). Statement. Botulinum toxin therapy of eye muscle disorders. Safety and effectiveness. *Ophthalmology* 1989; **2**: 37–41.

41 American Academy of Neurology. Assessment: the clinical usefulness of botulinum toxin-A in treating neurologic disorders. Report of the Therapeutics and Technology Assessment Subcommittee of the American Academy of Neurology. *Neurology* 1990; **40**, 1332–6.

42 AAO–HNS. American Academy of Otolaryngology–Head and Neck Surgery Policy Statement: Botox® for spasmodic dysphonia. *AAO–HNS Bull* 1990; **9**: 8.

43 National Institutes of Health Consensus Development Conference. Clinical use of botulinum toxin. National Institutes of Health Consensus Development Statement. *Arch Neurol* 1991; **48**: 1294–8.

44 Jankovic J, Hallett M. *Therapy with Botulinum Toxin*. New York: Marcel Dekker, 1994.

45 Moore AP. *Handbook of Botulinum Toxin Treatment*. Oxford: Blackwell Scientific, 1995.

46 Klawans HL. *Taking a Risk. Trials of an Expert Witness: Tales of Clinical Neurology and the Law*. Boston: Little Brown, 1991: 93–4.

47 Scott AB, Rosenbaum A, Collins CC. Pharmacologic weakening of extraocular muscles. *Invest Ophthalmol Vis Sci* 1973; **12**: 924–7.

48 Brin MF, The Spasticity Study Group. Dosing, administration, and a treatment algorithm for use of botulinum toxin A for adult-onset spasticity. *Muscle Nerve* 1997; **20** (Suppl. 6): S208–20.

49 Brin MF. Interventional neurology: treatment of neurological conditions with local injection of botulinum toxin. *Arch Neurobiol* 1991; **54**: 173–89.

50 Brin MF, Blitzer A, Herman S, Stewart C. Orofaciomandibular and lingual dystonia (Meige's syndrome). In: Moore P, ed. *Handbook of Botulinum Toxin Treatment*. London: Blackwell Science, 1995: 151–63.

51 Walsh FB, Hoyt WF. The ocular motor system: anatomy, physiology, and topographic diagnosis. In: *Clinical Neuro-Ophthalmology*. Baltimore: Williams & Wilkins, 1969: 130–349.

52 Hall A. The origin and purposes of blinking. *Br J Ophthalmol* 1945; **29**: 455–67.

53 Weinstein E, Bender MB. Integrated facial patterns elicited by stimulation of the brain stem. *Arch Neurol* 1943; **50**: 34–42.

54 Anderson RL, Patel BC, Holds JB, Jordan DR. Blepharospasm. Past, Present, Future. *Ophthal Plast Reconstr Surg* 1998; **14**: 305–17.

55 Chapman KL, Bartley GB, Waller RR, Hodge DO. Follow-up of patients with essential blepharospasm who underwent eyelid protractor myectomy at the Mayo Clinic from 1980 through 1995. *Ophthal Plast Reconstr Surg* 1999; **15**: 106–10.

56 Mauriello JAJ, Keswani R, Franklin M. Long-term enhancement of botulinum toxin injections by upper-eyelid surgery in 14 patients with facial dyskinesias. *Arch Otolaryngol Head Neck Surg* 1999; **125**: 627–31.

57 Berardelli A, Mercuri B, Priori A. Botulinum toxin for facial-oral-mandibular spasms and bruxism. In: Jankovic J, Hallett M, eds. *Therapy with Botulinum Toxin*. New York: Marcus Dekker, 1994: 361–7.

58 Ivanhoe CB, Lai JM, Francisco GE. Bruxism after brain injury: successful treatment with botulinum toxin A. *Arch Phys Med Rehabil* 1997; **78**: 1272–3.

59 Van Zandijcke M, Marchau MM. Treatment of bruxism with botulinum toxin injections. *J Neurol Neurosurg Psychiatry* 1990; **53**: 530.

60 Tan EK, Jankovic J. Treating severe bruxism with botulinum toxin. *J Am Dent Assoc* 2000; **131**: 211–6.

61 Brin MF, Blitzer A, Herman S, Stewart C. Oro-facio-mandibular and lingual dystonia (Meige's syndrome): botulinum toxin treatment. In: Moore AP, ed. *Handbook of Botulinum Toxin Treatment*. Oxford: Blackwell Scientific, 1994.

62 Adler CH, Factor SA, Brin MF, Sethi KD, Newman S. Secondary non-responsiveness to botulinum toxin type A in patients with oromandibular dysonia. *Mov Disord* 2002; **17**: 158–61.

63 Brin MF, Comella C, O'Brien C *et al*. An interim analysis of the clinical status of patients receiving current Botox® (lot 2024 or subsequent lots) for the treatment of cervical dystonia (CD). *Mov Disord* 2000; **15** (Suppl. 2): 28–9.

64 Brin MF. Botulinum toxin therapy: basic science and overview of other therapeutic applications. In: Blitzer A, Binder WJ, Boyd JB, Carruthers A, eds. *Management of Facial Lines and Wrinkles.* New York: Lippencott, Williams & Wilkins, 2000: 279–302.

65 Tan EK, Jankovic J. Botulinum toxin A in patients with oromandibular dystonia: long-term follow-up. *Neurology* 1999; **53**: 2102–7.

CHAPTER 7

The larynx and pharynx

LUCIAN SULICA, JEAN VERHEYDEN & ANDREW BLITZER

Introduction

Botulinum toxin type A (BtA) was used in the larynx for the first time in April 1984, to treat focal laryngeal dystonia. Although this remains the best documented use, BtA has since been used to treat a host of laryngeal disorders. These include neurological disorders like essential voice tremor, stuttering blocks and vocal tics; mucosal disorders such as vocal fold granuloma and glottic synechiae; and functional disorders such as muscle tension dysphonia (see below). In the pharynx, BtA has been used with some success as an alternative to surgery for upper oesophageal sphincter spasm and to relieve the clicking of palatal myoclonus.

The larynx

Relevant musculature

The larynx has both intrinsic and extrinsic muscles. The extrinsic muscles — the omohyoid, sternohyoid, sternothyroid, thyrohyoid, stylohyoid, digastric, geniohyoid and stylopharyngeus — act upon the larynx as a unit, elevating or lowering the organ as a whole (see Fig. 8.6). Denervation of these muscles has not been clinically useful, except in the special case of vocal tremor. In fact, since laryngeal elevation is an important mechanism in swallowing, inadvertent weakening of these muscles, as may happen in the treatment of cervical dystonia, may cause dysphagia.

The intrinsic laryngeal musculature consists of paired cricothyroid, posterior and lateral cricoarytenoid, thyroarytenoid and oblique arytenoid muscles, and an interarytenoid muscle. The recurrent laryngeal nerve serves all but the cricothyroid muscle. The cricothyroid is innervated by the external branch of the superior laryngeal nerve.

The posterior cricoarytenoid muscles are the principal abductors of the vocal folds and move the vocal fold margin away from the midline, increase the glottic aperture and enlarge the airway. The lateral cricoarytenoids, the interarytenoid and the thyroarytenoids adduct the vocal folds, bring them into apposition and close the glottis. The cricothyroid increases tension on the vocal folds, which is important for the modulation of vocal pitch.

Focal laryngeal dystonia/spasmodic dysphonia

Clinical characteristics

Dystonia is a chronic neurological disorder of central motor processing characterized by task-specific action-induced muscle spasms. It may be generalized or limited to one organ or group of muscles. When it affects the larynx it is usually isolated or focal. Overwhelmingly, laryngeal dystonia affects connected speech, although there are rare cases of breathing dystonia. Laryngeal dystonia typically begins in the mid-30s and is more common in women (63%) [1]. Eight out of 10 patients have adductor dysphonia, with inappropriate glottal closure producing characteristic strangled breaks in connected speech. Abductor dysphonia, in contrast, causes inappropriate glottal opening that produces breathy breaks. Typical speech patterns may be altered by compensatory manoeuvres resulting in pitch breaks, falsetto speech and disturbances in rhythm in either condition.

The diagnosis is clinical and based on careful history and visualization of the glottis during connected speech tasks. Clues in the history include deterioration of voice quality when under stress or on the telephone, and improvement with sedatives such as alcohol or benzodiazepines. Many patients find that certain manoeuvres, so-called 'sensory tricks', can improve speech. These include chewing, supporting the head, or adopting an accent or altered voice. Speaking with a sing-song intonation or while laughing can result in a more fluent voice, probably by taking advantage of the task-specific nature of the disorder.

The glottis is best visualized with a flexible nasopharyngoscope. Insertion of a transoral laryngeal mirror or rigid rod-lens endoscope, combined with traction on the tongue necessary to expose the vocal folds, makes connected speech impossible and may mask the typical laryngeal features. On endoscopic visualization, vocal folds of patients with abductor dysphonia open spasmodically during speech. In adductor dysphonia, there is irregular hyperadduction of variable force. This has been classified into four types arranged according to increasing force. In type 1, there is overcontraction of the vocal folds with compression of the vocal process and arytenoids (Fig. 7.1). In type 2, both true and false vocal folds close (Fig. 7.2). Type 3 features contact of the arytenoids to the petiole of the epiglottis and type 4, sphincteric closure of the glottis and supraglottis with arytenoid-epiglottic contact (Figs 7.3 & 7.4).

In addition to a complete otolaryngological examination, every patient should undergo a thorough neurological evaluation, even though laryngeal dystonia is not usually associated with other disease.

Occasionally, diagnosis of spasmodic dysphonia can be challenging. There is no single pathognomonic feature of the history or examination. Essential vocal tremor and muscle tension dysphonia, a functional disorder, can produce a similar-sounding voice, and form the most important entities of the differential diagnosis. Hyperadduction is a prominent feature in muscle tension dysphonia. Muscle tension dysphonia tends to be

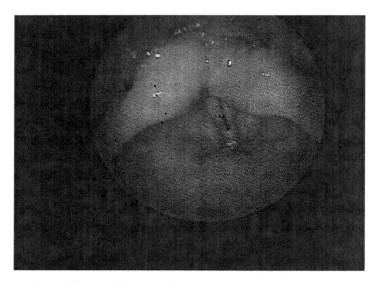

Fig. 7.1 Type 1 hyperadduction of the vocal folds.

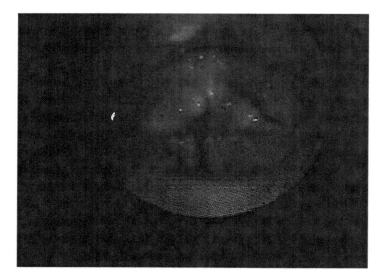

Fig. 7.2 Type 2 hyperadduction involves both true and false vocal folds.

less task-specific and has more sustained supraglottic contraction than dystonia, and spasticity is absent. Deterioration with stress is common. Further complicating the matter, some patients with abductor dysphonia develop muscle tension dysphonia in compensation for glottal opening. One-third of cases of spasmodic dysphonia have dystonic tremor [1]. These cases are difficult to distinguish from essential voice tremor.

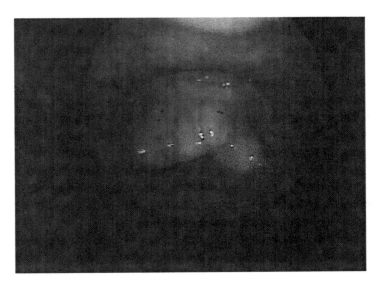

Fig. 7.3 Type 3 hyperadduction.

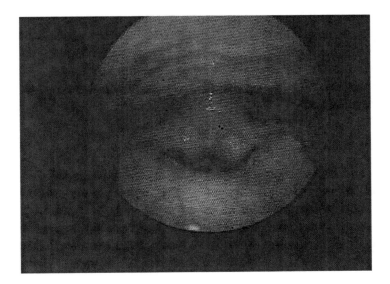

Fig. 7.4 Type 4 hyperadduction (sphincteric closure of the larynx).

Spasmodic dysphonia virtually never involves the extrinsic laryngeal muscles, whereas essential tremor (and muscle tension dysphonia) may. As there is no specific diagnostic test for spasmodic dysphonia, diagnosis of a difficult case remains a matter of expert opinion.

TREATMENT OF SPASMODIC DYSPHONIA

BtA is the primary therapy for spasmodic dysphonia. Speech therapy is sometimes useful in an adjunctive role, but does not yield marked improvement by itself [2]. Speech therapy can resolve muscle tension dysphonia, however, and a course may be useful as a diagnostic manoeuvre. We note with dismay that, even in the year 2001, we occasionally encounter a spasmodic dysphonia patient who has been undergoing psychotherapy for many years with a diagnosis of psychogenic dysphonia. Psychotherapy may help a patient manage the social stresses of the disorder, and thereby minimize the deterioration of voice with stress, but should not delay appropriate medical attention. There is no convincing evidence that psychotherapy or psychological intervention can relieve the symptoms of spasmodic dysphonia. Systemic pharmaceutical therapy is generally limited by the sedating side-effects of most medications, and no drug has been found to replace, or even consistently complement the effects of BtA.

Before the widespread adoption of BtA therapy for this disorder, treament was surgical. Reasoning that denervation of one vocal fold might diminish the symptoms of inappropriate contraction of laryngeal muscles, Dedo sectioned the recurrent laryngeal nerve on one side with satisfying initial results [3]. His procedure was duplicated at other centres, but over time, surgeons noticed a high rate of recurrence. Aronson and DeSanto reported a 64% failure rate at 3 years [4]. Various procedures were introduced to remedy this, including recurrent nerve avulsion/resection, superior laryngeal nerve section, thyroarytenoid muscle thinning, anterior commissure release, and lateralization thyroplasty, but none achieved consistently durable results. More specific adductor denervation has been recently reported [5], but long-term information is not yet available. Currently, we believe that surgery should be reserved for the very rare patient who does not benefit from BtA.

Treatment with BtA — review of the literature

BtA was used for spasmodic dysphonia after encouraging results in blepharospasm and torticollis. Previous experience in laryngeal electromyography allowed the senior author (A. Blitzer) to deliver the first injection of BtA into the human larynx in April of 1984, with significant relief of symptoms [6]. Since then, BtA has been widely and successfully used to manage spasmodic dysphonia. Today, the American Academy of Otolaryngology — Head and Neck Surgery endorses BtA as primary therapy for this disorder (Policy statement: botulinum toxin. Reaffirmed March 1, 1999).

The patients followed by Blitzer, Brin and colleagues since the first successful injection form the largest series for which data has been collected systematically, currently numbering over 1100 individuals. The most recent update was published in 1998, containing data on 901 patients treated over 12 years, and provides the basis for our observations regarding the clinical characteristics of the disorder and aspects of BtA treatment [1]. Information on treatment outcomes in these individuals was collected by prospective survey. Because speech fluency is ultimately a qualitative phenomenon, we rely on the patient as the ultimate arbiter of benefit. Using a Percent of Normal Function (PNF) Scale in which 100% represents normal speech function and 0% represents no ability to communicate at all, adductor spasmodic dysphonia patients reported that speech improves from a mean of 52% at baseline to 90% with treatment, with an average duration of benefit of about 15 weeks. Patients who have had recurrence of spasms following recurrent laryngeal nerve section also benefit, reporting an improvement in speech from approximately 46% to 84% (Sulica *et al.* unpublished data). Abductor spasmodic dysphonia patients have more modest benefit (improvement from approximately 55 to 67% on the same PNF scale) which is of shorter duration (10.5 weeks), probably because treatment is technically more difficult and is limited by respiratory complications if both posterior cricoarytenoids are over-aggressively denervated [1].

Since the aim of BtA therapy in spasmodic dysphonia is to provide symptomatic relief and not to cure, most investigators have found rating of function by the patient appropriate for measuring outcome. Prospective studies of smaller groups of patients confirmed subjective benefit in both adductor and abductor spasmodic dysphonia according to various scales of speech function [7–10]. The Voice Handicap Index (VHI) is a validated outcomes instrument for assessing patients with spasmodic dysphonia. In one study, 29 of 38 patients treated with BtA demonstrated significant improvement overall on the VHI, as well as improvement in subinventories addressing functional, physical and emotional handicap [11]. The (short-form) SF-36 is a more global outcomes inventory and, in these same patients, showed improvement in mental health and social functioning. Questionnaires have shown that BtA decreases depression and anxiety [12].

Analysis of acoustic parameters has provided more objective measures of treatment effectiveness, and findings have echoed the subjective data [9,13]. A meta-analysis attempted to bridge differences in treatment strategies and outcomes measures in 22 studies, and concluded that the average patient obtained significant improvement with BtA treatment [14].

To date, only one double-blind, placebo-controlled study of BtA in spasmodic dysphonia has been reported [15]. Compared to those injected with saline, patients treated with BtA showed marked improvement in both acoustic parameters and ratings by evaluators and by the patients themselves.

Various technical issues have been examined in limited patient series, especially the comparison of unilateral vs. bilateral injections into the thyroarytenoid muscle in adductor spasmodic dysphonia. Some analyses have suggested that swallowing difficulty and/or postinjection breathiness are reduced with unilateral treatment, but none found significant differences in benefit to voice [16–18].

Treatment with BtA — practical aspects

CLINICAL ASPECTS AND ADVERSE EFFECTS

Our injection treatment strategy for patients with spasmodic dysphonia, including those who have had recurrent laryngeal nerve section, has evolved as we have gained

Table 7.1 Botulinum toxin type A dose ranges (mu) for treatment of spasmodic dysphonia.

Type	Muscle	Botox®	Dysport®
Adductor spasmodic dysphonia	Thyroarytenoid m. (each side)	0.625–2.5	3.75–5
Abductor spasmodic dysphonia	Posterior cricoarytenoid m. (each side)	0.5–6.25	Approx. 30

experience. The standard treatment for adductor spasmodic dysphonia at our centre is a bilateral thyroarytenoid injection of equal amounts of BtA. Abductor spasmodic dysphonia is treated with bilateral posterior cricoarytenoid injections of BtA, which must be staggered for reasons discussed below. The rationale is that in most patients the motor control disorder is bilateral and symmetric. Based upon the response to initial treatment, we adjust the dose and reassess the value of bilateral vs. unilateral treatment. The effective dose is not proportional to the severity of voice disturbance, and varies considerably (Table 7.1).

DOSES: A HEALTH WARNING

Please read the warning on p. 35 about doses of Bt. There are three preparations available. *Dysport*® and *Botox*® are type A toxins (BtA), *NeuroBloc*®/*MYOBLOC*™ is type B (BtB). Even though the doses for each are quoted in mouse units (mu), the three preparations have different dose schedules: one mu of *Dysport*® is **not** the same as one mu of *Botox*®, and neither is equivalent to one mu of *NeuroBloc*®/*MYOBLOC*™.

We use a standard dilution of 4.0 mL of preservative-free saline/100 mu vial of Botox® (2.5 mu/0.1 mL) for all laryngeal and pharyngeal indications. We dilute this solution further in the injection syringe according to the requirements of each patient. Because injecting a large quantity of fluid into the vocal folds can cause dyspnea or even respiratory obstruction, we aim to limit the volume of each injection to 0.1 mL. We use a more concentrated solution for the unusual patients requiring more than 2.5 mu per injection for symptom control.

For adductor spasmodic dysphonia, our initial dose is approximately 1 mu Botox® per side. This represents a low average dose for our patient population. Although we prefer to maximize the interval between treatments, we may give a small additional dose a few weeks after the initial one if the voice does not become fluent. In an overwhelming majority of patients, dysphonia is well-controlled for 3 months or more with injections of 0.625–2.5 mu Botox® into each thyroarytenoid muscle. In abductor dysphonia, we initially inject 3.75 mu Botox® into one posterior cricoarytenoid muscle. Two weeks later, endoscopic evaluation of vocal fold mobility on the side injected allows us to estimate a safe dose for the contralateral side. A completely immobile vocal fold requires that the contralateral side be treated with a small dose to avoid airway obstruction, whereas a more mobile one permits a larger dose to be used. Asymmetric dosing in abductor dysphonia is the rule rather than the exception. Fluctuations in disease severity in both types of laryngeal dystonia may require small adjustments in dose from time to time.

As noted previously, bilateral injection is not essential to treatment success in adductor spasmodic dysphonia. In fact, some centres propose unilateral injection as the routine initial approach, having found that adverse effects are minimized [13,19]. The abnormal mechanism of dystonia may not be limited to abnormal neural signals to the muscles, but may also involve abnormal neuronal feedback via muscle spindles to the central nervous system. BtA may affect these afferent systems as well as simply weakening muscle. For instance, there is mounting evidence that in dystonia, BtA transiently changes mapping of muscle representation areas in the motor cortex, and reorganizes inhibitory and excitatory intracortical circuits, probably through peripheral mechanisms [20,21].

BtA treatment results in an initial period of marked muscle weakness lasting several days, followed by a months-long plateau of somewhat milder weakening that constitutes the principal therapeutic effect. In adductor spasmodic dysphonia, this is the cause of the breathy dysphonia that follows thyroarytenoid injection. We try to minimize the breathiness, though some is inevitable. The two phases of BtA effect are usually proportional. In adductor spasmodic dysphonia the duration of the breathiness can usually be shortened only by sacrificing the duration of benefit. Obviously, patients wish to minimize the frequency of injections, but each will have a different tolerance for breathy voice. A person to whom voice is crucial, such as a performer, may opt for smaller doses at more frequent intervals. Dyspnea is the equivalent adverse effect for abductor spasmodic dysphonia, since the posterior cricoarytenoid, a vocal fold abductor, is weakened. Since this is potentially life threatening, we treat only one side at a time, waiting approximately 2 weeks for the peak effect to pass before injecting the contralateral side. We usually use a flexible nasopharyngoscope to confirm that the vocal fold on the previously injected side is capable of some abduction before weakening the contralateral posterior cricoarytenoid muscle.

True complications of BtA treatment, such as dysphagia, result from spread of BtA to neighbouring muscles. This is related to dose and volume injected, and can be kept to a minimum using EMG or endoscopic visual guidance to place injections accurately in the muscle.

Because the clinical features of dystonia vary between patients, the physician must individualize the treatment of each patient. This includes selecting the muscles to be injected, adjusting doses, and varying the frequency of injection. There is often a balance between decreased spasms and loss of function, and the physician and the patient must arrive at an acceptable treatment plan together. Clinical experience and a detailed knowledge of anatomy are valuable in making these decisions.

INJECTION TECHNIQUES

The small size and proximity of the laryngeal muscles to one another place a premium on accuracy in BtA treatment of this region.

Electromyographic (EMG) guidance has proved very helpful in placing BtA precisely. We inject BtA through a 27-gauge Teflon®-coated needle attached to an EMG, functioning as a monopolar electrode, in virtually all laryngeal and pharyngeal applications. This allows the clinician to locate deep, small muscles that are impossible to palpate, and allows localization of the most electrically active areas of target muscles. EMG can minimize unwanted effects on neighbouring muscles, as well as maximize the benefit of each treatment by placing toxin close to its site of action at motor end plates, and allowing a smaller dose and volume to be used.

Endoscopic or endoscopic-assisted injection of BtA can be used in place of or in conjunction with EMG in BtA injection of all muscles of the larynx and pharynx. This may be done via the instrument port of a flexible endoscope inserted transnasally, via a curved needle inserted transorally under transnasal endoscopic guidance, or under direct or microscopic visualization in the operating room [22–25]. While we prefer EMG alone, we feel that whichever method delivers the safest, most effective treatment in a given physician's hands is acceptable.

Thyroarytenoid muscle. The patient lies supine with the neck extended. We do not routinely use local anaesthesia because it reduces the EMG signal, making it more difficult to identify the most active part of the muscle. We insert the needle through the neck skin and cricothyroid membrane in the anterior midline and, under EMG guidance, direct it superiorly and to the side of the target thyroarytenoid muscle. Often, it is helpful to bend the needle upwards to obtain a more anterior placement. Because of respiratory motion, laryngeal muscles are never truly at rest, and some motor unit potentials are always present. Once the needle is in an area that demonstrates crisp motor unit potentials, the patient is asked to phonate. A full interference pattern on EMG confirms placement, and toxin is injected. Experience will allow the physician to identify the characteristic acoustic signature of motor unit end plates, and make it unnecessary to refer to the visual signal (Fig. 7.5).

Posterior cricoarytenoid muscle. There are two methods of injecting the posterior cricoarytenoid. In younger patients in whom the laryngeal cartilages have not yet calcified, the posterior cricoarytenoid muscle may be reached through the posterior lamina of the cricoid cartilage [26]. An intratracheal injection of lidocaine helps to prevent the coughing which can occur as the needle crosses the lumen of the trachea. Because the target muscle lies on the opposite side of the cricoid cartilage, the local anaesthetic does not affect the EMG interference pattern. The needle is inserted through the skin and cricothyroid membrane in the midline and advanced across the airway until it meets the posterior lamina of the cricoid cartilage toward the side of the muscle to be injected. Gentle pressure pushes it through the cartilage, and the appearance of motor unit potentials identifies the posterior cricoarytenoid muscle. Because this is an abductor of the vocal fold, activation is seen with sniffing rather than phonation. Fragments of cartilage often plug the needle as it crosses the cricoid, and expelling them to begin the injection

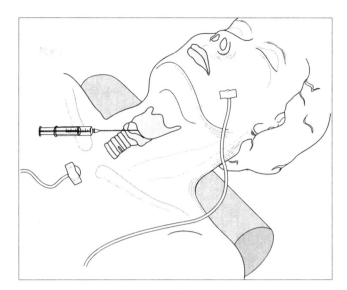

Fig. 7.5 Injection of the thyroarytenoid muscles for adductor spasmodic dysphonia.

may require considerable force on the plunger of the syringe. The injector should be aware of this in order to avoid misadventure.

We generally prefer to reach the posterior cricoarytenoid muscle via a retrolaryngeal approach. In this approach, the injector places his or her thumb at the posterior edge of the thyroid cartilage on the side to be injected and, using counter pressure from his or her other four fingers on the opposite side of the larynx, rotates the whole organ away from him or her. The needle penetrates the skin just behind the rotating thumb until it strikes the posterior aspect of the cricoid cartilage.

Withdrawing the needle slightly places it squarely into the belly of the posterior cricoarytenoid muscle. The patient sniffs to activate the EMG, and BtA is injected when the needle is in an area of brisk electrical activity (Fig. 7.6).

Other laryngeal uses

The success of BtA in the treatment of dystonia has led to investigational use in other disorders of inappropriate or excessive muscular contraction in the larynx.

Stuttering

Stuttering blocks, like dystonic spasms, are action-induced, task-specific movement abnormalities. They may involve respiratory, phonatory and/or articulatory mechanisms of speech. When the glottis is affected, bilateral thyroarytenoid muscle injections of BtA increase fluency as measured by both subjective and objective measures [27]. In

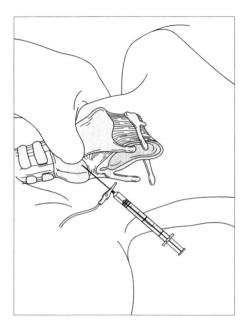

Fig. 7.6 Retrocricoid injection of the posterior cricoarytenoid muscle in abductor spasmodic dysphonia.

general, though, stutterers do not choose to undergo long-term BtA therapy, probably because reasonably effective behavioural therapy is available and their expectations are different from patients with spasmodic dysphonia [28].

Essential voice tremor

BtA can successfully treat both glottal and extralaryngeal essential voice tremor. In one study, BtA injection into one (15 mu Botox®) or both (2.5 mu Botox® each) thyroarytenoid muscles yielded objective benefit in only one-third of patients, although most patients reported subjective improvement [29]. This may have been due to less effortful voicing following BtA. However, vocal tremor is not exclusively a glottic phenomenon, and may involve extralaryngeal muscles, occasionally even more than intrinsic laryngeal muscles. Clinical and endoscopic examination can identify involved muscle groups and is necessary to tailor effective chemodenervation treatments. Another study, in which extralaryngeal strap muscles were sometimes injected in addition to bilateral thyroarytenoid muscles (1.25 mu Botox® each), noted both subjective and objective benefit more than half of patients [30]. Although tremor was not eliminated, its amplitude and consequently speech disturbance were decreased.

Vocal tics

Unilateral and bilateral BtA injections of the thyroarytenoid muscles have been successful in controlling vocal tics of Gilles de la Tourette syndrome, including coprolalia, in isolated cases [31–33]. Its success in this context again suggests an effect on the central nervous system, possibly mediated through afferent pathways.

Miscellaneous uses

Rontal and Rontal coined the term 'laryngeal rebalancing' to refer to chemodenervation of the interarytenoid muscle and the ipsilateral thyroarytenoid and lateral cricoarytenoid muscle to treat anteromedial cricoarytenoid dislocation resulting from external or intubation trauma [34]. Their term can be applied to an array of uses. BtA has been used to weaken adductors as an adjunct to treatment of vocal fold granuloma [35,36], and posterior glottic synechiae [37]. BtA has also been used in isolated cases of muscle tension dysphonia, a condition that results from unconscious hyperadduction of laryngeal muscles usually correctable with voice therapy [38].

The pharynx

Cricopharyngeal muscle spasm

Clinical characteristics

The cricopharyngeus muscle functions as the upper oesophageal sphincter. It is contracted and thus closed at rest, but it opens with swallowing to allow passage of the bolus. Failure of the upper oesophageal sphincter to relax with swallowing can cause severe dysphagia, and appears to be the cause of Zenker's diverticula. This spasm may occur in a myriad of neurological conditions such as stroke, postpolio syndrome, and amyotrophic lateral sclerosis, or it may be idiopathic [39,40]. The appearance of a postcricoid 'bar' on cineradiography is characteristic. The diagnosis may also be made by manometry.

Cricopharyngeal spasm can also develop following laryngectomy, interfering with swallowing and occasionally preventing the successful use of a tracheoesophageal speech prosthesis, which depends on the passage of air through the upper oesophageal sphincter for sound.

Traditionally, cricopharyngeal spasm has been treated surgically by dilatation, pharyngeal plexus neurectomy or cricopharyngeal myotomy. Because this is generally a disease of the elderly, or of patients with significant comorbidity, it may be preferable to avoid surgery.

BtA treatment — review of the literature

BtA permits non-surgical treatment of upper oesophageal sphincter spasm. In non-controlled prospective clinical studies, 70–100% of patients with dysphagia due to cricopharyngeal spasm benefited [22,41,42]. Decreased spasm was confirmed by cineradiography and sometimes manometry. Treatment permitted the consumption of solid food, removal of feeding tubes and weight gain. Benefit was greatest in patients who had cricopharyngeal spasm as the only abnormality, as opposed to those with associated dysmotility, or postsurgical defects, or dysphagia resulting from stroke. BtA injection can also be used as a diagnostic manoeuvre to identify patients who would benefit from myotomy [43]. Of note, some cricopharyngeal spasm is caused or aggravated by reflux of gastric acid and this must be treated before relaxing the sphincter, particularly in patients with associated neurogenic compromise of the larynx. Heartburn may complicate upper oesophageal sphincter weakening [22]. Often, gastroenterological evaluation is helpful in managing these patients.

BtA may help patients with cricopharyngeal spasm after laryngectomy, providing an alternative to surgery in the irradiated neck or debilitated patient. The majority of patients so treated are able to achieve tracheoesophageal voice [42–44].

Treatment with BtA — practical aspects

The cricopharyngeus muscle lies below the inferior pharyngeal constrictor muscle and above the muscles of the cervical oesophagus. The limits of the cricopharyngeus can be difficult to establish, and its fibres tend to blend with those of muscles above and below. The fibres of the cricopharyngeus, however, originate and insert into the cricoid cartilage, forming a semicircle encompassing the oesophageal lumen.

Injections may be performed endoscopically under general anaesthesia, with the contour of the contracted muscle directly observed via a rigid laryngoscope or oesophagoscope [22,45]. Alternately, it is possible to inject the muscle in the awake patient using electromyographic guidance [41].

Because the cricopharyngeus muscle originates and inserts into the cricoid cartilage, the position of the cricoid can be used as a guide to the level of this muscle in the neck. The larynx is rotated away from the side of the injection and the needle is inserted just lateral to the cricoid cartilage but medial to the carotid sheath, which is located by finding the carotid pulse. The characteristic electrical signal of the cricopharyngeus muscle appears once the EMG recording needle impales the muscle. The cricopharyngeus is contracted at rest, so it yields a loud and unambiguous EMG, generally demonstrating a full interference pattern. Even in patients with cricopharyngeal hypertonicity, swallowing relaxes the muscle and reduces the electrical signal. However, this elevates the larynx, and can displace the needle from the cricopharyngeus if the physician is not careful. Injection should be repeated on the opposite side of the larynx to treat the entire muscle.

The muscle can be somewhat more difficult to find in laryngectomized patients because the cricoid cartilage is absent, but both EMG and videofluoroscopy are helpful [44].

Recommended doses vary widely, depending on the technique used and the experi-

Table 7.2 Botulinum toxin type A dose ranges (mu) for treatment of cricopharyngeal spasm.

Muscle	Botox® Total dose (no. of injections)	Dysport® Total dose (no. of injections)
Cricopharyngeus	10–40 mu (3–4)	80–120 mu (3)

ence of the injector (Table 7.2). In the transcutaneous EMG-guided technique described above, four injections of 2.5 mu Botox® each suffice to improve swallowing. Other authors have used much larger doses with equally good clinical response [44,45].

Palatal myoclonus

Palatal myoclonus is a contraction of the palatal muscles that produces a characteristic clicking noise usually audible only to the patient. In a quiet room, this can sometimes be heard by the examining physician by placing the bell of a stethoscope to the auditory meatus. It is usually idiopathic, but may be associated with brainstem dysfunction or other neurological conditions. Contractions are usually bilateral and occur at rates of 40–240/min. BtA has relieved the clicking noise in several cases [46,47].

Injection is performed transorally, with or without electromyographic guidance, into the portion of the tensor veli palatini muscle just behind the posterior margin of the bony palate. Localizing the muscle can sometimes be difficult because mouth opening can suppress the contractions. Doses of 5–10 mu Botox® or 10–40 mu Dysport® have been found to be effective. The principal limitations of treatment are velopharyngeal incompetence, with resulting hypernasal voice and nasal regurgitation, and Eustachian tube dysfunction.

Conclusion

Judicious use of BtA in the larynx and pharynx has been of benefit in a wide variety of conditions. Most muscles of the region may be injected in the office, but their small size and proximity to one another makes detailed knowledge of the anatomy and physiology of the area essential in order to administer effective treatment and avoid adverse effects. As in other applications, the use of BtA has also provided insight into several disease processes, particularly with respect to the role of afferent systems in dystonia and other movement disorders.

References

1 Blitzer A, Brin MF, Stewart CF. Botulinum toxin management of spasmodic dysphonia (laryngeal dystonia): a 12-year experience in more than 900 patients. *Laryngoscope* 1998; **108**: 1435–41.

2 Murry T, Woodson GE. Combined-modality treatment of adductor spasmodic dysphonia with botulinum toxin and voice therapy. *J Voice* 1995; **9**: 460–5.

3 Dedo HH. Recurrent laryngeal nerve section for spastic dysphonia. *Ann Otol Rhinol Laryngol* 1976; **85**: 451–9.

4 Aronson AE, DeSanto LW. Adductor spastic dysphonia: 3 years after recurrent laryngeal nerve section. *Ann Otol Rhinol Laryngol* 1983; **93**: 1–8.

5 Berke GS, Blackwell KE, Gerratt BR *et al.* Selective laryngeal adductor denervation–reinnervation: a new surgical treatment for adductor spasmodic dysphonia. *Ann Otol Rhinol Laryngol* 1999; **8**: 227–31.

6 Blitzer A, Brin MF, Fahn S, Lange D, Lovelace RE. Botulinum toxin (BOTOX®) for the treatment of 'spastic dysphonia' as part of a trial of toxin injections for the treatment of other cranial dystonias. *Laryngoscope* 1986; **96**: 1300–1.

7 Liu TC, Irish JC, Adams SG, Durkin LC, Hunt EJ. Prospective study of patients' subjective responses to botulinum toxin injection for spasmodic dysphonia. *J Otolaryngol* 1996; **25**: 66–74.

8 Aronson AE, McCaffrey TV, Litchy WJ, Lipton RJ. Botulinum toxin injection for adductor spastic dysphonia. Patient self-ratings of voice and phonatory effort after three successive injections. *Laryngoscope* 1993; **103**: 683–92.

9 Whurr R, Lorch M, Fontana H *et al.* The use of botulinum toxin in the treatment of adductor spasmodic dysphonia. *J Neurol Neurosurg Psychiatry,* 1993; **56**: 526–30.

10 Ludlow CL, Naunton RF, Terada S, Anderson BJ. Successful treatment of selected cases of abductor spasmodic dysphonia using botulinum toxin injection. *Otolaryngol Head Neck Surg* 1991; **104**: 849–55.

11 Courey MS, Garrett CG, Billante CR *et al.* Outcomes assessment following treatment of spasmodic dysphonia with botulinum toxin. *Ann Otol Rhinol Laryngol* 2000; **109**: 819–22.

12 Murry T, Cannito MP, Woodson GE. Spasmodic dysphonia. Emotional status and botulinum toxin treatment. *Arch Otolaryngol Head Neck Surg* 1994; **120**: 310–6.

13 Ludlow CL, Naunton RF, Sedory SE, Schulz GM, Hallett M. Effects of botulinum toxin injections on speech in adductor spasmodic dysphonia. *Neurology* 1988; **38**: 1220–5.

14 Whurr R, Nye C, Lorch M. Meta-analysis of botulinum toxin treatment of spasmodic dysphonia: a review of 22 studies. *Int J Lang Commun Disord* 1998; **33** (Suppl.): 327–9.

15 Troung DD, Rontal M, Rolnick M, Aronson AE, Mistura K. Double-blind controlled study of botulinum toxin in adductor spasmodic dysphonia. *Laryngoscope* 1991; **101**: 630–4.

16 Zwirner P, Murry T, Woodson GE. A comparison of bilateral and unilateral botulinum toxin treatments for spasmodic dysphonia. *Eur Arch Otorhinolaryngol* 1993; **250**: 271–6.

17 Koriwchak MJ, Netterville JL, Snowden T, Courey M, Ossoff RH. Alternating unilateral botulinum toxin type A (BOTOX®) injections for spasmodic dysphonia. *Laryngoscope* 1996; **106**: 1476–81.

18 Langeveld TP, Drost HA, Baatenburg de Jong RJ. Unilateral versus bilateral botulinum toxin injections in adductor spasmodic dysphonia. *Ann Otol Rhinol Laryngol* 1998; **107**: 280–4.

19 Miller RH, Woodson GE, Jankovic J. Botulinum toxin injection of the vocal fold in spasmodic dysphonia: a preliminary report. *Arch Otolaryngol Head Neck Surg* 1987; **113**: 603–5.

20 Gilio F, Curra A, Lorenzano C *et al.* Effects of botulinum toxin type A on intracortical inhibition in patients with dystonia. *Ann Neurol* 2000; **48**: 20–6.

21 Byrnes ML, Thickbroom GW, Wilson SA *et al.* The corticomotor representation of upper limb muscles in writer's cramp and changes following botulinum toxin injection. *Brain* 1998; **121**: 977–88.

22 Schneider I, Thumfart WF, Pototschnig C, Eckel HE. Treatment of dysfunction of the cricopharyngeal muscle with botulinum A toxin: introduction of a new, non-invasive method. *Ann Otol Rhinol Laryngol* 1994; **103**: 31–5.

23 Ford CN, Bless DM, Lowery JD. Indirect laryngoscopic approach for injection of botulinum toxin in spasmodic dysphonia. *Otolaryngol Head Neck Surg* 1990; **103**: 752–8.

24 Green DC, Berke GS, Ward PH, Gerratt BR. Point-touch technique of botulinum toxin injection for the treatment of spasmodic dysphonia. *Ann Otol Rhinol Laryngol* 1992; **101**: 883–7.

25 Rhew K, Fiedler DA, Ludlow CL. Technique for injection of botulinum toxin through the flexible nasolaryngoscope. *Otolaryngol Head Neck Surg* 1994; **114**: 787–94.

26 Meleca RJ, Hogikyan ND, Bastian RW. A comparison of methods of botulinum toxin injection for abductory spasmodic dysphonia. *Otolaryngol Head Neck Surg* 1997; **117**: 487–92.

27 Brin MF, Stewart C, Blitzer A, Diamond B. Laryngeal botulinum toxin injections for disabling stuttering in adults. *Neurology* 1994; **44**: 2262–6.

28 Stager SV, Ludlow CL. Responses of stutterers and vocal tremor patients to treatment with botulinum toxin. In: Jankovic J, Hallett M, eds. *Therapy with Botulinum Toxin*. New York: Marcel Dekker Inc., 1994: 481–90.

29 Hertegard S, Granqvist S, Lindestad P. Botulinum toxin injections for essential voice tremor. *Ann Otol Rhinol Laryngol* 2000; **109**: 204–9.

30 Warrick P, Dromey C, Irish JC *et al.* Botulinum toxin for essential tremor of the voice with multiple anatomical sites of tremor: a crossover design study of unilateral versus bilateral injection. *Laryngoscope* 2000; **110**: 1366–74.

31 Salloway S, Stewart CF, Israeli L *et al.* Botulinum toxin for refractory vocal tics. *Mov Disord* 1996; **11**: 746–8.

32 Scott BL, Jankovic J, Donovan DT. Botulinum toxin injection into vocal cord in the treatment of malignant coprolalia associated with Tourette's syndrome. *Mov Disord* 1996; **11**: 431–3.

33 Trimble MR, Whurr R, Brookes G, Robertson MM. Vocal tics in Gilles de la Tourette syndrome treated with botulinum toxin injections. *Mov Disord* 1998; **13**: 617–9.

34 Rontal E, Rontal M. Laryngeal rebalancing for the treatment of arytenoid dislocation. *J Voice* 1998; **12**: 383–8.

35 Nasri S, Sercarz JA, McAlpin T, Berke GS. Treatment of vocal fold granuloma using botulinum toxin type A. *Laryngoscope* 1995; **105**: 585–8.

36 Orloff LA, Goldman SN. Vocal fold granuloma: successful treatment with botulinum toxin. *Otolaryngol Head Neck Surg* 1999; **121**: 410–3.

37 Nathan CO, Yin S, Stucker FJ. Botulinum toxin: adjunctive treatment for posterior glottic synechiae. *Laryngoscope* 1999; **109**: 855–7.

38 Kendall KA, Leonard RJ. Treatment of ventricular dysphonia with botulinum toxin. *Laryngoscope* 1997; **107**: 948–53.

39 McKenna JA, Dedo HH. Cricopharyngeal myotomy. Indications and technique. *Ann Otol Rhinol Laryngol* 1992; **101**: 216–21.

40 Blitzer A. Cricopharyngeal muscle spasm and dysphagia. *Op Tech Otolaryngol Head Neck Surg* 1997; **116**: 328–9.

41 Blitzer A, Brin MF. Use of botulinum toxin for diagnosis and management of cricopharyngeal achalasia. *Otolaryngol Head Neck Surg* 1997; **116**: 328–30.

42 Ahsan SF, Meleca RJ, Dworkin JP. Botulinum toxin injection of the cricopharyngeus muscle for the treatment of dysphagia. *Otolaryngol Head Neck Surg* 2000; **122**: 691–5.

43 Blitzer A, Komisar A, Baredes S, Brin MF, Stewart C. Voice failure after tracheoesophageal puncture: management with botulinum toxin. *Otolaryngol Head Neck Surg* 1995; **113**: 668–70.

44 Hoffman HT, Fischer H, VanDenmark D *et al.* Botulinum toxin injection after total laryngectomy. *Head Neck* 1997; **17**: 92–7.

45 Zormeier MM, Meleca RJ, Simpson ML *et al.* Botulinum toxin injection to improve tracheoesophageal speech after total laryngectomy. *Otolaryngol Head Neck Surg* 1999; **120**: 314–9.

46 Saeed SR, Brookes GB. The use of clostridium botulinum toxin in palatal myoclonus: a preliminary report. *J Laryngol Otol* 1993; **107**: 208–10.

47 Bryce GE, Morrison MD. Botulinum toxin treatment of essential palatal myoclonus tinnitus. *J Otolaryngol* 1998; **27**: 213–6.

Cervical and axial dystonia

REINER BENECKE, PETER MOORE, DIRK DRESSLER &
MARKUS NAUMANN

Introduction

Cervical dystonia is a predominantly motor syndrome of involuntary posturing of the head away from its normal central position. It may be dominated by sustained posture, spasms, jerks or tremor, or a combination of these features, and it is often painful. Nowadays, the term spasmodic torticollis is better reserved for one type of cervical dystonia, where there is both spasm and (usually) rotational torticollis. Cervical dystonia may be isolated or part of a wider segmental, multifocal or generalized idiopathic dystonia. Botulinum toxin A (BtA) injection into affected neck muscles has been the treatment of choice for cervical dystonia since the late 1980s, and gives significant relief of symptoms in most patients. Botulinum toxin B (BtB) has recently been introduced and is also effective.

Isolated *axial truncal dystonia* is rare. However, truncal dystonia often occurs as part of severe segmental and more generalized dystonia. Again, there may be sustained or slowly varying tilt or twist of the back, perhaps with superimposed myoclonic or other jerky movements. In the belly dancer form of truncal dystonia there is a prominent phasic component. As in cervical dystonia the combinations of muscles involved and the postures produced are highly individual. Bt therapy is less effective than for cervical dystonia and useful only in mild forms of truncal dystonia. Intrathecal baclofen and high frequency bilateral stimulation of globus pallidus internus are becoming treatments of choice for most patients who require more than oral medication.

This chapter focuses mainly on the use of botulinum toxin (Bt) in cervical dystonia, and briefly discusses treatment of axial or trunk dystonia at the end.

Epidemiology and disease course

Cervical dystonia is the most frequent form of idiopathic focal dystonia and the most common neurological indication for Bt treatment [1]. The average age of onset is in the early 40s, with over three-quarters of patients developing their cervical dystonia between the ages of 30 and 60 years. The prevalence of cervical dystonia is approximately 9/100 000 in Rochester, Minnesota, US. Cervical dystonia is slightly more common in females, with a male to female ratio of 1.0 : 1.2 [2]. The onset is usually insidious, although in some patients it may be abrupt. Most patients report deterioration over the initial 5 years and then symptoms tend to stabilize. In about one-third of patients with adult-onset idiopathic cervical dystonia there is progression to segmental dystonia, usually arm dystonia, writer's cramp or oromandibular dystonia. The arm dystonia is usually subtle, asymptomatic and may be apparent only to the diligent observer, appearing as an 'overflow' phenomenon most notably when the patient is walking or talking. Progression of adult-onset cervical dystonia to generalized dystonia should prompt the clinician to seek a secondary cause as it is extremely rare in idiopathic cases. About 5–20% of patients may experience spontaneous remission within 6 months after the first manifestation of cervical dystonia, but nearly all patients relapse within 5 years [2,3].

Clinical features

The clinical spectrum of abnormal head and neck posture is broad and depends on the pattern of dystonic activity of the more than 50 muscles which influence head and neck posture. There may be muscles active on one or both sides of the neck. Dystonic muscle activity can be mainly tonic, myoclonic, tremulous or a complex mixture. Secondary soft tissue and bony changes develop in some patients and contribute to abnormal postures. Sufferers seek treatment because of pain, functional disability or embarrassment.

Pain

At presentation about 70% of patients complain of pain. It usually affects the neck and/or shoulder, and aching pain and paraesthesiae may radiate into the arm and hand. These brachial symptoms have been termed 'radicular' [4] but they frequently do not conform to segmental dermatomes, and reflex and motor signs are absent. A true radiculopathy or not, the pain usually disappears after successful treatment of the cervical dystonia.

Disability

For many patients, the main incapacitating feature of their torticollis is functional impairment. Cervical dystonia may affect their work, leisure or activities of daily living. Head turning can prevent a proper view of the road during driving. It may curtail sedentary pursuits such as reading, writing and watching television, and sports such as cycling, tennis, squash or golf. In the street patients may bump into shop windows or into other pedestrians, and when crossing the road it can be difficult to look both ways. At the table the head may turn as the fork reaches the mouth, and in the bathroom cervical dystonia hinders toothbrushing and applying makeup.

Embarrassment

For a third group of cervical dystonia sufferers, embarrassment and anxiety provoke the major handicap, and often lead to social withdrawal and isolation. Public speaking or social engagements become a nightmare, and dealings with clients or customers are affected. In restaurants patients may spill food and drink and conversation is inhibited. Most patients perceive some or even severe stigma which may profoundly affect their social, private and working lives [5].

Quality of life

Quality of life is impaired in cervical dystonia. Generic instruments such as the SF-36, Beck anxiety and depression indexes, and measures of self-esteem, stigma, social support and acceptance of illness, reveal significant problems with reductions in quality of life comparable to patients with Parkinson's disease, mild to moderate multiple sclerosis and moderate epilepsy [6]. The intermittent and sometimes situation-specific appearance of objective abnormal posturing or spasms often makes it difficult to persuade others that sufferers have a genuine and disabling physical illness. Insurance companies and benefits agencies appear to have particular problems in understanding the concept.

Relieving and precipitating factors

Many patients with cervical dystonia can control the abnormal posture for a short time by using sensory tricks such as touching the head or neck, or other proprioceptive stimuli to modify the involuntary pulling. Such tricks are a characteristic and unique feature as well as a diagnostic clue present in about 70% of patients [7]. The most common trick is to place a finger or hand against the lower face as if trying to turn the head back to the midline, hence the term *geste antagonistique*. Other more subtle tricks include sucking on a pen or necklace, pulling on the end of the nose or at an earlobe, holding the back of the head, or resting the back of the head against a chair or wall. Interestingly, it can work just as well to touch the 'wrong' side of the face, and the acute observer will note that the restoration towards a more normal head posture frequently starts before the finger touches the face, indicating that it is not merely the tactile stimulus that is responsible.

Why tricks work in dystonia has been a mystery for more than a century. Tricks and other clues have sparked recent studies that suggest that dystonia may represent a primary sensory rather than a motor disorder [4,8–15]. Alternatively it could be a disorder of sensorimotor integration or of movement preparation [16]. Chapter 5 discusses these issues in more detail.

Emotional stress, self-consciousness, excitement, walking, fatigue or carrying objects may all aggravate cervical dystonia. On the other hand many sufferers find that their torticollis is not troublesome when they are absorbed or distracted, but infuriatingly their neck is at its worst when they relax, read or watch television. Lying supine, or on one side, relaxation and sleep helped spasmodic torticollis in 40% of 72 patients in one sample, but made it worse in 16–25% [17].

Differential diagnosis

Torticollis is a physical sign, not a diagnosis [3]. Several other disorders may mimic idiopathic cervical dystonia. These include lesions of the central nervous system, cranial nerves, cervical spine and surrounding soft tissues. About 8% of cervical dystonia patients suffer from secondary dystonia or symptomatic dystonia due to neurodegenerative diseases. Clinical and laboratory tests may be needed to exclude secondary dystonias, but in practice most of these are easily distinguished *clinically* from the true idiopathic cervical dystonia and no further investigation is needed. Nearly two-thirds of patients with cervical dystonia have bony degenerative changes apparent on plain cervical spine X-rays but there is no consistent relationship between symptoms and the X-ray picture. Magnetic resonance imaging (MRI) and/or computed tomography (CT) scans in a group of 149 patients with clinically idiopathic cervical dystonia found no abnormalities that altered management [18].

Neurological diseases and skeletal/soft-tissue abnormalities that may lead to abnormal head posture mimicking cervical dystonia are summarized in Table 8.1.

Neck injury may precede the development of cervical dystonia in up to 15% of patients, even when there has been no fracture. It is possible that local trauma triggers cervical dystonia and other focal dystonias in some genetically susceptible people.

Drug-induced cervical dystonia may follow treatment with drugs such as metoclopramide and other neuroleptics. Acute dystonic reactions may be dramatic and include oculogyric crisis. These usually settle, but most large series contain patients with tardive dystonia which is much more persistent. Women and the elderly are most at risk, particularly after high doses for prolonged periods. Eighty per cent of patients with tardive dystonia have torticollis and, unlike idiopathic torticollis, they are more likely to have retrocollis (49%) than rotational torticollis (34%).

Although cervical dystonia was considered psychogenic in the first part of the last century, psychogenic dystonia is rare and should only be diagnosed with caution. Clues suggesting a psychogenic aetiology are abrupt onset, accompanying bizarre movements, great variation of the clinical presentation and obvious psychiatric illness [19]. Neurophysiological studies may help [20].

Classification of cervical dystonia

Torticollis is classified according to the dominant head position (Fig. 8.1). For the muscles involved see Table 8.3.
- *Rotatory (simple) torticollis*. This is the most common type, present in over 50% of patients [21–23].

Table 8.1 Symptoms, syndromes and diseases mimicking cervical dystonia.

Skeletal abnormalities
Atlanto-axial dislocations
Fractures of cervical spine
Discopathy
Osteomyelitis of cervical spine
Klippel–Feil syndrome
Muscular and connective tissue abnormalities
Congenital torticollis with aplasia of sternocleidomastoid or fibrotic band
Fibrosis after X-ray therapy of chronic cervical syndrome
Local infection
Pharyngitis
Lymphadenitis
Neurological diseases
Vestibulo-ocular dysfunction
Tumours of posterior fossa
Arnold–Chiari syndrome
Sandifer syndrome
Cervical spinal cord tumours
Syringomyelia
Pareses of extraocular muscles
Strabismus
Oculomotor apraxia
Hemianopia
Spasmus nutans
Focal epilepsy

- *Laterocollis* or lateral head tilt (present in 10–15%).
- *Retrocollis* or backwards head tilt/neck extension (present in 10–15%).
- *Tremulous torticollis* with jerky tremor of the head, usually side to side in a 'no–no' fashion (present in 10–15%).
- *Complex torticollis* with variable head position, and no one predominant position (present in 10–15%).

Unusual variants include:

(a) *Pure anterocollis* with forward flexion of the neck. It is rarely idiopathic but may occur in multiple system atrophy [24].

(b) *Propulsion* with forwards shift of the head on the trunk.

(c) *Lateropulsion* with sideways shift of the head.

Cervical dystonia rating scales

There are many different rating scales for cervical dystonia and this suggests that none is ideal for all uses. This is partly because torticollis varies so much from hour to hour and day to day that a single 'objective' observation is insufficient. Some scales are

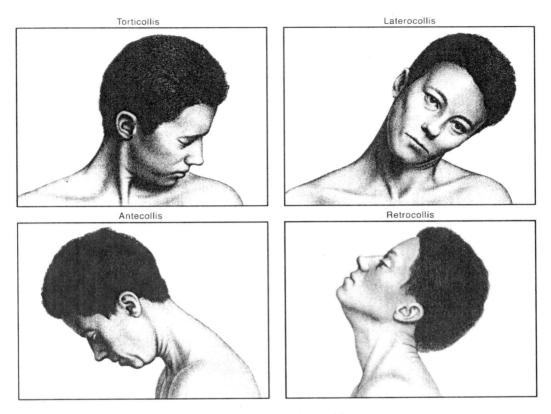

Fig. 8.1 Postural abnormalities in pure forms of cervical dystonia.

simple and suited to clinical service use; others are research instruments and are generally more complex. More scales are under development.

Subjective scales

As Bt is a symptomatic treatment the main assessment of success or failure should be based on the change in symptoms such as pain, pulling, spasms, neck position or embarrassment. The most pertinent questions are 'Did you notice any improvement and, if so, how much and for how long?' 'Did you have any side-effects?' 'Do you want another injection?' The injections themselves are mildly uncomfortable and patients will not come back repeatedly for further injections if they perceive no benefit. Brin's Global Clinical Rating Scale allows patients to assess and record their response continuously, giving an easily understood overview (see Chapter 3, Fig. 3.2). It is very quick to use in clinic.

Objective scales [25]

It is essential to document improvement after Bt injection, or lack of improvement in those patients who have developed antibodies. The first attempts to measure benefit objectively were made by Swash *et al.* who rated the effect of tetrabenazine on dystonic movement using videotapes [26]. Couch and Tolosa devised relatively simple rating scales [27,28]. Lang *et al.* proposed the first specific cervical dystonia rating scale. This scored the angles of abnormal head rotation and tilt and whether the abnormality was intermittent or continuous [29]. The Torticollis Rating Scale by Tsui *et al.* considered the amplitudes and persistence of tilt, turn and back/forward head movements, shoulder elevation and any added spasms, tremor or myoclonus in dystonic muscles [30]. It is quick and easy to perform in clinic, but takes no account of subjective distress or disability. Fahn's Columbia Torticollis Rating Scale measured subjective features such as pain and impairment of daily living activities as well as the objective severity of dystonia [31]. The currently popular Toronto Western Spasmodic Torticollis Rating Scale (TWSTRS) [32] also combines objective measures of the involuntary movements with assessments of pain and activities of daily life. Observers need more training (a video is available) and it takes longer to complete, but it is well validated. Another advantage is that each section can stand alone.

A new Cervical Dystonia Severity Scale (CDSS) is also under development [33]. Details of the Tsui Scale [30] and the TWSTRS [32], two of the most commonly used instruments, appear in the appendix to this chapter.

Treatment for cervical dystonia

The many different treatments tried over the years testify to both their relative ineffectiveness and the recalcitrance of cervical dystonia. Historically, the most effective therapies were oral drugs and surgery. There are no good controlled studies of many of the supposed remedies, which can be dramatic. Many patients have tried a series of non-proprietary remedies, even including exorcism. Most are expensive, although one patient found that wearing a close-fitting cardboard box on the head had an immediate 'positive effect' [34]! However, this novel and cheap solution cannot be considered aesthetic or entirely practical.

One recent survey attempted to rank treatments for mild, moderate and severe cervical dystonia according to the opinions of 12 movement disorders specialists. The experts felt that BtA treatment was first choice for each grade, followed by muscle relaxants, anticholinergic drugs, physical therapy and then a variety of other treatments depending on the severity of the cervical dystonia. The last resort was muscle resection [35]. Adler and Kumar give a useful summary of available treatments [36]. Many patients do well on combination treatments.

Physical and relaxation techniques

Physical therapies such as physiotherapy, acupuncture, osteopathy, chiropractic or the wearing of a neck collar are not consistently effective, but some patients find them helpful. Collars are sometimes counterproductive, and cervical dystonia can be powerful enough to break rigid collars or to create pressure sores. Neck manipulation is both ineffective and dangerous. There is a risk of vertebral or carotid artery dissection [37].

Relaxation therapies such as hypnosis, behaviour therapy, biofeedback and meditation may work more often than physical therapies and may help in up to 50% of patients [38]. Electromyographic (EMG) biofeedback is sometimes effective [39] and is a low cost, easily tolerated alternative or adjunct to the more predictably effective BtA, anticholinergic drugs and surgical treatments.

Pharmacotherapy

For many years, oral medications, including anticholinergic agents, γ-aminobutyric acid (GABA) mimetic agents, dopamine receptor antagonists, dopamine-depleting agents, and dopamine receptor agonists were the first choice for cervical dystonia [40,41]. Once it became available, BtA rapidly superceded oral drugs, so that they are now generally second-line treatments. Oral drugs remain important for patients with additional, more widespread dystonia which cannot all be treated with BtA or BtB. For a more extensive review see [36].

Anticholinergics

Traditionally, anticholinergic agents have been a first-line oral treatment for cervical dystonia. A double blind trial showed benefit [42]. In a retrospective analysis of open label trials of initial treatment with high-dose anticholinergic agents, 39% of cervical dystonia patients, particularly those with a disease duration of less than 5 years, reported a good response (defined as a slight, moderate, or marked improvement) [41]. In general, increase the dose slowly until there is either benefit or dose-limiting adverse effects appear. It is important to start at a low dose, such as 1–2 mg trihexyphenidyl daily, and to increase very gradually, perhaps at a rate of 2 mg weekly. Effective daily doses vary from 6 to 80 mg. Dose-limiting adverse effects of anticholinergic agents are common, and are related to peripheral and central actions including dry mouth, blurred vision, constipation, urinary retention, confusion, memory loss, hallucinations and behavioural changes.

Baclofen

Baclofen is less effective than anticholinergic agents, helping about 10% of patients with cervical dystonia. Dose-related adverse effects include muscle weakness, lethargy, dizziness, gastrointestinal complaints and urinary frequency [43]. Abrupt withdrawal of baclofen may provoke psychotic episodes and seizures. Patients with widespread dystonia may benefit from intrathecal baclofen, but it is rarely used in isolated cervical dystonia.

Tizanidine

Tizanidine is a recently introduced drug that is claimed to induce less muscle weakness than baclofen.

Benzodiazepines

Benzodiazepines potentiate the neuronal inhibition mediated by GABA. About 20% may respond to clonazepam [41]. It seems to be particularly effective in reducing dystonia-associated pain and exaggerated dystonic posturing related to anxiety or stress. Adverse effects of benzodiazepines include sedation and confusion.

Dopamine antagonists

Dopamine receptor antagonists, such as haloperidol, and dopamine-depleting agents, such as tetrabenazine, are probably less promising than anticholinergics [44]. Tetra-benazine appears to be more useful in tardive dystonia. Severe adverse events can occur with either, including parkinsonism, hypotension, depression, drowsiness and fatigue [45]. Clozapine appears not to be helpful in idiopathic cervical dystonia [46]. Do not use dopamine receptor antagonists in idiopathic cervical dystonia because of the potential to cause tardive dyskinesia.

Anticonvulsants

Anticonvulsants such as valproate or carbamazepine are occasionally useful.

Mexiletine

Mexiletine has been tried in a small, inconclusive study [47].

Levodopa and dopamine agonists

Levodopa and dopamine agonists are not useful in idiopathic dystonia except for rare cases of dopa-responsive dystonia.

Chemodenervation

Chemodenervation with Bt is discussed later in this chapter. Intramuscular phenol can also be effective, but is substantially more painful, and is probably best reserved for patients resistant to Bt [48]. Intramuscular doxorubicin remains experimental. It can certainly weaken rabbit sternomastoid muscles [49], and has successfully treated human hemifacial spasm and blepharospasm [50,51].

Surgery

Selective peripheral denervation of neck muscles [36]

A variety of peripheral surgical techniques may help cervical dystonia [52]. These include myotomy, microvascular decompression, and spinal accessory nerve section, with or without ventral rhizotomy. The most commonly performed operation is spinal accessory nerve section combined with selective dorsal ramisectomy. In general, these techniques have been poorly assessed. Several open label and uncontrolled studies yielded response rates ranging from 48 to 89% [53–55]. Less complex forms of cervical dystonia appear to respond better, and rotational torticollis is more responsive than laterocollis or retrocollis. In a recent retrospective analysis of 16 patients with BtA resistance undergoing selective ramisectomy to treat cervical dystonia, clinical rating scales showed a mean objective improvement of 32%. In about one-third there was modest long-term functional improvement [56]. Sixty-nine per cent of 46 patients who underwent highly individualized operations showed clinically meaningful improvement [57]. In another study, 60% of patients had functionally relevant improvement at a mean of 9.4 months, with return of pain in many at 18 months. Apart from improvement of pain by 30% at 6 months, TWSTRS scores did not improve significantly in patients with primary Bt failure [58]. Complications of selective dorsal ramisectomy include dysphagia, almost complete sensory loss over the distribution of the greater occipital nerve, occipital neuralgia, or hyperesthesia in the area governed by the greater auricular nerve. After the introduction of BtA, selective dorsal ramisectomy became a second line therapy mainly used when secondary resistance developed. Since BtB is now available and effective for some patients with secondary non-response due to neutralizing antibodies, selective dorsal ramisectomy may be regarded as a third line therapy for patients with antibodies against both BtA and BtB.

Brain lesioning and deep brain stimulation

STEREOTACTIC THALAMOTOMY

Stereotactic thalamotomy is more successful for limb than for axial dystonia. Sizeable bilateral thalamic lesions are usually necessary [59,60] and it has fallen out of favour chiefly because of the high rate of subsequent speech impediment. The most optimistic reports suggest that up to 60% of patients obtain satisfactory relief, although it may be delayed. Twenty to fifty-six per cent of patients experience troublesome dysarthria or dysphonia [59,60]. Results in cervical dystonia have been variable [61], with some studies reporting significant improvement and others little or no change.

PALLIDAL SURGERY

Older articles describe lesioning the anterior pallidum with highly variable results [62]. Lesioning declined rapidly after the introduction of Bt in the late 1980s, although in the mid-1990s technical improvements led to a resurgence of interest in surgery to relieve dystonia. In addition, better understanding of basal ganglia anatomy and pathophysiology has highlighted the role of the pallidum, which becomes overactive in dystonia, and potentially provides a target for more widespread suppression of dystonia through brain rather than selective peripheral surgery. Modern uncontrolled studies report striking benefit after unilateral or bilateral posteroventral pallidotomy in patients with primary generalized dystonia, many of whom also had cervical dystonia [63–65]. Most authors emphasize that dystonic patients improve after a delay and then slowly over several months after pallidotomy. Few patients have undergone this operation and the data are not conclusive.

DEEP BRAIN STIMULATION

Recently, bilateral deep brain stimulation of the globus pallidus internus has been performed in small numbers of patients with idiopathic generalized, segmental, or focal cervical dystonia [66–70]. There may be improvements in dystonic posture, associated pain and functional disability in severe complex cervical dystonia.

Deep brain stimulation appears to be as effective as pallidotomy. Benefits of deep brain stimulation for dystonia often accrue slowly, over some months. This may reflect gradual refashioning or reprogramming of the underlying physiological defect [71].

Deep brain stimulation has several advantages over lesioning. It is reversible and adjustable in that the electrodes can be turned off, adjusted for optimal effect or removed at any time. Many reports suggest that deep brain stimulation is safer than lesioning, especially when bilateral treatment is needed. The effects are easier to document objectively and in a double-blind manner when varying the stimulation parameters. It preserves options for the future should new treatments be developed. Disadvantages of deep brain stimulation revolve around the drawbacks of caring for a chronically implanted device—infection, migration of leads, battery replacement—and the extra cost of the device and follow up, including initial and periodic reprogramming to find the optimal stimulation parameters. Before we can recommend this treatment to severely affected and treatment resistant patients with cervical dystonia, we need the results from the larger and properly controlled studies which are underway on deep brain stimulation in dystonia.

Botulinum toxin review

In 1985, Tsui and colleagues [72] published the results of a successful pilot study in 12 patients with cervical dystonia treated with BtA, and followed this a year later with a report of a double blind, placebo-controlled trial in 21 patients [30]. Many open and randomized controlled trials have since confirmed that BtA and BtB are highly effective symptomatic treatments for cervical dystonia. Most of the studies used BtA (Botox® or Dysport®) [73–76], and there is an extensive literature showing that most patients derive long-term benefit [77]. Recent studies using BtB (NeuroBloc®/MYOBLOC™) have shown it is effective in A-responders and A-resistant patients [78–81]. Reviews [77,82] and guidelines [83,84] for treatment of cervical dystonia recommend Bt as first line therapy. BtA/BtB are not a cure, and patients need regular treatments, usually at 3–4 monthly intervals, to maintain control of symptoms.

Efficacy

The largest studies have been open label and generally show higher response rates than randomized controlled studies, partly due to a placebo effect and partly because they allow more flexibility in individualizing doses and patterns of muscles for injection. Open trials have recorded the benefits of repeated BtA injections into the neck muscle for up to 4 years in large numbers of patients [2,21,85,86]. Improvement usually begins within 1–3 weeks, averaging about 8 days with occasional delays of up to 8 weeks. Peak effect begins about 16 days following the injection. The reported average duration of benefit is 11–14 weeks and does not change significantly after repeat injections. The 'record' was 54 weeks, but such prolonged responses may be due to coincident natural remission. Perhaps the best guide is that most patients ask for reinjection at around 3 months. In one study improvement was generally most pronounced after the first injection and remained fairly constant after the sixth injection (Fig. 8.2). Figures 8.2 and 8.3 demonstrate that the relative improvement was similar for all patients irrespective of the severity and complexity of the cervical dystonia.

Cervical dystonia is the best-validated 'test-bed' for Bt, and there are a number of trials that examine responder rates, duration of action and dose-equivalence of individual preparations in cervical dystonia, in part because they are commercially sensitive issues. Duration is variously defined as duration of the plateau effect, time to return to preinjection state (usually 3–4 months after the last injection), or time to return to true baseline, equivalent to the patient's state before their first ever injection. This variation in definitions, combined with the obvious trade-off between benefits and adverse effects, makes it difficult to draw conclusions or to make comparisons between preparations based on open label studies or trials against placebo. Ideally, we need direct randomized and double blind controlled trial comparisons between the available preparations, using optimized doses. For further discussion of this issue see Chapter 3.

In long-term studies with BtA, 70–85% of patients benefit, with reduction in pain,

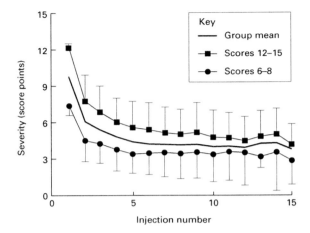

Fig. 8.2 Development of severity of cervical dystonia during the course of treatment, measured using the Tsui Scale. Ratings were performed prior to next injection, i.e. showing the residual effect (modified from Kessler [2]). *Squares:* mean scores +1 SD of the subgroup of patients with high severity (initial scores 12–15). *Circles:* mean scores (–1 SD) of the subgroup of patients with mild initial cervical dystonia (initial scores 6–8). *Line:* mean scores of the total group.

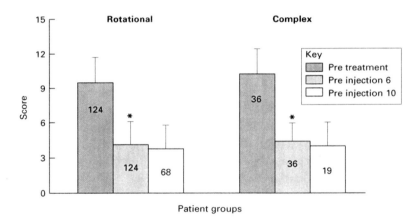

Fig. 8.3 Comparison of improvement (mean scores) between patients with pure rotational cervical dystonia (n = 124) and those with complex forms of cervical dystonia (n = 36). *P < 0.0001, reduction in score values (Wilcoxon's test for matched pairs); error bars, +1 SD. The number of observations is given in each bar (modified from Kessler [2]).

posturing and spasms. A few (4% in one study [2]) report worsening of the symptoms. Careful neuropsychiatric testing shows that quality of life improves [87]. Only rarely will a patient not show any improvement after repeated injections [2,21,85,88]. Indeed, in our experience, a patient who reports absolutely no improvement from repeated toxin treatments has either developed antibodies to the toxin, or has a condition other than

Table 8.2 Treatment effects of botulinum toxin injections in cervical dystonia.

Study	No. of patients	Dose (mu)	Responder Dystonia; pain	Scale (%)	Improvement (%)
Botox® (BtA)					
Tsui *et al.* [30]*	19	100	63;87	Tsui	30
Gelb *et al.* [75]*	20	280	15; 50	Tsui	20
Gelb *et al.* [91]*	28	280	32; 64	Tsui	20
Greene *et al.* [90]*	34	240	74; NA	GIR (0–3)	33
Jankovic & Schwartz [86]†	195	209	90; 93	GIR (0–4)	>50
Comella *et al.* [92]†	52	220	78; 86	TWSTRS	>25
Naumann *et al.* [76]†	133	155	100‡; 100‡	TWSTRS	35
Dysport® (BtA)					
Blackie & Lees [85]*	19	960	84; 75	Tsui	22
Blackie & Lees [85]†	50	875	83; 77	Tsui	22
Stell *et al.* [93]†	10	1200	90; 100	Tsui	47
Poewe *et al.* [94]†	37	632	86; 84	Tsui	>50
Wissel and Poewe [95]†	180	594	85; 85	Tsui	>50
Kessler *et al.* [2]†	616	778	89; 92	Tsui	>60
NeuroBloc®/MYOBLOC™ (BtB)					
Lew *et al.* [80]*	27	10 000	77; 83	TWSTRS	NA

*Double blind study. †Open study. ‡Comparative study of two Botox® preparations in known responders; pain reduction 52%.
GIR, Global Improvement Rating [Scale]; NA, not available; TWSTRS, Toronto Western Spasmodic Torticollis Rating Scale.

torticollis. Table 8.2 surveys the effects of BtA and BtB treatment in cervical dystonia described in a selection of open and double blind studies. It lists only studies that evaluated responder rates and percentage improvements [2, 30, 75, 76, 80, 85, 86, 90-95].

Patients with simple cervical dystonia, such as rotation or tilt, and with shorter duration of symptoms usually respond better. In complex cervical dystonia more muscles require injection and need bigger doses [96, 97]. Not all symptoms benefit equally. There may be complete relief of pain with no change in posturing or movement [96], and vice-versa. Benefit is dose related provided the dose is greater than a critical threshold for the patient. The usual trade-off between efficacy and adverse effects limits the maximum dose.

Efficacy compared to anticholinergics

One randomized double blind trial compared a mean dose of 292 mu Botox® against a mean dose of 16.25 mg/day oral trihexyphenidyl. BtA was clearly superior, with significant benefit in the TWSTRS disability subscale and the Tsui Scale [98].

Botulinum toxin type B

Three recent, double blind, placebo-controlled studies using BtB (NeuroBloc®/ MYOBLOC℗) for cervical dystonia are available [99]. The first tested BtB in unselected patients with cervical dystonia [80]. One subsequent study examined BtB in patients who were responsive to BtA injections, and compared placebo vs. BtB 5000 mu vs. BtB 10000 mu [78]. Another study tested BtB in patients who were A-resistant, comparing placebo vs. BtB 10000 mu [79]. In all studies TWSTRS total scores significantly improved from baseline to Week 4 after BtB, with the greatest improvements observed in the 10000 mu group. The benefits lasted 12–16 weeks before patients returned to their preinjection baseline. As an entry criterion was that baseline must be at least 16 weeks after the most recent BtA injection, it is difficult to know from these studies whether the duration of action is any different from BtA. The benefits and adverse effects reported were otherwise comparable with those seen in similar BtA trials. There is currently at least one randomized, controlled trial underway to compare BtA against BtB directly, and this may decide some of the issues around dose equivalence, responder rates and duration of action. Open label studies suggest that NeuroBloc®/MYOBLOC℗ is safe and well tolerated at doses up to 15000 mu [100].

BtB clearly has a role in treating patients with cervical dystonia who have become resistant to BtA. There are theoretical differences between BtB and BtA preparations in ease of storage, duration of response, and ability to focus weakness and minimize adverse events such as antibody formation. When these theoretical advantages are clarified in randomized clinical trials they will combine with commercial factors such as cost to decide its place as a primary treatment.

Risks of botulinum toxin A and botulinum toxin B in cervical dystonia

The incidence of adverse effects of Bt in cervical dystonia varies widely, and depends on the dose, muscles injected and the experience of the injector. Most studies report side-effects in 20–30% of patients per treatment cycle and about 50% of patients experience such events at some time during their therapy. Dysphagia, neck weakness and local pain at the injection site are the most frequent adverse effects.

Antitoxin antibody formation may render patients resistant to Bt. In patients with mild cervical dystonia already being treated successfully for blepharospasm or spasmodic dysphonia it may sometimes be wise to withhold Bt for torticollis in order to preserve its benefit if the blepharospasm/dysphonia is more disabling.

Dysphagia

Dysphagia is by far the most common and troublesome adverse effect and occurs in about 10–30% of patients. It is probably caused by direct diffusion of toxin through fascial boundaries into the pharyngeal muscles. Dysphagia is more likely if the sternomastoid is injected (especially if both are injected) and is related to both total dose and the dose delivered into the sternomastoid. It is less frequent if multiple small-volume injections are given instead of a large-volume bolus. Patients with pre-existing swallowing abnormalities do not appear to get worse after toxin therapy. Dysphagia usually starts about 7 days after toxin injections and typically persists for 14 days (range: 1–56 days). Exclude other causes if dysphagia begins much later or persists for longer than 2 months.

Dysphagia is usually minor, defined as not requiring a change of diet. Reassure patients that it will resolve within a few days or weeks and advise them to sip water with their food and take small, well-chewed mouthfuls or pureed food. In up to 5% moderate dysphagia occurs and necessitates a change to a soft diet. Severe dysphagia occurs with fewer than 5% of treatments, most often after sternomastoid injection in women with slim necks. Drinking may be difficult, with choking, aspiration and weight loss. Rarely, patients with severe dysphagia may need hospitalization for a few days for hydration, feeding tube or airway protection.

Care is needed especially when there is pre-existing bulbar or respiratory embarrassment. One patient with severe chronic bronchitis died after BtA treatment for his or her torticollis was followed by a chest infection [101], and one of our own patients who had severe secondary dystonia with bulbar and diaphragmatic involvement developed chest infections after each of his injections.

Neck muscle weakness

Bt injections in cervical dystonia may cause transient weakness of neck muscles in about 5% patients. This side-effect is usually mild and resolves usually within a few weeks. Occasionally it manifests as vertigo, usually in motor vehicles and presumably caused by a mismatch of sensory and motor information within the vestibular system. If neck muscle weakness is disabling a collar may be helpful during the day.

Pain

Although the injections themselves are uncomfortable (particularly the deeper splenius, levator scapulae and semispinalis injections) and injection related pain sometimes persists for some days, none of our patients have stopped treatment for this reason. Pain occurs in about 1–5% of patients.

Dry mouth

Dry mouth is a relatively frequent side-effect when NeuroBloc®/MYOBLOC™ is used at a total dose of 10 000 mu. In one report the prevalence was 44% [79], whereas the frequency of dry mouth or sore throat with BtA (Botox® or Dysport®) is generally under 10%. It usually resolves within 3 weeks and does usually not require treatment. Dry mouth may be confused with or aggravate pre-existing or Bt induced dysphagia. It may be that BtB has a higher affinity and efficacy at autonomic cholinergic synapses than BtA at doses with similar effects at neuromuscular junctions.

Other side-effects

Other side-effects are less worrying, but include dysphonia (6%), jaw stiffness or weakness after bilateral splenius injections (3%), back pain after trapezius injections (2%), dyspnoea (2%), and lethargy (1–9%). Some patients report flu-like symptoms or generalized weakness. These side-effects wear off within a few weeks and require no specific treatment. Rarely, brachial neuritis may occur [102,103].

Distant or widespread weakness may follow Bt injections in disorders of neuromuscular transmission such as Lambert–Eaton myasthenic syndrome and myasthenia gravis, in myopathies, neuropathies and anterior horn cell diseases (for example, one patient with old crural polio reported increasing leg weakness with successive injections [21]). However, with care torticollis can be successfully and safely treated in myasthenia gravis [104,105]

Practical treatment of cervical dystonia with botulinum toxin

General remarks

Start treatment with Bt as early as possible to minimize secondary changes in the muscles involved (contractures) and in other connective tissues, such as bone, joints and cervical discs. Indications for Bt treatment of cervical dystonia are:
- Obviously abnormal head and neck posture or spasms.
- Pain.
- Impairment of daily activities at home or at work.
- Secondary changes in the cervical spine.
- Impaired self-confidence and reactive depression.

Rarely, patients with slight postural abnormalities refrain from Bt therapy once they know about its potential good and bad effects. They can always reconsider if their cervical dystonia worsens.

Local anatomy

This section describes the actions of the principal neck muscles involved in torticollis and the relevant anatomy including injection points. See Figs 8.4–8.6. Be aware that neck muscle activation patterns can change spontaneously in cervical dystonia despite constant dystonic head position [106].

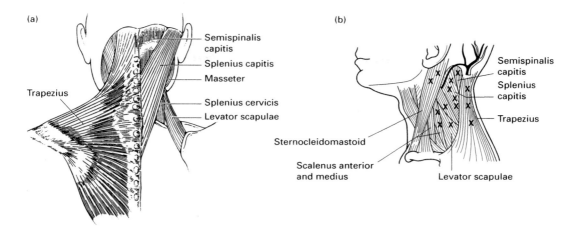

Fig. 8.4 (a) Diagram of the more important muscles in the posterior neck. (b) Injection sites (x) within various muscles treated with botulinum toxin in cervical dystonia. Dependent on type of cervical dystonia, muscles are injected on one side or some ipsilaterally and some contralaterally.

STERNOMASTOID

Its main action in rotational torticollis is to rotate the neck (and hence chin) to the opposite side. In laterocollis it may pull the head over towards the ipsilateral shoulder. In propulsion it propels the head forwards, and in anterocollis it pulls the chin directly downwards.

Above, the sternomastoid arises from the mastoid process and to a lesser extent the lateral half of the superior nuchal line. Below, it inserts onto the manubrium sterni and the medial third of the clavicle. It is superficial and is the easiest neck muscle to identify.

SPLENIUS CAPITIS

Splenius capitis rotates the head in the ipsilateral direction in rotatory torticollis, tilts the head ipsilaterally in laterocollis and tilts the head backwards in retrocollis.

Above, it attaches to the mastoid process and the rough surface of the occipital bone just below the lateral third of the superior nuchal line. It passes downwards, medially and posteriorly to attach into the lower half of the ligamentum nuchae, the spine of the seventh cervical vertebra, and the spines of the upper thoracic vertebrae. It lies fairly deeply in the neck beneath a fascial carpet but in the untreated patient it can usually be palpated just behind the upper posterior border of the sternomastoid. After previous splenius injections the thinned muscle can be difficult to palpate. Branches of the lesser occipital nerve may course over the muscle (external to the

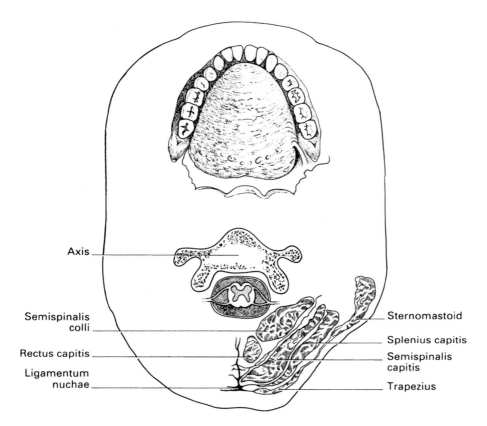

Fig. 8.5 Anatomy of neck muscles at the C2/3 level.

fascia) and on occasion may be encountered during injection, causing brief but excruciating neuralgic pain.

LEVATOR SCAPULAE

Levator scapulae elevates the ipsilateral shoulder or, with the shoulder fixed it tilts the neck ipsilaterally in laterocollis.

Above, it attaches to the transverse processes of the axis, atlas and third and fourth cervical vertebrae. Below, it attaches to the superior third of the medial border of the scapula. It is found behind the posterior border of the sternomastoid just inferior to the splenius and superior to the scalenus complex. When hyperactive it is relatively easily palpated, but like splenius capitis it can be difficult to feel after previous toxin injections.

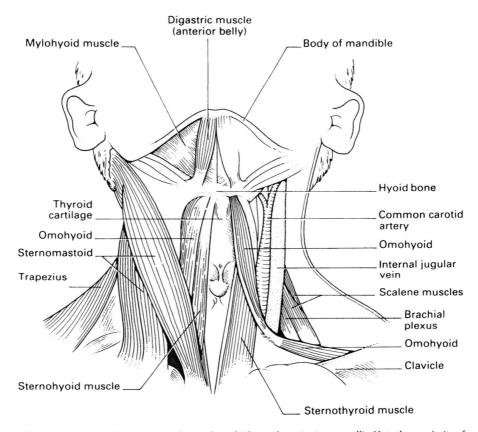

Fig. 8.6 Diagram of the anterior neck muscles, which may be active in antecollis. Note the proximity of the carotid artery and internal jugular vein to these muscles.

TRAPEZIUS

Trapezius elevates the shoulder. If the shoulder is fixed, it pulls the neck ipsilaterally in laterocollis and extends the neck backwards in retrocollis. In rotatory torticollis it may act in concert with the contralateral splenius to rotate the head to the contralateral side.

Above, the superior fibres of trapezius attach to the medial third of the superior nuchal line of the occipital bone, the external occipital protuberance and the ligamentum nuchae. These fibres pass down to attach to the lateral third of the clavicle. The middle and inferior fibres are less important in torticollis. They arise from the thoracic vertebrae and attach to the acromium and scapula. Because it is superficial, it is easy to palpate and grasp trapezius particularly at the base of the neck.

SEMISPINALIS CAPITIS

Semispinalis capitis extends the neck in retrocollis. It can also be weakly active in tilting the head ipsilaterally in laterocollis or rotating the head contralaterally in rotatory torticollis.

Above, it attaches to the medial aspect of the area between the inferior and superior nuchal lines of the occipital bone. Below, it attaches to the lower cervical vertebrae (C4–C7) and the upper seven thoracic vertebrae (T1–T7). It lies deep to the trapezius and splenius muscles and this three-muscle complex is easy to see and palpate posteriorly on either side of the midline (nuchal furrow). It may be markedly asymmetric in normal subjects so that apparent hypertrophy in torticollis does not prove it is responsible for the dystonic spasms.

ANTERIOR NECK MUSCLES

Anterior neck muscles pull the chin downwards or forwards in anterocollis or propulsion. They include the anterior vertebral muscles comprising longus colli, longus capitis, rectus capitis anterior and rectus capitis lateralis. These muscles are deep seated and apart from longus capitis are not readily accessible to Bt injection. The suprahyoid and infrahyoid muscles are chiefly involved in speech, swallowing and respiration, but it is possible that spasms of these muscles may contribute to anterocollis.

Sometimes dystonic spasm of the platysma influences head posture. Unilateral platysma overactivity may pull the chin downwards and cause anterocollis, or it may pull the head laterally and downwards to produce a combined laterocollis and anterocollis. Spasms of the platysma are easy to recognize since it is very superficial and its thickened cords stand out from the normal neck contour with puckering of the overlying skin.

The first botulinum toxin injection

Before treatment, inform the patient about Bt treatment in general, the nature and time course of its benefits and side-effects, and alternative treatments. Stress that Bt is a symptomatic treatment and not a cure. Patients should give written informed consent at least for the first injection cycle.

CLINICAL MUSCLE SELECTION

The first and most crucial step is to select the best pattern of muscles to inject. History and examination are both important, and can sometimes unearth conflicting information. Examine the patient to define the type and severity of cervical dystonia while you listen to the history. This gives much more time to observe the patient acting more naturally, without making your close scrutiny too obvious. Experienced observers can also use the time to score the severity of the torticollis.

We recommend that you:
- Sit directly in front of the patient, who in turn should sit straight in a comfortable

chair that does not have a headrest, and preferably no armrests. Do not let the patient sit sideways on. It can be useful to sit any relative or companion in the room on the patient's less favoured side to maximize the chance of observing the torticollis and the difficulties that it produces. Make sure you can see the neck—many patients habitually cover it with a scarf or roll-neck pullover. Encourage the patient, repeatedly if necessary, to keep his or her hands away from the head and to avoid using compensatory tricks that might modify or hide the torticollis. This arrangement makes it much easier to detect even subtle postural change and involuntary movement, and to clarify the dominant abnormality if the posture is varying or particularly spasmodic. It can also be uncomfortable and distressing for the patient, who may not have realized just how much he or she had been compensating for the dystonia.

• Consider the various patterns of muscle activation that could produce the dominant activity. Remember that some movements may be compensatory. Occasionally, cocontracting antagonists are able to overcome the active primary agonists to produce a pseudo or counter-dystonic posture for short periods. Clarify this from the history, evidence from a companion or the effects of a *geste*. For instance, the patient may have difficulty seeing traffic on the difficult side. Ask whether he or she prefers to sit on the left or right of a group.

In any convenient order, ask the patient to:

• Demonstrate the most common posture and the most and least comfortable positions.

• Look both ways. The more easily attained and sustained direction of gaze usually indicates the more active muscles.

• Show his or her favourite trick manoeuvre. Often this will be touching the chin with one hand—but it is not always the hand on the side of the primary movement. It may appear to be the *wrong* hand. Remember it is a sensory trick, not a forceful corrective action. Activity in the primary dystonic muscles melts away while the *geste* is working.

• Set the head straight using the *geste* if necessary. Then hold it still for as long as possible, without using the *geste*. The first movements away from the midline are often most informative.

• Turn, tilt and tip the head back and forwards slowly, and through as full a range as possible.

• Perform a finger–nose test, and an arm-hold test.

• Point to painful spots, which often indicate muscles in spasm. For clarity, make sure he or she points with one finger.

• Depending on the history, watch the patient writing, standing, walking about or lying down.

Palpate the muscles to pick out the most active. For instance, trapezius and levator scapulae both elevate the shoulder. It is often straightforward to define their relative contributions by palpation.

A videotape of the examination can be invaluable for immediate study and as a record.

In general, select muscles that are painful or tender or that are visibly or palpably hyperactive, and muscles that cause the dominant movements identified. It is easy to define the dystonic muscles in simple and pure forms of cervical dystonia and can require considerable experience in more complex or fluctuating torticollis, especially as some head postures may arise from several different patterns of activation. Try to restrict injections to a limited number of the more important and powerfully dystonic muscles. Table 8.3 lists common patterns for injection in the main subtypes of cervical dystonia. Not all muscles need injection each time.

ELECTROMYOGRAPHIC RECORDINGS
Physiologists had been studying the pathophysiological basis of cervical dystonia using careful EMG recordings even before Bt treatment was available [107–111]. Nowadays, EMG may be used to:
1 Examine the patterns of muscle activation and the relative contributions of individual muscles. Combining EMG and clinical information may be very powerful in difficult cases, but can sometimes be misleading. EMG is not a substitute for the clinical process of defining the optimum pattern for injection.
2 Assist in localizing previously selected target muscles and ensuring accurate placement of Bt. It can be most helpful in obese patients.
3 Detect muscle weakness after Bt therapy, through a reduced M-wave response, denervated muscle fibres (positive sharp waves and fibrillation potentials) and electrically silent areas with loss of motor unit action potentials. These changes are important because they demonstrate a biological response to Bt therapy and exclude primary or secondary resistance due to antibody formation.
4 Allow the injector to direct the toxin into more susceptible parts of the muscle. This mainly applies in subsequent injection cycles, when EMG can help to avoid reinjecting residual, inactive, silent regions. The strategy is intuitively reasonable, but not proven to have a clinically useful effect.

Thus EMG may be helpful in some patients for selection of muscles for injection, or for accurate placement of injections. EMG-assisted (both in selection and injection) toxin injections do result in a higher proportion of patients gaining greater improvement than injections based solely on clinical examination and injected without EMG assistance [92,97,112–114]. However, EMG can be time-consuming and adds to the discomfort and expense of Bt treatment. Many centres reserve EMG-assisted injections for patients who are technically difficult to assess or inject, for the few patients who have not responded to clinically directed injections, or when there is an obvious change of the pattern of abnormal posturing under continuous Bt treatment.

As an aid to learning, trainees and less experienced physicians may choose to record surface EMG from sternocleidomastoid, splenius capitis, levator scapulae and the upper portion of trapezius to inform their clinical impressions of the pattern of muscles involved, especially for the patients' first Bt injections. EMG pattern interpretation is

Table 8.3 Muscles that may be involved and worth injecting in various types of cervical dystonia.

Anterocollis (head tips forward)
Bilateral injection of:
Sternocleidomastoid
Scalenus medius
Infrahyoid muscles

Retrocollis (head tips back)
Bilateral injection of:
Splenius capitis
Semispinalis capitis
Capitis trapezius (cervical part)

Laterocollis (tilt)
Ipsilateral injection of:
Sternocleidomastoid
Trapezius (cervical part)
Scalenus medius
Scalenus posterior
Splenius capitis

Torticollis (rotation or turn)
Ipsilateral injection of:
Splenius capitis
Levator scapulae
Trapezius (cervical part)

Contralateral injection of:
Sternocleidomastoid

Head protrusion (anterior shift)
Bilateral injection of:
Sternocleidomastoid

Head retraction (posterior shift)
Bilateral injection of:
Splenius capitis
Levator scapulae

Torticollis (turn) plus laterocollis (tilt) to same side
Ipsilateral injection of:
Splenius capitis
Semispinalis capitis
Trapezius (cervical part)
Levator scapulae
Scalenus medius
Scalenus posterior
Sternocleidomastoid

Contralateral injection of:
Sternocleidomastoid

Torticollis (turn) plus laterocollis (tilt) to the opposite side
(e.g. torticollis to the left and laterocollis to the right)
Injection of:

Sternocleidomastoid	Right
Scalenus medius	Right
Scalenus posterior	Right
Splenius capitis	Right
Levator scapulae	Right
Trapezius (cervical part)	Right
Splenius capitis	Left

Combination of anterocollis (head tips forward) and laterocollis (tilt)
Ipsilateral injection of:
Sternocleidomastoid (on the side of the tilt)
Infrahyoid muscles
Scalenus anterior
Scalenus medius
Scalenus posterior
Levator scapulae
Splenius capitis
Trapezius (cervical part)

Contralateral injection of:
Sternocleidomastoid

Combination of retrocollis (head tips back) and laterocollis (tilt)
Ipsilateral injection of:
Scalenus medius
Scalenus posterior
Levator scapulae
Splenius capitis
Trapezius (cervical part)

Contralateral injection of:
Splenius capitis

Combination of retrocollis and torticollis
Ipsilateral injection of:
Splenius capitis
Semispinalis capitis
Trapezius (cervical part)

Contralateral injection of:
Sternocleidomastoid
Splenius capitis

more difficult in subsequent injection cycles because lingering Bt toxicity may contaminate the recordings even when the muscles have recovered clinically.

Full diagnostic EMG analyses are more complex. EMG activity in a muscle can either be dystonic or compensatory. Many patients cannot easily relax compensatory activity, so it may be mistaken as being dystonic.

Surface electrodes can record only sternocleidomastoid, splenius capitis and the upper portion of trapezius without crosstalk from neighbouring muscles. Recording from deeper muscles requires the more time-consuming and painful needle electrodes. It is difficult to identify deeply lying cervical muscles and patients need to be very cooperative. It is not clear whether careful EMG identification and precise injection of these muscles is beneficial, especially as there may be diffusion of toxin anyway from larger, more superficial muscles. The theoretical advantage of Bt injection at the sites of motor points, which EMG can identify, may also be irrelevant because of toxin diffusion.

Chapter 4 discusses this topic in more detail.

Toxin dilution and dose

DOSES: A HEALTH WARNING

Please read the warning on p. 35 about doses of Bt. There are three preparations available. *Dysport®* and *Botox®* are type A toxins (BtA), *NeuroBloc®/MYOBLOC™* is type B (BtB). Even though the doses for each are quoted in mouse units (mu), the three preparations have different dose schedules: one mu of *Dysport®* is **not** the same as one mu of *Botox®*, and neither is equivalent to one mu of *NeuroBloc®/MYOBLOC™*.

Based on clinical experience there is a rough relationship in doses between the three preparations on the market (Botox® vs. Dysport® vs. NeuroBloc®/MYOBLOC™ = 1 : 3–4 : 50). There are no decisive studies establishing clear advantages of one preparation of BtA over the other regarding effectiveness, frequency/severity of side-effects, and risk of antibody formation. We do not yet know the risk of antibody formation after repeated injections of BtB.

It is not appropriate to recommend a single fixed dose for each situation, not least because patients and muscles vary in their susceptibility to Bt. Choosing the right dose may be difficult for a patient's first injection, but trial and error soon establish the optimum dose. Suitable initial total doses in average cases are Botox® 120 mu, Dysport® 500 mu and NeuroBloc®/MYOBLOC™ 7500 mu. Some centres recommend a sliding scale as shown in Table 8.4.

Suggested doses for individual muscles appear in Table 8.5. Note that Tables 8.4 and 8.5 give recommended doses for the *initial* injection. Adjust subsequent doses and distribution according to the response. If the response is inadequate, increase the dose — with caution up to twice the starting dose — and/or inject additional muscles selected from the groups shown in Table 8.3. Side-effects may dictate lower doses or a different distri-

Table 8.4 Sliding scale recommendations for total Bt dose depending on the severity of the cervical dystonia as measured by the Tsui score.

Score	Total Bt dose (mu)		
	Botox®	Dysport®	NeuroBloc®
12–15	200	800	10 000
9–12	150–200	600–800	7500–10 000
6–9	100–150	400–600	5000–7500
3–6	80–120	320–480	4000–6000

Table 8.5 Recommended dose ranges for individual muscles involved in cervical dystonia (for the first treatment the lowest dose/muscle is usually injected).

Muscle	Recommended dose ranges (mu)		
	Botox®	Dysport®	NeuroBloc®
Sternocleidomastoid	20–50	80–200	1000–2500
Splenius capitis	50–100	200–400	2500–5000
Semispinalis capitis	15–30	60–120	750–1500
Levator scapulae	10–25	40–100	500–1250
Trapezius (upper portion)	20–50	80–200	1000–2500
Scalenus anterior	10–20	40–80	500–1000
Scalenus medius	10–20	40–80	500–1000
Scalenus posterior	10–20	40–80	500–1000
Infrahyoid muscles	10–15	40–60	500–750

Note: in bilateral injections of some muscles dose reduction is necessary (see text).

bution. The total dose in any one injection cycle should not exceed 300 mu Botox®, 1200 mu Dysport® or 15 000 mu NeuroBloc®/MYOBLOC™.

Modify the basic recommendations using the following principles:

1 Give higher doses in men and in young, athletic, heavily built or more severely affected patients.

2 Divide the toxin between the muscles according to their perceived contribution to the torticollis.

3 Minimize dysphagia by giving sternocleidomastoid injections into the upper third of the muscle. Halve the dose per muscle for bilateral injections of the sternocleidomastoid and the hyoid muscles.

4 For bilateral injections into the splenius capitis and semispinalis capitis reduce the individual dose per muscle to 60%. This will also minimize any undue difficulty lifting the head up.

5 Reduce the dose for muscles already weakened by previous injections, or where there is special risk of side-effects.

Most injectors use a 2–5 mL syringe and a 27 gauge hypodermic needle. Dilute 100 mu Botox® or 500 mu Dysport®/2.5 mL normal saline. NeuroBloc®/MYOBLOC™ is offered in a solution of 5000 mu/mL, and can be diluted but not concentrated. There are no definitive systematic studies of the best concentration to use in cervical dystonia. Experts suggest that higher concentrations may decrease the prevalence of side-effects [2,115, 116], perhaps because of less toxin diffusion at lower volumes. Dysphagia is the most relevant side-effect and is presumably induced by diffusion into the pharyngeal muscles. However, in a study in animals and in extensor digitorum brevis in human volunteers, lower concentrations were more effective and produced fewer local side-effects [117].

Injecting individual muscles

Figures 8.4–8.6 show the anatomy of some of the important neck muscles. Always draw back briefly on the plunger to avoid injecting into a vessel. Relax the muscle a little before injecting as this reduces the pressure required and any discomfort. Bulkier or long muscles deserve several smaller injections.

STERNOCLEIDOMASTOID

Identify the muscle by asking the patient to press his or her opposite hand against his or her chin on the opposite side to tonically activate the muscle. Ensure he or she is not pushing on the cheek and that he or she rotates the head initially rather than tilting or pushing laterally. It can then be helpful to 'point the chin up' and 'point the (ipsilateral) ear down'. Hold the now prominent muscle firmly between your fingers, reaching behind the muscle. These manoeuvres are especially important in patients with obese necks, or when previous injections have left a relatively atrophic muscle. Inject into the upper-third of the muscle, angling the needle upwards and at an oblique angle along its axis.

TRAPEZIUS

A dystonic trapezius may be obvious. If not, ask the patient to hold the head straight and elevate the shoulder, if necessary against resistance from your hand. The flat, sheet-like muscle is easy to pin between two fingers to prevent it slipping away from the needle. Inject along the plane of the sheet.

LEVATOR SCAPULAE

The same manoeuvres will make levator scapulae prominent and easily felt just anterior to trapezius. Inject directly into it.

SPLENIUS CAPITIS

Activate sternomastoid as above. Splenius capitis is just posterior and deep to sternomastoid at the level of the angle of the jaw, and you may be able to palpate or roll it beneath your finger. Inject directly into it at a depth of 1.0–2.5 cm.

SEMISPINALIS CAPITIS

Ask the patient to press his or her head back against the heel of your hand while you palpate these paired muscles with fingers of the same hand to delineate the obvious midline gap between them, and their lateral borders. Give the injections directly into the muscle.

After the injection

Remind the patient about the likely delay in response, how to monitor it, and what to do about side-effects. Make sure there is an identified physician to consult in case of any major problems, and arrange a follow-up visit. The best time to clarify the response is 4 weeks later, during the plateau phase. Once a pattern is established such interim visits are unnecessary.

Repeat injections

The patient should report on the benefits of the injection and their time course, and the severity and duration of side-effects. Repeat any clinical ratings and compare with previous scores. Aim to reinject the patient when the toxin is wearing off, and defer reinjection if the toxin is still working well. Individual patient-clinician pairs will negotiate their own compromises about how much it should be wearing off. Typically, if peak effect equals 100%, the severity of the cervical dystonia will be 20–50% above baseline, usually 10–14 weeks after injection. Remember the last dose will continue to wear off before the next one takes effect. Do not reinject your patients within 8–10 weeks because of the risk of antibody formation.

For each injection cycle, review muscle selection, total dose, and dose per individual muscle, as described above. A special trap is a shoulder still drooping from the last injections, when it is easy to assume that the other side is abnormally high. Ask the patient which shoulder has spasms. Reduce the total dose or the dose to sternocleidomastoid if there was important dysphagia. After prominent neck pain and/or weakness reduce the dose for the splenius capitis muscle(s). Provided there were no major side-effects, increase the total dose if benefit was fleeting or inadequate—although these can be difficult to define. Do not increase the total dose or dose per muscle by more than 20% each time. If high doses produce major side-effects and little benefit, reconsider the indications for injection and review the pattern of muscles and doses. Consider using EMG.

Botulinum toxin treatment of axial dystonia

The term axial dystonia describes dystonic hyperactivity in muscles of the trunk including the paraspinal and abdominal wall muscles. There is truncal extension or flexion, and lateral flexion or scoliosis. Although it may be isolated, axial dystonia occurs most often as part of idiopathic segmental or generalized dystonia but it can also appear in neuroleptic-induced acute and tardive dystonia. Some clinicians use the term 'Pisa syndrome' when dystonia leads to tonic lateral flexion of the trunk, others consider this to be pejorative and avoid it. When phasic dystonia is most pronounced in abdominal wall muscles the so-called 'belly dancers dyskinesia' may result. Axial dystonia induces malpositioning of the axial skeleton and can cause discopathies with radicular lesions as well as arthroses of vertebral joints. After prolonged and severe disease, permanent deformations of the thoracic and abdominal cavities may occur and may give rise recurrent pneumonia and cardiac arrhythmias.

There are no systematic analyses of the effects of Bt, but axial dystonia rarely responds convincingly to local Bt injections. In most cases there are so many powerful muscles involved that the necessary total dose would be too high and would cause severe systemic side-effects. These patients may respond to oral medication or intrathecal baclofen. Deep brain stimulation of the globus pallidus also appears promising for axial dystonia.

It may be worth trying Bt in selected patients with less severe axial dystonia who need injections into a limited number of muscles. Four women and one man with severe idiopathic or tardive truncal and cervical dystonia received open label BtA (Botox®) injections into lumbar paravertebral muscles in 4–6 sites using 25–50 mu per site. The mean total dose of BtA was 201 mu. Blinded videotape evaluation showed objective improvement in three patients with the mean truncal dystonia score improving by 37%. Pain improved substantially. None of the patients was worse and no adverse effects occurred. Most cases needed additional oral medication [118]. Recommended doses for paraspinal muscles (thoracic or lumbar portion) on one side range from 60 to 100 mu Botox® or 240–400 mu Dysport®. Excessive weakness is unlikely.

Suggested doses for muscles of the abdominal wall range from 40 to 80 mu Botox® or 160–320 mu Dysport® per site. Prolapse of the abdominal wall may occur, and at total doses above 400 mu Botox® or 1500 mu Dysport® there may be systemic side-effects with general weakness and dysphagia.

References

1 Stacy M. Idiopathic cervical dystonia: an overview. *Neurology* 2000; **55**: S2–S8.
2 Kessler KR, Skutta M, Benecke R. Long-term treatment of cervical dystonia with botulinum toxin A. efficacy, safety, and antibody frequency. *J Neurol* 1999; **246**: 265–74.
3 Dauer WT, Burke RE, Greene P, Fahn S. Current concepts on the clinical features, aetiology and management of idiopathic cervical dystonia. *Brain* 1998; **121**: 547–60.

4 Lekhel H, Popov K, Anastasopoulos D *et al.* Postural responses to vibration of neck muscles in patients with idiopathic torticollis. *Brain* 1997; **120**: 583–91.

5 Papathanasiou I, MacDonald L, Whurr R, Jahanshahi M. Perceived stigma in spasmodic torticollis. *Mov Disord* 2001; **16**: 280–5.

6 Camfiels L, Ben-Schlomo Y, Warner T, Warner T. The impact of cervical dystonia on quality of life. *Mov Disord* 2000; **15**: 143.

7 Naumann M, Magyar S, Reiners K, Erbguth F, Leenders K. Sensory tricks in cervical dystonia. perceptual dysbalance of parietal cortex modulates frontal motor programming. *Ann Neurol* 2000; **47**: 322–8.

8 Grünewald RA, Yoneda Y, Shipman JM, Sagar HJ. Idiopathic focal dystonia. a disorder of muscle spindle afferent processing? *Brain* 1997; **120**: 2179–85.

9 Berardelli A, Rothwell JC, Hallett M *et al.* The pathophysiology of primary dystonia. *Brain* 1998; **121**: 1195–212.

10 Lenz FA, Suarez JI, Metman LV *et al.* Pallidal activity during dystonia: somatosensory reorganization and changes with severity. *J Neurol Neurosurg Psychiatry* 1998; **65**: 767–70.

11 Bara-Jimenez W, Catalan MJ, Hallett M, Gerloff C. Abnormal somatosensory homunculus in dystonia of the hand. *Ann Neurol* 1998; **44**: 828–31.

12 Rome S, Grünewald R. Abnormal perception of vibration-induced illusion of movement in dystonia. *Neurology* 1999; **53**: 1794–800.

13 Kaji R, Murase N. Sensory function of basal ganglia. *Mov Disord* 2001; **16**: 593–4.

14 Murase N, Kaji R, Shimazu H *et al.* Abnormal premovement gating of somatosensory input in writer's cramp. *Brain* 2000; **123**: 1813–29.

15 Tinazzi M, Priori A, Bertolasi L *et al.* Abnormal central integration of a dual somatosensory input in dystonia. Evidence for sensory overflow. *Brain* 2000; **123**: 42–50.

16 Hallett M. Disorder of movement preparation in dystonia. *Brain* 2000; **123**: 1765–6.

17 Jahanshahi M. Factors that ameliorate or aggravate spasmodic torticollis. *J Neurol Neurosurg Psychiatry* 2000; **68**: 227–9.

18 Risvoll H, Kerty E. To test or not? The value of diagnostic tests in cervical dystonia. *Mov Disord* 2001; **16**: 286–9.

19 Factor SA, Podskalny GD, Molho ES. Psychogenic movement disorders. frequency, clinical profile, and characteristics. *J Neurol Neurosurg Psychiatry* 1995; **59**: 406–12.

20 Brown PTP. Electrophysiological aids to the diagnosis of psychogenic jerks, spasms and tremor. *Mov Disord* 2001; **16**: 595–9.

21 Anderson TJ, Rivest J, Stell R *et al.* Botulinum-toxin treatment of spasmodic torticollis. *J R Soc Med* 1992; **85**: 524–9.

22 Jankovic J, Leder S, Warner D, Schwartz K. Cervical dystonia. clinical findings and associated movement disorders. *Neurology* 1991; **41**: 1088–91.

23 Chan J, Brin MF, Fahn S. Idiopathic cervical dystonia: clinical characteristics. *Mov Disord* 1991; **6**: 119–26.

24 Quinn N. Multiple system atrophy—the nature of the beast. *J Neurol Neurosurg Psychiatry* 1989; **June**: 78–89.

25 Lindeboom R, Brans JWM, Aramideh M, Speelman SD, De Haan RJ. Treatment of cervical dystonia: a comparison of measures for outcome assessment. *Mov Disord* 1998; **13**: 706–12.

26 Swash M, Roberts AH, Zakko H, Heathfield KW. Treatment of involuntary disorders with tetrabenazine. *J Neurol Neurosurg Psychiatry* 1972; **35**: 186–91.

27 Couch JR. Dystonia and tremor in spasmodic torticollis. *Adv Neurol* 1976; **14**: 245–58.

28 Tolosa ES. Modification of tardive dyskinesia and spasmodic torticollis by apomorphine. *Arch Neurol* 1978; **35**: 459–62.

29 Lang AE, Sheehy MP, Marsden CD. Anticholinergics in adult-onset dystonia. *Can J Neurol Sci* 1982; **9**: 313–19.

30 Tsui JK, Eisen A, Stoesl AJ, Calne S, Calne DB. Double blind study of botulinum toxin in spasmodic torticollis. *Lancet* 1986; **2**: 245–7.

31 Fahn S. Assessment of the primary dystonias. In: Munsat T, ed. *Quantification of Neurological Deficits*. Boston: Butterworths, 1989: 241–70.

32 Consky E, Basinski A, Belle L, Ranawaya R, Lang A. The Toronto Western Spasmodic Torticollis Rating Scale (TWSTRS). *Neurology* 1990; **40** (Suppl. 1): 445.

33 O'Brien C, Brashear A, Cullis P *et al.* Cervical dystonia severity scale reliability study. *Mov Disord* 2001; **16**: 1086–90.

34 Christensen JEJ. New treatment for spasmodic torticollis? *Lancet* 1991; **338**: 573.

35 Marchetti A, Magar R, Lau H *et al.* Treatment algorithm for cervical dystonia. *Mov Disord* 2000; **15**: 150.

36 Adler C, Kumar R. Pharmacological and surgical options for the treatment of cervical dystonia. *Neurology* 2000; **55**: S9–S14.

37 Sherman DG, Hart RG, Easton JD. Abrupt change of head position and cerebral infarction. *Stroke* 1981; **12**: 2–6.

38 Jahanshahi M, Marsden C. Treatments for torticollis. *J Neurol Neurosurg Psychiatry* 1989; **52**: 1212.

39 Jahanshahi M, Sartory G, Marsden C. EMG biofeedback treatment of torticollis: a controlled outcome study. *Biofeedback Self Regulation* 1991; **16**: 413–38.

40 Fahn S, Marsden CD, Calne DB. Classification and investigation of dystonia. In: Marsden CD, Fahn S eds. *Movement Disorders 2*. London: Butterworths, 1987: 332–58.

41 Greene P, Shale H, Fahn S. Analysis of open label trials in torsion dystonia using high dosages of anticholinergics and other drugs. *Mov Disord* 1988; **3**: 46–60.

42 Burke R, Fahn S, Marsden C. Torsion dystonia. a double blind, prospective trial of high-dosage trihexyphenidyl. *Neurology* 1986; **36**: 160–4.

43 Greene P. Baclofen in the treatment of dystonia. *Clin Neuropharmacol* 1992; **15**: 276–88.

44 Lang AE. Dopamine agonists and antagonists in the treatment of idiopathic dystonia. *Adv Neurol* 1988; **50**: 561–70.

45 Jankovic J, Orman J. Tetrabenazine therapy of dystonia, chorea, tics, and other dyskinesias. *Neurology* 1988; **38**: 391–4.

46 Thiel A, Dressler D, Kistel C, Ruther E. Clozapine treatment of spasmodic torticollis. *Neurology* 1994; **44**: 957–8.

47 Ohara S, Hayashi R, Momoi H, Miki J, Yanagisawa N. Mexiletine in the treatment of spasmodic torticollis. *Mov Disord* 1998; **13**: 934–40.

48 Massey J. Treatment of spasmodic torticollis with intramuscular phenol injection. *J Neurol Neurosurg Psychiatry* 1995; **58**: 258–9.

49 Falkenberg J, Iaizzo P, McLonn L. Physiological assessment of muscle strength in vitro after direct injection of doxorubicin into rabbit sternocleidomastoid muscle. *Mov Disord* 2001; **16**: 683–92.

50 Wirtschafter JD. Chemomyectomy of the orbicularis oculi muscles for the treatment of localized hemifacial spasm. *J Neuroophthalmol* 1994; **14**: 199–204.

51 Wirtschafter JD. Clinical doxorubicin chemomyectomy. An experimental treatment for benign essential blepharospasm and hemifacial spasm. *Ophthalmology* 1991; **98**: 357–66.

52 Lang AE. Surgical treatment of dystonia. In: Fahn S, Marsden CD, DeLong M, eds. *Dystonia 3: Advances in Neurology*. Philadelphia: Lippincott-Raven Publications, 1998: 185–98.

53 Bertrand CM. Selective peripheral denervation for spasmodic torticollis. surgical technique, results, and observations in 260 cases. *Surg Neurol* 1993; **40**: 96–103.

54 Davis DH, Ahlskog JE, Litchy WJ, Root LM. Selective peripheral denervation for torticollis: preliminary results. *Mayo Clin Proc* 1991; **66**: 365–71.

55 Braun V, Richter H-P. Selective peripheral denervation for the treatment of spasmodic torticollis. *Neurosurgery* 1994; **35**: 58–63.

56 Ford B, Louis ED, Greene P, Fahn S. Outcome of selective ramisectomy for botulinum toxin resistant torticollis. *J Neurol Neurosurg Psychiatry* 1998; **65**: 472–8.

57 Krauss JK, Toups EG, Jankovic J, Grossman RG. Symptomatic and functional outcome of surgical treatment of cervical dystonia. *J Neurol Neurosurg Psychiatry* 1997; **63**: 642–8.

58 Münchau A, Palmer J, Dressler D *et al*. Prospective study of selective peripheral denervation for botulinum-toxin resistant patients with cervical dystonia. *Mov Disord* 2000; **15**: 141.

59 Cooper IS. Neurosurgical treatment of the dyskinesias. *Clin Neurosurg* 1977; **24**: 367–9.

60 Andrew J, Fowler CJ, Harrison MJG. Stereotaxic thalamotomy in 55 cases of dystonia. *Brain* 1983; **106**: 981–1000.

61 Vitek J. Surgery for dystonia. *Neurosurg Clin N Am* 1998; **9**: 345–66.

62 Vitek JL, Chockkan V, Zhang JY *et al*. Neuronal activity in the basal ganglia in patients with generalized dystonia and hemiballismus. *Ann Neurol* 1999; **46**: 22–35.

63 Lozano AM, Kumar R, Gross RE *et al*. Globus pallidus internus pallidotomy for generalized dystonia. *Mov Disord* 1997; **12**: 865–70.

64 Lin J-J, Lin G-Y, Shih G, Lin S-Z, Chang D-C, Lee C-C. Benefit of bilateral pallidotomy in the treatment of generalized dystonia. *J Neurosurg* 1999; **90**: 974–6.

65 Ondo WG, Desaloms JM, Jankovic J, Grossman RG. Pallidotomy for generalized dystonia. *Mov Disord* 1998; **13**: 693–8.

66 Tronnier V, Fogel W. Pallidal stimulation for generalized dystonia. Report of three cases. *J Neurosurg* 2000; **92**: 453–6.

67 Bötzel K, Bereznai B, Steude U, Jäger M, Dasser T. Chronic high frequency stimulation of globus pallidus internus in different types of dystonia: a clinical, video and MRI report of three patients. *Mov Disord* 2000; **15**: 168.

68 Roubertie A, Cif L, Vayssiere N *et al*. Symptomatic generalized dystonia: neurosurgical treatment by continuous bilateral stimulation of the internal globus pallidus in eight patients. *Mov Disord* 2000; **15**: 156.

69 Krauss JK, Pohle T, Weber S, Ozdoba C, Burgunder JM. Bilateral stimulation of globus pallidus internus for treatment of cervical dystonia. *Lancet* 1999; **354**: 837–8.

70 Islekel S, Zileli M, Zileli B. Unilateral pallidal stimulation in cervical dystonia. *Stereotact Funct Neurosurg* 1999; **72**: 248–52.

71 Kumar R, Dagher A, Hutchison W, Lang A, Lozano A. Globus pallidus deep brain stimulation for generalized dystonia. *Neurology* 1999; **53**: 871–4.

72 Tsui JK, Eisen A, Mak E *et al*. A pilot study on the use of botulinum toxin in spasmodic torticollis. *Can J Neurol Sci* 1985; **12**: 314–16.

73 Jankovic J, Orman J. Botulinum A toxin for cranial-cervical dystonia: a double blind, placebo-controlled study. *Neurology* 1987; **37**: 616–23.

74 Lorentz IT, Subramaniam SS, Yiannikas C. Treatment of idiopathic spasmodic torticollis with botulinum toxin A. a double blind study on twenty-three patients. *Mov Disord* 1991; **6**: 145–50.

75 Gelb DJ, Lowenstein DH, Aminoff MJ. Controlled trial of botulinum toxin injections in the treatment of spasmodic torticollis. *Neurology* 1989; **39**: 80–4.

76 Naumann M, Yakovleff A, Durif F. A randomized, double-masked, crossover comparison of the efficacy and safety of botulinum toxin type A produced from the original bulk toxin source and current toxin source for the treatment of cervical dystonia. *J Neurol* 2002; **249**: 57–63.

77 Comella C, Jankovic J, Brin M. Use of botulinum toxin type A in the treatment of cervical dystonia. *Neurology* 2000; **55**: S15–21.

78 Brashear A, Lew MF, Dykstra DD *et al*. Safety and efficacy of NeuroBloc® (botulinum toxin type B) in type A-responsive cervical dystonia. *Neurology* 1999; **53**: 1439–46.

79 Brin MF, Lew MF, Adler MD *et al*. Safety and efficacy of NeuroBloc® (botulinum toxin type B) in type A-resistant cervical dystonia. *Neurology* 1999; **53**: 1431–8.

80 Lew MF, Adornato BT, Duane DD *et al*. Botulinum toxin type B. A double blind, placebo-controlled, safety and efficacy study in cervical dystonia. *Neurology* 1997; **49**: 701–7.

81 Cullis PA, O'Brien CF, Truong DD *et al*. Botulinum toxin type B: an open-label, dose-escalation, safety and preliminary efficacy study in cervical dystonia patients. *Adv Neurol* 1998; **78**: 227–30.

82 Adler C. *Botulinum Toxin Treatment of Movement Disorders Neurobase*, 3rd edn. San Diego, CA: Arbor Publishing, 2001.

83 Williams A. Consensus statement for the management of focal dystonias. *Br J Hosp Med* 1993; **50**: 655–9.

84 Report of the Therapeutics and Technology Assessment Subcommittee of the American Academy of Neurology. Training guidelines for the use of botulinum toxin for the treatment of neurological disorders. *Neurology* 1994; **44**: 2401–3.

85 Blackie JD, Lees AJ. Botulinum toxin treatment in spasmodic torticollis. *J Neurol Neurosurg Psychiatry* 1990; **53**: 640–3.

86 Jankovic J, Schwartz PA. Botulinum toxin injections for cervical dystonia. *Neurology* 1990; **40**: 277–80.

87 Jahanshahi M, Marsden CD. Psychological functioning before and after treatment of torticollis with botulinum toxin. *J Neurol Neurosurg Psychiatry* 1992; **55**: 229–31.

88 Jahanshahi M, Marion MH, Marsden C. Natural history of adult-onset idiopathic torticollis. *Arch Neurol* 1990; **47**: 548–52.

89 Blackie JD, Lees AJ. Botulinum toxin treatment in spasmodic torticollis. *J Neurol Neurosurg Psychiatry* 1990; **53**: 640–3.

90 Greene P, Kang U, Fahn S *et al*. Double blind, placebo-controlled trial of botulinum toxin injections for the treatment of spasmodic torticollis. *Neurology* 1990; **40**: 1213–18.

91 Gelb DJ, Yoshimura DM, Olney RK, Lowenstein DH, Aminoff MJ. Change in pattern of muscle activity following botulinum toxin injections for torticollis. *Ann Neurol* 1991; **29**: 370–6.

92 Comella CL, Tanner CM, DeFoor-Hill L, Smith C. Dysphagia after botulinum toxin injections for spasmodic torticollis. Clinical and radiologic findings. *Neurology* 1992; **42**: 1307–10.

93 Stell R, Thompson PD, Marsden CD. Botulinum toxin in spasmodic torticollis. *J Neurol Neurosurg Psychiatry* 1988; **51**: 920–3.

94 Poewe W, Schelowsky L, Kleedorfer B *et al*. Treatment of spasmodic torticollis with local injections of botulinum toxin. One-year follow-up in thirty-seven patients. *J Neurol* 1992; **239**: 21–5.

95 Wissel J, Poewe W. Dystonia—a clinical, neuropathological and therapeutic review. *J Neurol Transm* 1992; **38** (Suppl.): 91–104.

96 Lu CS, Chen RS, Tsai CH. Double blind, placebo-controlled study of botulinum toxin injections in the treatment of cervical dystonia. *J Formos Med Assoc* 1995; **94**: 189–92.

97 Jankovic J, Schwartz KS. Clinical correlates of response to botulinum toxin injections. *Arch Neurol* 1991; **48**: 1253–6.

98 Brans JWM, Speelman JD & members of the BOVAS. Botulinum toxin vs. trihexyphenidyl in cervical dystonia: a prospective, randomized, placebo controlled study. *Mov Disord* 1994; **9**: 43.

99 Lew M, Brashear A, Factor S. The safety and efficacy of botulinum toxin type B in the treatment of patients with cervical dystonia: summary of three controlled clinical trials. *Neurology* 2000; **55**: S29–35.

100 Lew MF, Brashear A, Factor S. The safety and efficacy of botulinum toxin type B in the treatment of patients with cervical dystonia: summary of three controlled clinical trials. *Neurology* 2000; **55**: S29–S35.

101 Committee on Safety of Medicines. Reminder: botulinum type A toxin (Dysport®)—severe dysphagia with unlicensed route of administration. *Current Problems Pharmacovigilance* 1993; **19**: 11.

102 Sampaio C, Castro-Caldas A, Sales-Luis MI *et al*. Brachial plexopathy after botulinum toxin administration for cervical dystonia [letter]. *J Neurol, Neurosurg Psychiatry* 1993; **56**: 220.

103 Glanzman RL, Gelb DJ, Drury I, Bromberg MB, Truong DD. Brachial plexopathy after botulinum toxin injections. *Neurology* 1990; **40**: 1143.

104 Emmerson J. Botulinum toxin for spasmodic torticollis in a patient with myasthenia gravis. *Mov Disord* 1994; **9**; 367–79.

105 Duane D, Stuart S, Case J, LaPointe L. Successful and safe use of botulinum toxin A in a patient with subclinical myasthenia gravis and lingual/brachial/manual dystonia. *Mov Disord* 2000; **15**: 149.

106 Münchau A, Filipovic S, Oester-Barkey A *et al.* Spontaneously changing muscular activation pattern in patients with cervical dystonia. *Mov Disord* 2001; **16**: 1091–7.

107 Nakashima K, Thompson PD, Rothwell JC *et al.* An exteroceptive reflex in the sternocleidomastoid muscle produced by electrical stimulation of the supraorbital nerve in normal subjects and patients with spasmodic torticollis. *Neurology* 1989; **39**: 1354–8.

108 Podivinski F. Torticollis. In: Vinken PF, Bruyn GW, eds. *Handbook of Clinical Neurology*, Vol. 6. Amsterdam: North Holland, 1968: 567–603.

109 Rondot PMMP, Dellatolas G. Spasmodic torticollis—review of 220 patients. *Can J Neurol Sci* 1991; **18**: 143–51.

110 Stejskal L. Counterpressure in torticollis. *J Neurol Sci* 1980; **48**: 9–19.

111 Tournay A, Paillard J. Torticollis spasmodique et électromyographie. *Rev Neurol* 1955; **93**: 347–55.

112 Dubinski RM, Grey CS, Vetere-Overfield B, Koller WC. Electromyographic guidance of botulinum toxin treatment in cervical dystonia. *Clin Neuropharmacol* 1991; **14**: 262–7.

113 Jankovic J, Brin MF. Therapeutic uses of botulinum toxin. *N Engl J Med* 1991; **324**: 1186–94.

114 Stell R, Bronstein AM, Marsden CD. Vestibulo-ocular abnormalities in spasmodic torticollis before and after botulinum toxin injections. *J Neurol Neurosurg Psychiatry* 1989; **52**: 57–62.

115 Benecke R. Botulinum toxin A in der Behandlung der zervikalen Dystonien. In: Richter HP, Braun V, eds. *Schiefhals. Behandlungskonzepte des Torticollis Spasmodicus*. Berlin: Springer, 1993: 63–78.

116 Benecke R. Zervikale Dystonie. In: Laskawi R, Roggenkaemper P, eds. *Botulinum Toxin Therapie im Kopf Hals Bereich*. Munich: Urban & Vogel, 1999: 171–212.

117 Bigalke H, Wohlfarth K, Irmer A, Dengler R. Botulinum A toxin Dysport$^{\text{®}}$ improvement of biological availability. *Exp Neurol* 2001; **168**: 162–70.

118 Comella CL, Shannon KM, Jaglin J. Extensor truncal dystonia: successful treatment with botulinum toxin injections. *Mov Disord* 1998; **13**: 552–5.

Cervical dystonia rating scales

The Toronto Western Spasmodic Torticollis Rating Scale (TWSTRS)

A. Maximal excursion

Rate maximum amplitude of excursion, asking the patient not to oppose the abnormal
movements; examiner may use distracting or aggravating manoeuvre. When degree of
deviation is between two scores, choose the higher of the two.

1   Rotation (turn: right or left)

None	0	Moderate (1/2–3/4 range)(46–67°)	3
Slight (<1/4 range) (1–22°)	1	Severe (>3/4 range)(68–90°)	4
Mild (1/4–1/2 range) (23–45°)	2		

2   Laterocollis (tilt: right or left; exclude shoulder elevation)

None	0	Moderate (16–35°)	2
Mild (1–15°)	1	Severe (>35°)	3

3   Anterocollis/retrocollis

Anterocollis		*Retrocollis*	
None	0	None	0
Mild downward deviation of chin	1	Mild backward deviation of vertex with upward deviation of chin	1
Moderate downward deviation (approx. 1/2 possible range)	2	Moderate backward deviation (approx. 1/2 possible range)	2
Severe (chin approx. chest)	3	Severe (approx. full range)	3

4   Lateral shift (right or left)

Absent	0	Present	1

5   Sagittal shift (forward or backward)

Absent	0	Present	1

Sum A (add the numbers: maximum = 12)

B   Duration factor

Provide an overall score estimated through the course of the standardized examination after
estimating maximum excursion (exclusive of asking patient to allow head to deviate
maximally).

None	0
Occasional deviation (<25% of the time), most often submaximal	1

Occasional deviation (<25% of the time), often maximal or intermittent
deviation (25–50% of the time), most often submaximal   2

Intermittent deviation (25–50% of the time), often maximal or frequent deviation
(50–75% of the time), most often submaximal   3

Frequent deviation (50–75% of the time), often maximal or constant deviation
(>75% of the time), most often submaximal   4

Constant deviation (>75% of the time), often maximal   5

Score (×2)/maximum = 10

C Effect of sensory tricks
Complete relief by one or more tricks   0
Partial or only limited relief by tricks   1
Little or no benefit from tricks   2

D Shoulder elevation/anterior displacement
Absent   0
Mild (<1/3 possible range), intermittent or constant   1
Moderate (1/3–2/3 possible range) and constant (>75% of the time) or severe
(2/3 possible range) and intermittent   2
Severe and constant   3

E Range of motion (without aid of sensory tricks)
If limitation occurs in more than one plane of motion use individual score that is highest.
Able to move to extreme opposite position   0
Able to move head well past midline but not to extreme opposite position 1
Able to move head barely past midline   2
Able to move head toward but not past midline   3
Barely able to move head beyond abnormal posture   4

F Time
Time (up to 60 s) for which patient is able to maintain head within 10° of neutral position
without the use 'of sensory tricks' (mean of two attempts).
>60 s   0
46–60 s   1
31–45 s   2
16–30 s   3
<15 s   4

Total severity score   **Sum A–F. (Maximum = 35)**

Tsui Rating Scale

Rotation

Lateral rotation	0–3	0 = normal
Head-tilting	0–3	1 = <15°
Flexion or extension	0–3	2 = 15–45°
		3 = >45°
Subtotal	0–9 (A)	
Frequency	0–2 (B)	0 = normal
		1 = intermittent
		2 = continuous

Shoulder displacement

	0–3 (C)	0 = normal
		1 = mild
		2 = moderate
		3 = severe

Intermittent movements

Amplitude	0–2 (D)	0 = normal
		1 = mild
		2 = severe
Frequency	0–2 (E)	0 = normal
		1 = intermittent
		2 = continuous

Total torticollis score = (A × B) + C + (D × E)

CHAPTER 9

Limb and occupational dystonia

GEOFF SHEEAN

Introduction

Dystonia can affect any group of muscles under voluntary control. The limbs are affected in generalized dystonias, whether primary or secondary to some recognized disease, including neurodegenerative (e.g. Huntington's disease, Wilson's disease, corticobasal degeneration) and other diseases (e.g. anoxic-ischaemic brain injury, head injury) that affect control of movement. Focal limb dystonia, especially of the foot and ankle, is a complication of levodopa treatment of Parkinson's disease. Dystonic muscle overactivity can occur at rest and be aggravated by movement, or occur only during voluntary movement, a so-called action dystonia. An intriguing form of focal action dystonia of the arm is that restricted to a single task, often an occupational or recreational activity (Table 9.1 [1]), for example, writing, typing or playing a musical instrument: these are labelled task-specific dystonias. Later, other manual actions can become affected, and the dystonia is then called non-task specific or complex. In the focal dystonia that is brought on by writing, writer's cramp, these two forms have been called 'simple' (task-specific) or 'dystonic' (complex), although the label 'dystonic' is confusing. In some patients, the initial task remains by far the most affected and I call these task-dominant complex dystonias.

This chapter will deal mostly with action dystonias of the limb. Because writer's cramp is so well-known and has been the most thoroughly studied of the arm dystonias, I will discuss it in more detail to serve as a model for other occupational or recreational focal arm action dystonias; the principles apply to all. They have in common difficulty in performing a task because of excessive muscular contraction, typically involving cocontraction of antagonist muscle pairs that are used in the task. This muscle overactivity leads to abnormal postures and movements, discomfort, and sometimes tremor and myoclonic jerks, which interfere with performance of the task.

Writer's cramp: a model for arm action dystonia

Epidemiology

Writer's cramp was first described in the medical literature in the first half of the 19th century (see [2] for historical details), when it was known as scrivener's palsy: a

Table 9.1 Occupational and recreational task-specific dystonias (adapted from [1]).

Musicians	Sportsmen	Professions
Pianists	Snooker players	Telegraphers
Violinists	Golfers (yips)	Typists
Guitarists	Dart players	Watchmakers
Drummers		Engravers
Harpists		Seam-mistresses and tailors
Trumpeters (mouth)		Knitters
Saxophonists (mouth)		Stonemasons
Horn players (mouth)		Ironmongers
Cellists (thigh)		Turners
		Smiths
		Cigarette makers
		Milkers
		Painters
		Enamellers
		Compositors
		Money counters
		Letter sorters
		Shoemakers
		Artificial flower makers
		Dancers

scrivener copied business documents by hand. The word 'cramp' emphasizes that there is often intense muscle contraction that locks the wrist and fingers, twisting them into abnormal postures, and interfering with handwriting. The estimated prevalence of writer's cramp is 69/million [3], which is probably too low; I suspect writer's cramp is much more common. Sheehy and Marsden [2] published the first detailed study of writer's cramp in 1982, describing 29 patients and dividing them into three groups. Task-specific forms were called 'simple' and patients in whom tasks other than writing were affected from the start were called 'dystonic'. The third category was 'progressive' writer's cramp, in which patients began as task-specific but later became non-task specific. I find the progressive category helpful mainly to warn patients with simple writer's cramp that there is a chance of it affecting other manual actions. I refer to both the progressive and dystonic forms as 'complex' writer's cramp. By 1988, they had collected 91 patients [4]. In the larger group, men were affected more often than women (55 : 36). The complex form was as common as the simple forms (44 : 47) but more common in men than in women (31 : 13). The age of onset ranged from 8 to 67 years, most commonly around the age of 40 years. A family history of writer's cramp is uncommon, occurring in about 5% of patients [4].

Clinical features [5]

The symptoms usually begin gradually but can come on rapidly over a few weeks. Often there is no precipitant but about 5% of patients report antecedent trauma to the limb. Others say that their symptoms began during a period of intense writing, such as studying for an exam or when they were under pressure to write more or more quickly. Once begun, the symptoms usually continue, often worsening despite reduction in the need or pressure to write.

Patients usually describe difficulty writing and might recognize muscle tension or spasm in their hand or forearm. This muscle tension can spread to the arm, shoulder and neck muscles. Mild discomfort from muscle spasm is common but pain is not [4] and suggests additional nerve or nerve root entrapment, or soft-tissue inflammation. Patients might report abnormal postures of the wrist or fingers, tremor, or myoclonic jerks. Many say that their hand seems to 'freeze' or 'lock-up'. The muscle spasms can cause the pen to fall from their hand. Early in the course of the disease the symptoms develop only after the patient has been writing for a while, and this latency period becomes gradually shorter until spasms begin immediately or even when simply putting pen to paper. The patient might be able to persist and finish the writing task, but often writing must be suspended for a rest or discontinued altogether, with the duration of continuous writing becoming increasingly shorter. Writing becomes slow, difficult, an effort, possibly uncomfortable, and penmanship often suffers. Some patients manage to maintain the quality of their script but at a cost. There might be a sensory trick or *geste antagonistique*, as in cervical dystonia, that improves writing, such as lightly touching the hand or forearm with the other hand. Patients may try to change pens, often preferring thicker pens with felt tips. Others alter their pen grip or their writing style to adapt to the problem, usually with little or only temporary success. Most patients try to cope by limiting their writing in favour of typing or dictating. Unfortunately, for many these strategies are incompatible with their jobs. Some try to write with the other hand but this is difficult for most people, and about a quarter of patients eventually develops writer's cramp in that hand [4]. Some patients blame their dystonia on a poor writing style. Normal left-handers seem to write awkwardly, but in one study [2] the handedness ratio was 27 : 2 right-handed : left-handed; probably no greater than expected.

Prognosis

The degree of disability produced by writer's cramp is variable and depends on the severity of the writing difficulty itself and on the individual's requirements for writing. Many patients' livelihoods depend upon being able to write, and some writing tasks cannot be performed through keyboard devices. Many avoid writing as much as possible and some lose their jobs. The chance of remission is very poor. However, only about 15% of patients are forced to completely give up writing with the affected hand [4]. About 40% of patients who begin with simple writer's cramp develop complex cramps [4]. The dystonia does not usually spread beyond the hands to involve other areas of the body but those who change to writing with the other hand have a one in four chance of developing writer's cramp in that hand. One patient of mine with writer's cramp in the left hand developed typist's cramp in the right; different muscles were involved for each hand.

Differential diagnosis

The differential diagnosis of writer's cramp includes focal nerve entrapments (carpal tunnel syndrome, ulnar neuropathy, thoracic outlet syndrome), cervical root entrapments, and soft-tissue disorders (e.g. tendinitis and epicondylitis). Sometimes these conditions are coincidental or appear secondary to the muscle spasms and dystonic postures. Treating them may help some of the symptoms but does not cure the dystonia or writing difficulties. Other neurological disorders can begin with similar symptoms, including multiple sclerosis and neurodegenerative disorders such as Parkinson's disease [4]. There have been cases of writer's cramp due to focal brain lesions such as tumours and haemangiomas, but generally there are no brain imaging abnormalities.

Tremor occurs in about a fifth of patients [4]. In primary writing tremor, where writing is the only task that brings on tremor, it is difficult to distinguish variants of essential tremor from dystonia. A very tight pen-grip, and abnormal postures that arise as a compensatory 'trick' to control the tremor, can misleadingly suggest dystonia. Asking the patient to write with the grip used before symptoms began may help to distinguish between the two.

Other task-specific focal dystonias

Another frequently studied task-specific focal hand dystonia affects musicians. Newmark and Hochberg [6] reported on 59 affected musicians and found a male dominance (possibly selection bias) and three stereotypic patterns: flexion of digits four and five in pianists, flexion of digit three in guitarists, and extension of digit three in clarinetists. Possible triggers found in 37 (63%) patients were trauma, inflammation (tenosynovitis and tendinitis) or intense practice. As with writer's cramp, the authors found no progression of dystonia beyond the hand.

Whenever practical, examine musicians and patients with other occupational or recreational dystonias while they perform the relevant task. Look for the same basic clinical features—dystonic posturing, cocontraction, tremor, myoclonus, mirror movements and a sensory trick.

Pathophysiology

For many years, writer's cramp was considered a psychosomatic condition and was treated as such. This continued until Sheehy and Marsden's paper was published in

1982 [2], which stated their belief that it is a focal dystonia. Psychological testing supports this view. Their paper [2] was highly influential; there was an abrupt change from the publication of nearly all papers on writer's cramp in psychiatric or psychology journals to publication in neurological or physiological journals.

It is very likely that all forms of task-specific hand dystonias share the same pathophysiology.

The techniques used to study the pathophysiology of other forms of dystonia have been applied also to writer's cramp and other task-specific dystonias. Electromyography (EMG) of muscles during performance of the inciting task, including writing and mimicking instrument playing, shows five abnormal motor patterns [7]: cocontraction of agonist-antagonist muscle pairs, prolonged EMG bursts, tremor, lack of selectivity during attempted independent finger movements and 'failure of willed activity'. Cocontraction is probably explained by impaired reciprocal inhibition [8].

Premovement cortical potentials (contingent negative variation [CNV]) are abnormal suggesting that sensory-motor integration, which is a necessary part of a motor subroutine, is impaired [9]. Transcranial magnetic stimulation studies of the motor cortex have shown abnormalities of cortical excitability [10] and inhibition [11]. This might explain the activation of muscles not needed in the task, the excessive activity of those that are needed, and the spreading of muscle overactivity from the hand and forearm to the arm and shoulder, known as dystonic 'overflow'. Positron emission tomography (PET) studies show abnormalities of cortical activation in writer's cramp [12] and musician's cramp [13].

Several observations suggest that focal dystonia, including writer's cramp, might have a sensory component [14,15]. High-frequency vibration stimulates Ia sensory afferents preferentially, and when applied to the affected limb produces in some patients with writer's cramp a tonic vibration reflex causing dystonic posturing, similar to that which occurs during writing. Injection of involved muscles with a mixture of alcohol and local anaesthetic blocks the tonic vibration reflex and H-reflexes, and can improve the dystonia without causing muscle weakness [16]. There are two possible explanations for this. The first is that the local anaesthetic-alcohol injection blocks muscle Ia afferents, reducing sensory input. The second is that the injection blocks overactive spindle gamma efferents that increase spindle sensitivity thereby reducing Ia afferent activity [17]. The clinical phenomenon of the 'sensory trick' also suggests a role for the sensory system in the pathophysiology of dystonia. Finally, there are abnormalities of the N30 potential of the median somatosensory evoked potentials (SEP), which represents early sensory processing in the cortex [17].

That focal hand dystonias most often affect tasks like writing or playing a musical instrument might simply reflect the facts that that they are complex and require considerable training. When first learning these tasks, performance is slow, an effort and difficult, with the need for frequent rests. There is often excessive cocontraction, activation of proximal muscles and postures that resemble dystonia. With practice, the movements become easier, more fluid and less of an effort, with greater economy of muscle activation. Such training involves forming motor subroutines requiring integration of sensory input with complex patterns of motor inhibition and activation. If predisposed, perhaps genetically, this could all break down and cause an action dystonia. Peripheral trauma is becoming more accepted as a trigger or even a cause of dystonia and other movement disorders, and there is much circumstantial evidence to support this [18]. However, only about 5% of patients with writer's cramp have a history of trauma that could be considered relevant [4], although it might occur more frequently in musicians [6].

Focal hand dystonia is a central nervous system disorder, probably based in the basal ganglia, leading to dysfunction of the planning and execution of motor commands. The result is activation of muscles normally involved in the task that is excessive, either in amount, duration or timing, and/or activation of muscles not normally involved in the task.

Diagnosis

The diagnosis of writer's cramp is usually made from the history and watching the patient write and draw (Table 9.2 & Fig. 9.1). For the other occupational or recreational dystonias, study the affected task. The history and neurological examination should exclude most neurological diseases that can mimic writer's cramp—focal nerve entrapments, radiculopathies, generalized dystonia, dopa-responsive dystonia, movement disorders such as Parkinson's disease, and other neurological diseases. The hardest condition to separate from writer's cramp is an overuse disorder, such as tenosynovitis or tendinitis. Severe pain and focal tenderness over tendons or bony attachments can help.

Occasionally tests are needed, such as nerve conduction studies and EMG (Table 9.3). Magnetic resonance imaging (MRI) of the brain is usually unnecessary in straightforward task-specific dystonia. I recommend testing for Wilson's disease with serum copper and caeruloplasmin levels. Although patients with the *DYT1* gene have presented with writer's cramp, based on published recommendations [19] it is not necessary to test for this unless there is a strong family history of dystonia and the patient's condition began under the age of 26 years. I do not prescribe levodopa routinely for all patients with writer's cramp as a test for dopa-responsive dystonia.

Conventional treatment

Standard medications for dystonia are the anticholinergic drugs, such as trihexyphenidyl and benzodiazepines, such as clonazepam. These have the same poor response rate in writer's cramp and other limb dystonias of about 10–20% [1,2]. Side-effects probably prevent reaching an effective dose. Other drugs tried for focal dystonia include baclofen, valproate, gabapentin, and tizanidine. Specialist physiotherapists have had some success, and there have been case reports of successful treatment with acupuncture and hypnotherapy, biofeedback, relaxation techniques, and writing

Table 9.2 History and examination points for writer's cramp.

History questions

1 Duration of problem and course (progressive?)
2 General problem: difficulty writing, e.g. slow, an effort, poor script? Pain or discomfort?
3 Specific problem: cramping, abnormal postures, tremor, myoclonic jerks?
4 Latency (time after starting to write that symptoms appear), getting shorter?
5 Amount of writing before forced to stop, getting shorter?
6 Tried using non-dominant hand to write? If so, for how long?
7 Blackboard or whiteboard writing affected?
8 Sensory trick? (E.g. touching writing hand or forearm with other hand)
9 Onset after trauma, or during a period of stress, or intense writing?
10 Family history of similar problems, tremor, Parkinson's disease, other movement disorders?
11 Task-specific, now or in the past, or non-task specific? (Especially with other fine movements, such as typing, playing a musical instrument, painting, knitting, buttoning)

Examination

1 Resting posture of the hand
2 Picking up a pen
3 Pen on paper poised to write, relaxed and then with firm grip
4 Writing standard material (phrase, address, poem, etc.)
5 Drawing tasks (spirals, joined loops, saw-tooth vertical lines)
6 Left-hand writing (mirror movements)
7 Blackboard or whiteboard writing
8 Other tasks—doing up buttons, drinking from a glass, using a spoon, etc.
9 Palpation for tenderness, muscle contraction (including cocontraction)
10 'Movement disorders examination: gait, coordination, muscle tone, postural stability, resting, postural or action tremors, eye movements, evidence of dystonia elsewhere
11 General neurological examination

retraining [1,2]. None of these treatments has been tested in blinded trials and any benefits do not last [2]. A trial of levodopa should be considered when dopa-responsive dystonia is possible, especially for dystonia beginning in the leg.

Botulinum toxin treatment of focal limb dystonia

Rationale

EMG studies of focal hand dystonia [7] indicate that the abnormal motor command generated centrally leads to muscle activity in the wrong place and at the wrong time. Botulinum toxin (Bt) is a natural choice because it can reduce muscle overactivity selectively, and to a controllable degree. We have no conclusive evidence that Bt exerts its beneficial effect in any other way, despite suspicions of the contrary.

Dystonic muscle overactivity may interfere with writing function in several ways. First, writing may be impaired mechanically by an abnormal posture, such as flexion or

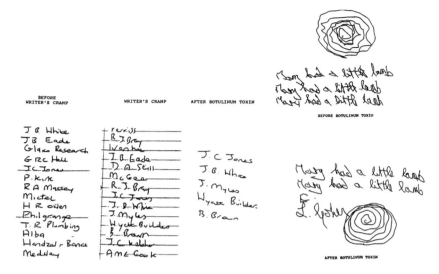

Fig. 9.1 Writing and drawing tasks in the evaluation of writer's cramp.

Table 9.3 Investigations for writer's cramp.

Routine
Serum copper and caerulopalsmin (and more detailed testing for Wilson's disease when indicated)

When indicated
Nerve conduction and EMG studies — for focal nerve entrapments and root disease, etc.
MRI brain
Polyelectromyography — for diagnosis and selection of muscles
DYT1 gene test

EMG, electromyography; MRI, magnetic resonance imaging.

extension of the wrist or pronation of the forearm. Similarly, there may be flexion of a finger or thumb, pushing it against the pen, or extension of a finger or thumb, which lifts off the pen. Writing becomes difficult because the hand is not in the best position for writing or because of loss of control of the pen. Second, because writing involves a carefully controlled sequence of agonist and antagonist muscle contractions, failure of one or both muscles of an agonist-antagonist pair to relax appropriately (in time and amount) will interfere with this process. In some patients, the wrist and fingers appear to 'lock' or 'seize up' with intense cocontraction preventing normal writing. An abnormal posture need not necessarily be seen but some patients can feel and describe the sensation that their muscles 'want' to draw the hand into such a posture. Third, tremor and myoclonic jerks will impair writing. Fourth, and less commonly, discomfort interferes with writing. Mild pain can arise within the dystonic muscles, in compensatory muscles fighting against them, or within the soft tissues. Extreme pain is unusual and might suggest tenosynovitis or similar soft tissue inflammation.

There seem to be three types of muscle overactivity in writer's cramp and other task-specific dystonias. The first is the primary dystonic activity occurring in the forearm and hand (as described earlier). The second is an 'overflow' dystonia involving more proximal muscles, accounting for the abnormal elbow and shoulder movements such as shoulder abduction with elbow elevation and extension. It is triggered by, or is in some way associated with, the primary dystonic movement. The third is voluntary or semivoluntary, non-dystonic, compensatory muscle activity which represents an attempt to overcome the dystonic activity or to counteract its effects in order to gain better control of the pen. I suspect that even this compensatory muscle activity can become distorted by dystonia. One patient with dystonic extension of the index finger during writing developed progressive hyperflexion of the other fingers and thumb, as though her compensatory index finger flexion command had spread to the other fingers.

Literature review

Open label studies of the treatment of focal hand dystonia with botulinum toxin A (BtA) have generally shown good results. Rivest and colleagues [20] produced subjective improvement in 11 of 12 (92%) patients, seven of whom (58%) thought it was significant. Others have obtained similar degrees of subjective improvement: Cohen and colleagues, 84% [21]; Wissel and colleagues, 76% [22]. Other studies [23,24] also report 'significant' improvements. Turjanski and colleagues [25] found that 27 of 44 patients improved on at least one occasion after an injection. Only 16 patients continued receiving injections, all with good response over 4 years. The reasons for dropping out were side-effects (four patients), poor response (10 patients) and lack of sustained response (six patients). Nine patients were lost to follow-up, five of whom had obtained 'clear benefit'. Thus, only 16 (36%) remained on treatment. Others have found that good long-term results can be achieved [26]. In one study of musician's dystonia [27], 83% (15 of 18 patients) reported some degree of benefit, with only six patients considering it major improvement, enough to continue professional performance.

Although there have been numerous placebo-controlled, blinded trials of Bt treatment for other focal dystonias, there have been only three for writer's cramp [28–30]. In one placebo-controlled crossover study, only six out of 20 patients reported improvement after a single dose of BtA, four with definite improvement and two with slight improvement [28]. Blind ratings of their writing were better in only four of the 20 patients, all of whom reported improvement. Twelve patients improved in a computerized test of pen control, contrasting with the low number with subjective improvement. A placebo-controlled crossover study of 10 patients with occupational hand dystonia found subjective benefit in eight patients, confirmed by objective tests of performance [30]. However, these were not naive patients; all had responded to BtA in the past. In another study of focal hand dystonia [29], seven of the nine patients with writer's cramp improved with at least one of the three doses of Bt that were given: one patient also improved substantially with placebo.

The better results in open label studies compared with the placebo studies might be due to the study design and the choice of outcome measures. Many of the open label studies involved one or only a few injection sessions but Turjanski's [25] experience tells us that an initial good response might not be maintained.

While encouraging, the blinded studies do not show convincing objective improvement in writing. Objective benefit could be difficult to achieve. Some qualities of writing, such as comfort, degree of effort, or the patient's confidence are not easily measured or suitable for objective evaluation. The more readily quantifiable parameters, such as speed, duration and possibly legibility of writing, might not be impaired or considered significant by the patient. Wissel and colleagues [22] used computerized analysis of writing speed to show a significant improvement after BtA in their open label study. Tsui and colleagues [28] also used computerized analysis of the speed and accuracy of pen movement and found statistically significant improvement compared with placebo. However, this contrasted with relatively rare subjective improvement in writing. The discrepancy might have occurred because the computerized test was not of writing. Blind reviews of video recordings of handwriting did not show improvement with BtA in one placebo-controlled study [29] but did in an open study [22]. The individuality of the writing problem argues against standardized outcome measures. Likewise, the individual sensitivity to the toxin and the wide range of degree of muscle overactivity argues against using standardized doses. Furthermore, it often takes several treatment sessions to find the best dose and muscle combination; studies evaluating response after a single treatment are less likely to show a benefit. The question of true blinding in placebo-controlled studies of BtA is especially relevant in writer's cramp because patients easily notice even slight weakness in their hand. All of this makes it extremely difficult to show a clear objective benefit of BtA therapy in writer's cramp.

Patient satisfaction is the ultimate goal of therapy but can be misleading. Some patients need a very high level of writing ability (or musical performance) that BtA treatment cannot provide, and rate their response poorly. One patient, who could only write a few lines before treatment, could afterwards write up to two pages; he still rated his response as poor because he wanted to write continuously for half an hour or more. Professional musicians with a focal hand dystonia who want to be able to continue solo concert performances are hard to satisfy, perhaps because they usually need both normal power and normal control.

Treatment

The assessment and treatment proceeds in several stages:

1 Identification of overactive muscles.
2 Selection of overactive muscles for injection.
3 Choosing the dose.

4 Injection.

5 Follow-up.

Identification of overactive muscles

A short examination of the act of writing is usually enough to make the diagnosis of writer's cramp. However, choosing the muscles for injection requires a more detailed examination before treatment with Bt. Just as with other occupational or recreational focal limb dystonias, examine the particular task involved. Take a video recording for comparison after treatment. The location of any muscular discomfort and palpation of muscles can be a clue to muscle overactivity but cannot distinguish between dystonic and compensatory overactivity.

Most important is observation during various writing and drawing tasks, watching for any abnormal postures and movements. I use some standard writing tasks (e.g. the poem 'Mary had a little lamb', their name and address) and drawing tasks (e.g. a spiral, loops) (Fig. 9.1). Initially, I look for dystonic postures of the fingers or wrist that might only develop after prolonged writing, the cramp delay or latency. Common patterns include flexion of the wrist, especially with ulnar deviation, excessive flexion of one (especially the index finger) or more fingers, or of the thumb (Figs 9.2a,b & 9.3). Corresponding extensor patterns are also common (Figs 9.2c & 9.3). Patients may begin to perform these tasks using an altered writing technique they have adopted to compensate for their problem, for example, a different pen grip or arm and hand posture, and many of these look quite unnatural. This can either mask their dystonia or else give the false impression of dystonic posturing when the problem is, say, a pure writing tremor. Ask the patients try to write using their 'normal', premorbid technique, even though this can be difficult because many have forgotten how they used to hold the pen. They should avoid fighting any dystonic movement and should disregard the quality of the writing they produce. However, the adaptive postures can sometimes reveal the dystonic features. For instance, if a patient no longer involves the index finger in writing it could be because its action is dystonic.

Dystonic posturing can develop gradually during writing, with progressive addition of muscles. For example, the index finger might flex first, followed by the thumb, then the other fingers, and finally the wrist. This could indicate that the flexion of index finger is the primary dystonic movement and that the others represent dystonic overflow. Resolution of all abnormal postures with selective treatment of the index finger flexors would confirm this. Having identified a dystonic movement or posture, remember that several muscles may control a particular action, acting in synergy. For example, flexion of the index finger may be due to activity of the deep or superficial finger flexor, or some combination of the two: rarely, the lumbrical-interosseous muscles are important. Given that task-specific dystonia represents disordered control of normal movement, which is programmed as an action rather than movements of individual muscles, several muscles could be acting abnormally. Observation alone might reveal the muscle that is chiefly re-

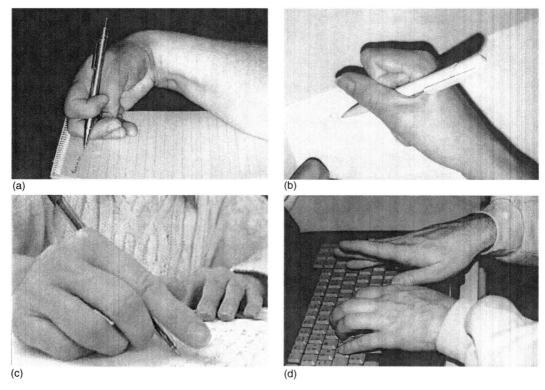

Fig. 9.2 Some examples of dystonic postures during writing or typing. (a) Hyperflexion of the wrist and dystonic posturing of the thumb and fingers (especially digit 2). (b) Dystonic flexion of the right index finger during writing. (c) Dystonic extension of the index finger during writing. The finger eventually lifts off the pen. (d) Dystonic extension of the right index finger during typing. (a,b,d Courtesy of Markus Naumann, Würzburg.)

sponsible. A helpful trick [I learned recently from David Simpson (Mt. Sinai Hospital, New York)] is to ask the patient to 'freeze' their hand position when the dystonic posture has occurred during writing and to turn the hand over to examine the position of the wrist and fingers.

Proximal abnormal postures might occur, such as a rising elbow due to shoulder abduction or even truncal twisting. This has been attributed to spread of dystonic activity to more proximal muscles, dystonic 'overflow', but in some cases it seems compensatory, to counteract the dystonic posture. For example, with dystonic wrist extension, which takes the pen away from the paper, shoulder abduction raises the elbow and helps bring the pen back to the paper. Such proximal movements nearly always disappear with successful treatment of the distal dystonic movements.

One may also see tremor and infrequently, myoclonic jerks. Drawing tasks, especially the spiral, show tremor quite well. Making small, rapid circular movements with the pen will often reveal the extent of the loss of fine control of the pen and impaired

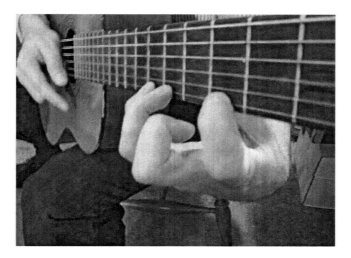

Fig. 9.3 Musician's dystonia in a professional guitarist. The middle finger tended to flex dystonically forcing it to miss strings or leave the fretboard. Fighting this tendency caused dystonic flexion of the index and middle fingers, possibly a dystonic overflow from the middle finger extensors. This forced the guitarist to stop performing. Injections of botulinum toxin to the middle finger fascicle of flexor digitorum profundus and flexor digitorum superficialis resulted in, according to the patient, 100% restoration of his guitar playing ability for 3 months.

ability to perform rapid alternating movements with the pen. It is also a continuous task that allows a longer period of time to identify the dystonic activity compared with writing, which is discontinuous.

On occasions there is no dystonic posture; the patient simply seems to have great difficulty writing and there may be cocontraction. Writing with the other hand might bring out a dystonic movement or posture on the affected side, known as a mirror movement. This can be very helpful when choosing muscles for Bt injection. When looking for mirror movements while writing with the unaffected hand, it is important for the affected hand to be relaxed and resting on its ulnar border. Use the same writing and drawing tasks. Other clues that might come from the drawing tasks include greater difficulty making an extensor movement compared with a flexor movement, such as during the vertical strokes. This could indicate a flexor pattern of dystonia.

Observant patients might report a sensation which the examiner cannot see, such as an involuntary tendency for the wrist or a particular digit to move in a certain direction. For example, they may feel that their thumb or index finger is involuntarily pushing down (flexing) excessively on the pen, perhaps indicating flexor dystonic activity. Having the patient hold the pen poised to write and gripping it firmly will, after a lag period, sometimes provoke dystonic activity such as an abnormal movement or posture. For example, this manoeuvre may provoke flexion of the thumb at the interphalangeal joint, just as it does during writing. However, because the patient is not trying to write it is easier to see and the patient has less inclination to overcome it, or it is easier for them to resist opposing it. In some cases, the patient reports that something 'takes over' and they begin to involuntarily grip the pen harder than they intend to. Palpation of the muscles will reveal intense cocontraction. Performing these same manoeuvres with the unaffected hand will make the difference between the two sides obvious.

Rating the severity of writer's cramp

Assess the many aspects of handwriting that can be affected by writer's cramp—the quality of script, the speed, duration, comfort, fluency, and ease of writing, and the patient's confidence in writing. Most patients report that their script has deteriorated for at least some of the time. There are rating scales for clinical and research use but the specific aspects of writing affected in a patient must be considered when judging the response to treatment and a standard assessment is not appropriate. Some of these characteristics are not easily quantified objectively and must remain subjective.

Electromyographic assessment

Sometimes it is hard to select target muscles for injection with clinical examination alone and EMG recording may help. Some physicians who treat writer's cramp and similar disorders routinely use EMG for this purpose, looking for abnormal patterns of muscle activation, as described by Cohen and Hallet [6]. I do not routinely use EMG to *choose* muscles for injection in my clinic, except for writing tremor, but EMG or electrical stimulation is essential in guiding the injection to the target muscles. Rivest and colleagues [20] reported high rates of success without using EMG to select muscles. However, the value of EMG in selecting muscles for injection has not yet been formally studied.

Record EMG during the writing or drawing tasks mentioned earlier, using surface electrodes placed over the wrist flexors and extensors. Short, fine needle electrodes can be used in other muscles (pronator teres, pronator quadratus, supinator, flexor pollicis longus). However, recording during writing from some of the muscles commonly involved (deep finger flexors) is not possible or not practical with surface or needle electrodes, and implanted wire electrodes are somewhat impractical for busy clinics [6]. Occasionally it proves useful to show abnormal cocontraction that is not obvious clinically, or tonic spasm, or a loss of the normal alternating patterns. Even with EMG it can be difficult to know whether activity in a muscle represents the primary dystonia, cocontraction or compensatory activity.

EMG recording can be more useful in cases with substantial tremor. The wrist flexors and extensors are all suitable for surface electrode recording and satisfactory recordings can be made from supinator, pronator teres and pronator quadratus using fine, short concentric needle electrodes during writing or drawing. One often finds that not all of the four wrist flexors and extensors are active in producing a flexion/extension type tremor. Only three or even two of these muscles might be active and, surprisingly, antagonist muscles may not be involved; it may be the flexors alone or the extensors alone, or only one of the wrist flexor or extensor muscle pairs. In the same way, when there is a component of pronation-supination, I have seen cases where pronator teres was not involved but pronator quadratus was very active: in one patient, this was the only muscle active from the pronator-supinator group in what appeared clinically to be a purely flexion-extension tremor. EMG recording in tremor is not only educational but allows selection of muscles for injection; there is no point injecting muscles not active in the tremor.

As noted by Cohen and Hallet [6], some patients with writer's cramp appear to not have excessive muscle contraction but rather a failure of voluntary movement, akin to the hypokinesia of Parkinson's disease. One patient of mine had a tendency for excessive flexion of the thumb which, when treated with BtA, improved his writing. However, he continued to have difficulty writing and EMG recording revealed a paucity of EMG activity whilst attempting to write, suggesting a failure of central motor drive. Such patients are not suitable for Bt therapy.

Selection of muscles for injection

It can be difficult to distinguish between dystonic and compensatory muscular hyperactivity. With experience, clinical patterns become familiar and mirror movements might help. Once a dystonic action is identified, I prefer to begin by injecting only one of the agonists that could produce the action. For example, with dystonic index finger flexion, I might choose to start with flexor digitorum profundus or flexor digitorum superficialis, depending upon the appearance of the movement. If the response to an adequate weakening of the first muscle is unsatisfactory, the other can be added or substituted. Table 9.4 provides some guidelines. One frequently finds that some seemingly dystonic movements disappear when a primary dystonic muscle is injected. In one patient, the index

Table 9.4 Guidelines for the injection of muscles according to the dystonic action.

Dystonic posture	Muscles
Finger flexion	Flexor digitorum profundus, flexor digitorum superficialis, lumbricales
Finger extension	Extensor digitorum communis, extensor indicis proprius, palmar interosseous
Thumb flexion	Flexor pollicis longus, flexor pollicis brevis
Thumb extension	Extensor pollicis brevis, extensor pollicis longus
Wrist flexion	Flexor carpi radialis, flexor carpi ulnaris
Wrist extension	Extensor carpi radialis, extensor carpi ulnaris
Thumb adduction	Adductor pollicis
Ankle plantarflexion	Gastrocnemius, soleus (tibialis posterior, flexor digitorum longus, flexor hallucis longus)
Ankle inversion	Tibialis posterior, medial gastrocnemius (tibialis anterior, flexor digitorum longus, flexor hallucis longus)
Great toe dorsiflexion	Extensor hallucis longus
Toe flexion	Flexor digitorum brevis, flexor digitorum longus

finger would flex first, then the thumb and wrist. Injection of the index finger prevented all dystonic movements. The proximal 'overflow' dystonic postures do not usually require treatment as they also frequently improve with treatment of the distal muscles. A stepwise approach has the advantage of clarifying which of the muscles injected are responsible for the clinical benefit and of limiting the dose and side-effects of BtA. Another reason for not injecting all overactive muscles is that some might not be functionally important. For example, all fingers may flex excessively but flexion of the fourth and fifth fingers usually does not impair writing, while flexion of the thumb, index and middle fingers does.

Dose selection

DOSES: A HEALTH WARNING

Please read the warning on p. 35 about doses of Bt. There are three preparations available. *Dysport®* and *Botox®* are type A toxins (BtA), *NeuroBloc®/MYOBLOC™* is type B (BtB). Even though the doses for each are quoted in mouse units (mu), the three preparations have different dose schedules: one mu of *Dysport®* is **not** the same as one mu of *Botox®*, and neither is equivalent to one mu of *NeuroBloc®/MYOBLOC™*.

For the first injection, I take a typical starting dose (Table 9.5) and modify it according to several factors. These include the degree of muscle overactivity, the patient's likely tolerance of excessive weakness of the muscle (consider personality, profession, hobbies, level of concern about weakness), and the size of the muscle in that patient. In general, it is best to begin with a conservative dose because patients tolerate excessive weakness poorly and it could discourage the patient from continuing with treatment. Note that the doses used are generally less than those used to treat the same muscles in spasticity.

Table 9.5 Suggested starting doses (mu) of botulinum toxin for task-specific hand dystonia.

Muscle	Usual number of injection sites (range)	Botox®	Dysport®
Extensor carpi radialis/ulnaris	2 (1–2)	10	40
Flexor carpi radialis/ulnaris	2 (1–2)	15	60
Flexor digitorum profundus	1 per fascicle	5–10 per fascicle	30–40 per fascicle
Extensor indicis proprius	1	5	20–30
Flexor pollicis longus	1	10	40
Extensor pollicis longus/brevis	1	5	10–15
Flexor digitorum superficialis	1 per fascicle	10	30–40 per fascicle

Injection technique

To treat focal dystonia using BtA, I dilute 1 vial of Dysport® (500 mu) with 2.5 mL saline (=20 mu/0.1 mL) or 1 vial of Botox® (100 mu) with 1 mL saline (=10 mu/0.1 mL); BtB (MYOBLOC®) is a solution of 5000 mu/mL. Diffusion increases with volume and hence dilution [31]. The number of muscles and the anatomical complexity of the forearm demands highly accurate placement and if diffusion is a problem the toxin might need to be more concentrated (e.g. half the volume); this is not possible with MYOBLOC®, which can only be diluted.

The injection is given with a needle that can also record EMG or deliver electrical stimuli. I use disposable Teflon®-coated hollow 26G needles (Myoject®, TECA®). Anatomical guides [32] are very helpful but do not guarantee accurate localization because there is much individual variation. Using EMG guidance check placement by having the patient voluntarily contract the target muscle as well as those nearby. However, it is sometimes difficult to voluntarily contract one without the other, even in the normal patient, and lack of selectivity is a feature of dystonia [6]. Localization by electrical stimulation of the muscle through the injection needle overcomes this problem, as it causes the muscle to contract and move the attached body part. Although it is not proven in clinical practice, accurate localization should help the success of the injection, produce consistent responses, and limit unwanted diffusion. A fairly standard injection technique will also help reproducibility. A standard EMG machine will perform both EMG and electrical stimulation but there are small devices that only stimulate or only record audio EMG. I use a single injection site for small muscles, like extensor indicis proprius and flexor pollicis longus, and two or more injection sites for larger muscles, like flexor carpi radialis and biceps and most of the leg muscles.

Bt readily diffuses across fascial planes, leading to less weakness of the injected muscle and causing weakness of adjacent muscles. This is common in the forearm and is one reason for a poor result [33]. Common patterns of diffusion in the arms are listed in Table 9.4. Choosing the right approach to the muscle may help to reduce weakness in adjacent muscles. For example, an approach from the radial aspect of extensor carpi radialis might avoid weakness of extensor digitorum communis. Diffusion is less of a problem in the leg.

Postinjection instructions and follow-up

I neither encourage nor discourage activity of the injected arm after the injection. Although exercise immediately afterwards produces more weakness, the clinical results are not better than enforced rest [34]. Weakness begins within a week, usually within a few days, but the clinical benefit can be delayed for some weeks.

I ask patients to report by telephone about 2–3 weeks later, when the response is usually apparent. Review in person is better but not always possible because of distance or other restrictions. Poor responses without excessive weakness could warrant a small 'top-up' injection, but these must be used cautiously. I usually reserve top-ups for the first injection only, as they might increase the risk of clinical resistance (see Chapter 3). The top-up dose is determined by the degree of weakness produced by the initial injection and is usually 25–50% of the initial dose. If this injection subsequently proves successful, injection of the total dose given (initial plus top-up) on the next occasion may sometimes be excessive and so I may inject only 75–80% of this total. The usual treatment interval is 3 months and responses usually last 2.5–3.0 months, although some patients obtain longer benefit, occasionally up to 6 months. Some patients need oral medications, such as trihexyphenidyl or clonazepam, to help them through the period after the benefit has worn off and until the next injection begins to work.

At each review, I ask the time to the onset and to the peak of response, the duration of the weakness and benefit, the degree of benefit at maximum (as a percentage of normal), and any side-effects. Patients also rate their writing ability at the time of review, for example, 70% of normal. I ask about changes in speed, legibility, duration, comfort, and ease of writing. I test the strength of the injected and adjacent muscles, and examine writing and drawing. Wissel and colleagues [22] developed a standardized rating scale for a clinical trial but I prefer an individualized evaluation. Keep samples of writing and drawing. Video recordings are ideal. Use these assessments to decide on subsequent injection sites and doses. It usually takes a few injection sessions to find the best treatment regimen.

Some degree of weakness seems necessary for success, but it is difficult to say how much is desirable. I aim for the least amount of weakness that gives a satisfactory response. Some patients obtain benefit with remarkably little weakness whereas others only obtain good results with a degree of weakness that interferes with other actions of the hand. The trick is so seek a balance between enough weakness to help the dystonia and too much weakness that makes overall hand function deteriorate unacceptably.

A poor response could be due to incorrect muscle selection such as a compensatory muscle, or injection of only one of the agonist muscles producing the dystonic movement. There may be insufficient weakness, excessive weakness, or weakness of adjacent muscles. Given the inherent variability in the potency of the toxin and in the injection technique, I advise against making too large a change in dose based upon the outcome of a single injection.

Continuing treatment in the longer term

When repeated injection cycles produce consistent responses, consider trying to lower the dose by 10–20%. Similarly, muscles that no longer seem dystonic could be omitted from the injection session as a test. Often, patients doing well have diminishing dystonic posturing at each subsequent injection; whilst this is clearly a good thing, it does mean that the best chance to see the problem is before Bt is given. Without that experience or history it can be hard to understand why certain muscles have been injected. Continuity of care is important, especially as it can be difficult to relate the full flavour of treatment decisions in the written notes. Occasionally, patients report that the injections are becoming less helpful. Before immediately fearing secondary non-response, consider the patient's altered perception; the first injection often seems the best, in its contrast with the untreated state. Withholding the toxin for a while might clarify the situation.

The pattern of the dystonia can change after the first injection [25]. One of my patients who appeared to have an isolated problem of excessive thumb flexion improved dramatically after injection into flexor pollicis longus but then noticed that her index finger was also flexing excessively. Another patient improved after injection of the deep flexor of the index finger but after a few treatments also developed a tendency for the middle finger to flex. Whether these changes reflect progression of the disease or an unmasking of a covert dystonic muscle is unknown, but given the rapidity with which it develops after beginning BtA treatment, I suspect the latter.

When the duration of benefit and weakness is short, a higher dose might produce a more prolonged response. There is a risk of provoking excessive weakness without any prolongation of benefit. Some patients notice a biphasic profile of weakness, with an initial period of more profound weakness lasting a few weeks that partially recovers. This might be due to reinnervation of some muscle fibres by collaterals [35]. Thereafter, strength remains stable until BtA gradually starts to wear off at about 2.5–3.0 months. One patient needed this initial period of excessive weakness in order to obtain a satisfactory duration of benefit subsequently.

Side-effects

The main side-effect is excessive weakness of the injected muscle. This is more common after the first injection when the patients' particular sensitivity to the toxin is unknown. Weakness of adjacent muscles (Table 9.6 [33]) occurs because of diffusion. It is common and can cause a poor outcome [33], but it is usually not disabling. Rashes and flu-like symptoms are very uncommon. I have not yet seen secondary clinical resistance, suggesting the development of immunity, possibly because of the lower doses of toxin used compared with torticollis. A very rare complication is a condition resembling neuralgic amyotrophy [36]. Some target muscles are close to blood vessels or nerves, such as the pronator teres and flexor carpi radialis (brachial artery and median nerve) and the flexor pollicis longus (radial artery), and there is the potential for damage to these structures.

Table 9.6 Common patterns of diffusion in the upper limb (compiled from personal experience and [33]).

Muscle injected	Diffusion to
Extensor carpi radialis	Extensor digitorum communis
Flexor pollicis longus	Flexor digitorum superficialis to digit 2, flexor digitorum profundus to digit 2
Flexor carpi ulnaris	Flexor digitorum profundus to digits 4 and 5
Extensor indicis proprius	Extensor pollicis longus, extensor pollicis brevis
Extensor carpi ulnaris	Extensor pollicis longus, extensor digitorum communis to digit 5
Flexor digitorum superficialis	Flexor digitorum profundus

Predicting and assessing outcome

It is difficult to predict who will benefit from treatment. Tsui and colleagues [28] suggested that those with wrist-joint deviation did better than those without. In my experience, those that do best are those with very clear dystonic postures involving few muscles. The outcome is worse when it is difficult to identify target muscles. Because of the delicate and sometimes impossible balance between dystonia suppression and weakness it is harder to satisfy patients such as musicians [27] and those who need to write a lot or very quickly.

Other limb dystonias

The treatment of limb dystonia not related to an occupational or recreational task is similar and less complicated [36]. The overactive muscles are usually not hard to identify because the dystonic postures are often present at rest (Figs 9.4 & 9.5). Common patterns in the arms are finger and elbow flexion or extension, wrist flexion (less often extension), and shoulder flexion, adduction or extension. There may be inversion or plantarflexion of the ankle, or dorsiflexion of the great toe ('striatal toe'). Some postures are induced or aggravated by action such as walking or attempting to pick up an object. Using these dystonic postures to choose muscles for injection requires only knowledge of functional anatomy. EMG is occasionally helpful. As with all dystonia, there may also be tremor or myoclonus. Leg muscles need higher doses than the arm and it can be more difficult to achieve the weakness needed for a good response (Table 9.7). On the other hand, excessive weakness occurs less often.

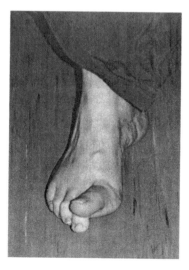

Fig. 9.4 'Striatal toe' due to dystonic activation of the extensor hallucis longus muscle. (Courtesy of Markus Naumann, Würzburg.)

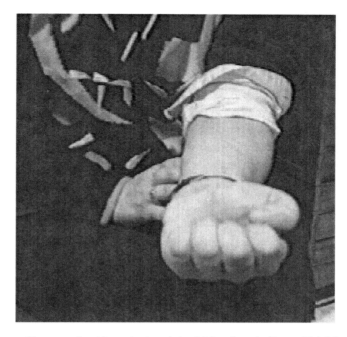

Fig. 9.5 A case of late-onset hemidystonia. A stroke in childhood resulted in a stable left hemiparesis with little spasticity. Many years later, the woman developed painful dystonic spasms of her left wrist and fingers, most often in flexion, that prevented her from typing.

Table 9.7 Suggested starting doses (mu) for some muscles in the lower limbs.

Muscle	Usual number of injection sites (range)	Botox®	Dysport®
Tibialis posterior	2 (1–4)	100	250
Gastrocnemius (one belly)	2 (1–2)	100	200
Soleus	2 (1–2)	100	200
Flexor hallucis longus	1	50	150
Flexor digitorum longus	2 (1–2)	75	200
Extensor hallucis longus	1	50	150
Flexor digitorum brevis	2 (1–2)	100	250

Unlike the occupational or recreational limb dystonias, the goal here is less often to restore active function and more often to reduce pain, improve hygiene, prevent contractures, or make activities of daily living easier for the patient and their carer. However, BtA treatment of dystonic equinovarus deformity can improve gait substantially. When the dystonia is so severe that there is very little active function to preserve in the limb, the dose of BtA can be more liberal as there is less concern about worsening function with excessive weakness. As with spasticity, some of the hypertonia might be due to soft tissue changes rather than muscle contraction.

Future directions

We should try to find a way to prolong the duration of the toxin's action. Like most dystonia, limb dystonia is usually life-long. A prolonged action would mean fewer injections, which would be more convenient for the patient and would expose them to less toxin, reducing side-effects and perhaps secondary resistance. One of the most frustrating parts of treating task-specific dystonias is that several injection sessions are often needed to get the best result. With the usual 3-month minimal interval between injections, this could mean 9–12 months of trial and error. If there were no risk of immunogenicity and secondary clinical resistance, patients could receive more frequent injections, speeding up the process. We have no clear way to separate dystonic from compensatory muscle overactivity, and no definitive way to determine which dystonic muscle activity is primary, and therefore a target for injection, and which is secondary. Electrophysiological or other tests to tease out this puzzle would be welcome.

Summary

Three double blind clinical trials [28–30] and many open label trials [20–27] give relatively strong support for the use of Bt in occupational hand dystonia. However, many neurologists are reluctant to use botulinum toxin in hand dystonias. I suspect it is because they are difficult and time-consuming to evaluate and treat. Novice injectors often have poor results, with excessive weakness and little or no benefit, which discourages them from trying again. It is challenging to select the muscles for injection and localize the target muscle accurately. However, persistence is often rewarding, and for some patients the result is almost miraculous. More than other forms of focal dystonia, this condition should perhaps be treated only by those with a special interest.

References

1 Thompson PD. Writer's cramp. *Br J Hosp Med* 1993; **50**: 91–4.
2 Sheehy MP, Marsden CD. Writer's cramp—a focal dystonia. *Brain* 1982; **105**: 461–80.
3 Nutt JG, Muenter MD, Melton LJ, Aronson A, Kurlkand LT. Epidemiology of dystonia in Rochester. *Minnesota Adv Neurol* 1988; **50**: 361–6.
4 Sheehy MP, Rothwell JC, Marsden CD. Writer's cramp. In: Fahn, S *et al.*, eds. *Dystonia 2, Adv Neurology*, Vol. 50. Raven Press: New York, 1988: 457–72.
5 Jedynak P, Tranchant C, Zegers de Beyl D. Prospective clinical study of writer's cramp. *Mov Disord* 2001; **16**: 494–9.
6 Newmark JA, Hochberg FH. Isolated painless manual incoordination in 57 musicians. *J Neurol Neurosurg Psychiatry* 1987; **50**: 291–5.
7 Cohen LG, Hallett M. Hand cramps: clinical features and electromyographic patterns in a focal dystonia. *Neurology* 1988; **38**: 1005–12.
8 Nakashima K, Rothwell JC, Day BL *et al.* Reciprocal inhibition between forearm muscles in patients with writer's cramp and other occupational cramps, symptomatic hemidystonia and hemiparesis due to stroke. *Brain* 1989; **112**: 681–97.

9   HamanoT, Kaji R, Katayama M *et al*. Abnormal contingent negative variation in writer's cramp. *Clin Neurophysiol* 1999; **110**: 508–15.

10 Ikoma K, Samii A, Mercuri B, Wassermann EM, Hallett M. Abnormal cortical motor excitability in dystonia. *Neurology*; Year?; **46**: 1371–6.

11 Ridding MC, Sheean G, Rothwell JC, Inzelberg R, Kujirai T. Changes in the balance between motor cortical excitation and inhibition in focal task-specific dystonia. *J Neurol Neurosurg Psychiatry* 1995; **59**: 493–8.

12 Ceballos-Baumann AO, Sheean G, Passingham RE, Marsden CD, Brooks DJ. Botulinum toxin does not reverse the cortical dysfunction associated with writer's cramp: a PET study. *Brain* 1997; **120**: 571–82.

13 Pujol J, Roset-Llobet J, Rosines-Cubells D *et al*. Brain cortical activation during guitar-induced hand dystonia studied by functional MRI. *Neuroimage* 2000; **12**: 257–67.

14 Hallet 1995 Hallett M. Is dystonia a sensory disorder [Editorial]? *Ann Neurol* 1995; **38**: 139–40.

15 Kaji R, Rothwell JC, Katayma M *et al*. Tonic vibration reflex and muscle afferent block in writer's cramp. *Ann Neurol* 1995; **38**: 155–62.

16 Kaji R. Facts and fancies on writer's cramp. *Muscle Nerve* 2000; **23**: 1313–5.

17 Hallet M. Disorder of movement preparation in dystonia [Editorial]. *Brain* 2000; **123**: 1765–6.

18 Jankovic J. Post-traumatic movement disorders. Central and peripheral mechanisms. *Neurology* 1994; **44**: 2006–14.

19 Bressman SB, Sabatti C, Raymond D *et al*. The DYT1 phenotype and guidelines for diagnostic testing. *Neurology* 2000; **54**: 1746–52.

20 Rivest J, Lees AJ, Marsden CD. Writer's cramp, treatment with botulinum toxin injections. *Mov Disord* 1991; **6**: 55–9.

21 Cohen LG, Hallett M, Geller BD, Hochberg F. Treatment of focal dystonias of the hand with botulinum toxin injections. *J Neurol Neurosurg Psychiatry* 1989; **52**: 355–63.

22 Wissel J, Kabus C, Wenzel R *et al*. Botulinum toxin treatment in writer's cramp: objective response evaluation in 31 patients. *J Neurol Neurosurg Psychiatry* 1996; **61**: 172–5.

23 Jankovic J, Schwatrz KS. Use of botulinum toxin treatment of hand dystonia. *J Hand Surg* 1993; **18A**: 883–7.

24 Behari M. Botulinum toxin in the treatment of writer's cramp. *J Assoc Physicians India* 1999; **47**: 694–8.

25 Turjanski N, Pirtosek Z, Quirk J *et al*. Botulinum toxin in the treatment of writer's cramp. *Clin Neuropharmacol* 1996; **19**: 314–20.

26 Karp BI, Cole RA, Cohen LG *et al*. Long-term botulinum toxin treatment of focal hand dystonia. *Neurology* 1994; **44**: 70–6.

27 Cole RA, Cohen LG, Hallett M. Treatment of musician's cramp with botulinum toxin. *Med Probl Peform Art* 1991; **6**: 137–43.

28 Tsui JK, Bhatt M, Calne S, Calne DB. Botulinum toxin in the treatment of writer's cramp: a double blind study. *Neurology* 1993; **43**: 183–5.

29 Yoshimura DM, Aminoff MJ, Olney RK. Botulinum toxin therapy for limb dystonias. *Neurology* 1992; **42**: 627–30.

30 Cole R, Hallett M, Cohen LG. Double blind trial of botulinum toxin for treatment of focal hand dystonia. *Mov Disord* 1995; **4**: 466–71.

31 Shaari CM, Sanders I. Quantifying how location and dose of botulinum toxin injections affect muscle paralysis. *Muscle Nerve* 1993; **16**: 964–9.

32 Perotto A. *Anatomical Guide for the Electromyographer: the Limbs and Trunk*, 3rd edn. Springfield, IL: Charles C. Thomas, 1994.

33 Ross MH, Charness ME, Sudarsky L, Logigian EL. Treatment of occupational cramp with botulinum toxin: diffusion of toxin to adjacent non-injected muscles. *Muscle Nerve* 1997; **20**: 593–8.

34 Chen R, Karp B, Goldstein S *et al*. Effect of muscle activity immediately after botulinum toxin injection for writer's cramp. *Mov Disord* 1999; **14**: 307–12.

35 de Paiva A, Meunier FA, Molgo J, Aoki KR, Dolly JO. Functional repair of motor endplates after botulinum neurotoxin type A poisoning: biphasic switch of synaptic activity between nerve sprouts and their parent terminals. *Proc Natl Acad Sci U S A* 1999; **96**: 3200–5.

36 Sheean GL, Murray NMF, Marsden CD. Pain and remote weakness in limbs injected with botulinum toxin for writer's cramp. *Lancet* 1995; **346**: 154–6.

37 A. Quirk JA, Sheean GL, Marsden CD, Lees AJ. Treatment of non-occupational limb and trunk dystonia with botulinum toxin. *Mov Disord* 1996; **11**: 377–83.

Spasticity in adults

JEAN-MICHEL GRACIES, HARALD HEFTER,
DAVID M SIMPSON & PETER MOORE

Introduction

Muscle overactivity is one of the three cardinal disabling features in patients with spasticity, accompanying motor weakness and muscle shortening. Muscle overactivity is not evenly distributed throughout the muscles, and across joints there is usually imbalance between agonists and antagonists. Local treatment targeting overactivity in specific muscles is therefore often preferable to systemic approaches.

Das and Park were the first to report the use of botulinum toxin (Bt) in the treatment of spasticity in adults. They observed improvement in six patients with stroke-related spasticity treated with Bt in an open study [1]. However, the idea was not entirely new. Justinus Kerner (1786–1862), the German physician and poet who wrote the first accurate and comprehensive description of botulism, proposed a variety of therapeutic uses for the toxin, including muscle hyperactivity.

Regulatory agencies in some European countries have approved botulinum toxin A (BtA) for the treatment of childhood and adult spasticity, but it still awaits approval for spasticity by the Food and Drug Administration (FDA) in the US. Strictly speaking, a large amount of expert practice with Bt remains 'off-licence' and unproven, especially in the field of spasticity [2]. Where relevant, patients and caregivers must understand and accept that Bt remains off-licence (i.e. off-label).

There has been considerable experience with BtA in spasticity over the last decade, through pragmatic clinical practice and open studies, supported by randomized controlled trials (RCTs). This chapter blends these streams of information and emphasizes the importance of using BtA for spasticity in the setting of the wider rehabilitation goals. When treating spasticity *BtA should not be used outside a combination with physical treatments.* This chapter reviews the evidence supporting the use of Bt in spasticity. It then presents practical guidelines on when and how to use Bt, and provides direction for future research.

What is spasticity, and how does it produce impairment?

Spasticity is a velocity-sensitive hyperreflexia. It is caused by disease of the *central nervous system* (CNS), i.e. the brain or spinal cord. Clinically, spasticity is a feature often associated with hypertonia, increased resistance to passive muscle stretch and limb movement. It is usually associated with other features such as weakness or poor control of voluntary muscle activation, altered sensation or sensory inattention. Spasticity is often compounded by additional brain disturbance affecting arousal, mood, language and other functions, any of which may profoundly disrupt rehabilitation.

The pathophysiology of spasticity is complex [3]. In the early stages neural components may predominate, and as spasticity evolves and becomes more persistent, immobilized muscles may remain in a contracted state for long periods. This aggravates the soft tissue changes due to immobilization, and may generate further biomechanical resistance to passive movement. Eventually, the shortening of the muscle-tendon complex may produce limb deformity. In many 'spastic' muscles there is little electromyographic (EMG) activity, and the resistance to passive movement is due mainly to the biomechanical component.

A primary aim of the treatment of spastic muscles is to maintain length and allow normal positioning of the limbs to prevent secondary soft tissue changes. Bt can facilitate this by relaxing targeted muscles, allowing them to be stretched and thus reducing both the neurogenic and biomechanical components of spasticity.

To appreciate the role of local treatments such as Bt in spasticity, it is useful to understand in more detail how spasticity is associated with functional impairment. Damage to central motor pathways results in two series of events in the neural-muscular-skeletal chain contributing to movement [4].

Acute events: paralysis, flaccidity, and muscle shortening

These acute events begin immediately or within hours of injury, often while the patient is still at the site of the accident, in the emergency room or the acute care unit. The injury to motor centres disrupts the function of several descending pathways, including the corticospinal pathway involved in the execution of voluntary commands. The resulting paralysis immediately leaves the muscles immobilized. In the acute care setting, patients typically lie supine in stretchers continuously, usually with the paralysed legs in full extension and the paralysed arms positioned with internal rotation of the shoulder, elbow flexion and pronation, and often wrist and finger flexion. Thus, some of the paralysed muscles are commonly immobilized in a short position, including leg extensors, and internal rotators, pronators and flexors in the arms. This immobilization in a shortened position is the initial mechanism for muscle contracture, which progresses in animals and humans through loss of sarcomeres (shortening), accumulation of connective tissue, and loss of protein mass [5,6]. The injury to motor centres and descending pathways also disrupts the descending flow that normally influences spinal cord reflex circuitry. At first, this commonly extinguishes many spinal reflex responses, including stretch reflexes, and translates into muscle flaccidity.

Subacute events: plastic neural rearrangements, muscle overactivity, changes in passive and active muscle properties, and muscle contracture

This second cascade of events unfolds in the several weeks following injury, and mostly consists of plastic neural rearrangements, a consequence of both the injury and paralysis-related disuse. As interrupted descending fibers degenerate, extensive sprouting occurs at segmental spinal levels. Interneuronal endings branch out onto other interneurones or somatic motorneuronal membranes to occupy the spaces left empty by the missing descending fibers [7]. The physiological result is the gradual emergence of abnormal and often excessive reflex responses to peripheral inputs such as cutaneous stimuli [8] or muscle stretch [9]. All contribute to global muscle overactivity [10]. In addition to these *spinal* plastic rearrangements, *higher* centres select replacement strategies to elicit movement, involving the remaining intact descending pathways (e.g. reticulospinal, rubrospinal, vestibulospinal), intact corticospinal fibers that may branch and sprout abnormally at the motorneurone level [11,12], or ipsilateral motor cortex activation [13]. Both mechanisms generate abnormal patterns of supraspinal descending drive, which contribute to muscle overactivity.

Muscle overactivity

It is useful to group muscle overactivity into two types [4,14], depending upon whether it involves prominent stretch-sensitivity, i.e. excessive reflex motor unit recruitment through activation of stretch-receptors in the overactive muscle.

In the first type there is stretch-sensitive muscle overactivity. Examples include *spasticity*, *spastic dystonia*, and *spastic cocontraction*. These are distinguished by their primary triggering factors, which are phasic muscle stretch, tonic muscle stretch, or volitional command, respectively [4].

Spasticity is a velocity-dependent increase in stretch reflex, i.e. excessive muscle contraction in response to *phasic* stretch in the absence of volitional motor command [15]. Spasticity is thus measured at rest.

Spastic dystonia, described by Denny-Brown [16], is tonic muscle contraction in the absence of phasic stretch or volitional command. Spastic dystonia is primarily due to an abnormal pattern of supraspinal descending drive that is characterized by the inability to relax muscles despite efforts to do so. Spastic dystonia is sensitive to the degree of *tonic* stretch imposed on the dystonic muscle [16].

Spastic cocontraction is the inappropriate recruitment of an antagonist, triggered by *willed command* of an agonist. This pathologic segmental cocontraction occurs in the absence of phasic stretch and is sensitive to the degree of tonic stretch of the cocontracting antagonist [17]. Like spastic dystonia, spastic cocontraction is primarily due to an abnormal pattern of supraspinal descending drive. Both can be aggravated by abnormal peripheral reflex reactions, in particular the degree of tonic stretch imposed on the overactive muscle.

The second category of muscle overactivity comprises forms that are not prominently stretch-sensitive. They include pathologic extrasegmental cocontraction (i.e. synkinesis, overflow, chorea, athetosis), excessive cutaneous or nociceptive responses, and inappropriate muscle recruitment during autonomic or reflex activities such as sneezing, coughing, and yawning. These forms of overactivity are also likely to involve some stretch-sensitivity, but this has not been established as a major feature.

Other factors in spastic hypertonia: changes in passive and active muscle properties

In patients with damage to the central motor pathways, clinicians often record increased tone (increased resistance to passive movement) even with slow movements [18]. Resistance to stretch may result from changes in passive muscle properties that are caused by prolonged immobilization and overactivity [6,19–21], and involve decreased passive extensibility of muscle. In patients with spasticity, even with no electrical or EMG activity *resting* muscle passively resists being stretched, and compared with normal muscle generates abnormally increased torque for the same degree of lengthening [5]. Immobilization or overactivity [22] also change *active* muscle properties [23–25], and increase the torque developed per motor unit recruited.

In conclusion, patients with spasticity are impaired by muscle weakness, inappropriate muscle overactivity and soft tissue contracture. We discuss now how a weakening agent such as Bt may promote functional improvement in these patients.

How does Bt work in spasticity?

Knowledge of the mechanism of action of Bt injections helps clinicians understand how it might influence the unfolding sequence of developing spasticity. Most of our knowledge comes from work with BtA although serotypes B, C, D, and F have also been studied [26–31].

In brief

The most obvious effect of intramuscular BtA is the induced muscle weakness and atrophy. Logically, the controlled, temporary weakness could reduce the available force of spastic contraction. A more subtle effect was suggested by animal studies showing that muscle spindle afferent activity may be reduced even before any detectable weakness (see below). Remote spread of the toxin to distant muscle spindles could contribute to this effect even with no detectable distant weakness. There may be direct or indirect central effects, as Bt receptors occur on a variety of cells within the brain and spinal cord. Patients given selective injections of BtA often gain more widespread relaxation of spasticity, but this could simply be due to the removal of a major focus of spasticity with its attendant pain, spasm and other discomforts which act to provoke the more widespread spasticity.

A protective effect?

There is some evidence that BtA may have a direct effect within the CNS (see below). However, it is possible that altering reflex activity and the force of contraction influences the evolution of central circuitry indirectly. Early treatment of spasticity could in theory break a cycle of spasm, pain, fibrosis and contracture and influence remodelling of central circuits. Bt treatment assists physiotherapy by easing manipulation of limbs and training of antagonists. It also allows more comfortable and better tolerated splinting.

In early studies using the hereditary spastic rat, Cosgrove and Graham injected BtA into the gastrocnemius muscle of infant rats, *before* they developed spasticity. They showed that BtA blocked the development of the expected biomechanical changes of spasticity, of overall shortening of the muscle-tendon unit, and increase in the tendon : muscle ratio [32]. Notably this experiment was performed in growing rats and perhaps is more relevant to human paediatric practice than to adult medicine, but it supports the possibility of a therapeutic window early in the development of spasticity, even in adults.

In depth

The various serotypes of Bt are structurally and functionally similar. They are high molecular weight protein complexes consisting of the neurotoxin and additional non-toxic proteins that protect the toxin molecule [33]. The A and B neurotoxin molecules are di-chain proteins, in which the heavy-chain binds to two distinct acceptors on nerve terminal membranes [34]. The ensuing uptake of Bt is energy and temperature-dependent and is accelerated by nerve stimulation, a treatment that also shortens the time course of the toxin-induced neuroparalysis [35]. The light-chain is a zinc-dependent endoprotease that cleaves synaptic proteins implicated in docking and fusion of vesicles, which in turn blocks transmission at all cholinergic synapses in the nervous system, and potentially other types of synapses [29,30]. The main physiological consequence in muscle is inhibition of spontaneous and evoked quantal neurotransmitter acetylcholine release at the α-motorneurone ending [33–37]. This results in reduced muscle activity, whatever the stimulus, including voluntary activation or electrical nerve stimulation.

The neurophysiological consequences of Bt action after intramuscular injection may involve the following factors:

CNS action

There is evidence for central effects after intramuscular injection of Bt. *In vivo* animal studies have shown that Bt can enter the CNS following peripheral administration [38]. Binding sites for Bt heavy-chain occur in several areas of CNS grey matter for all serotypes of Bt analysed, including A, B and C, particularly in the hippocampus and cerebellum [39–46]. Bt binding sites in animal brain synaptosomes are relatively serotype-specific [47]. In addition, Bt can inhibit release of acetylcholine from rat cerebrocortical synaptosomes, confirming that Bt affects synapses in the CNS [48].

Histoautoradiography shows that after intramuscular injection of Bt in animals, Bt or its fragments pass to the ventral roots and to the adjacent spinal cord by retrograde axonal transport, and spread to the contralateral spinal cord and ventral roots [49]. Direct stimulation of the injected muscle increases the retrograde transport to the ipsilateral spinal cord half segments [49]. Similar observations of intraxonal movement of toxin have been made with tetanus toxin [50]. Synthesis and/or proximo-distal axonal transport of other tracers may also change after intramuscular injection of Bt [51–53].

Retrograde axonal transport and central spread probably contribute to the significant impairments of central synaptic transmission, central reflexes and motoneuronal firing pattern observed in animals after high-dose injections or in experimental botulism [54–60]. Animal studies indicate that Bt blocks recurrent Renshaw inhibition when applied directly to the spinal cord (recurrent axon collaterals of α-motorneurones form cholinergic synapses with Renshaw cells), and central synaptic blocking may also occur in other spinal or supraspinal cholinergic pathways [59,61].

Intramuscular Bt injection may have central effects in humans, including decreased Renshaw inhibition and increased presynaptic inhibition exerted on the motorneurones supplying the injected muscle, and reduction of their overall excitability. H-wave reflexes persist in weakened muscles in human botulism, even when the stimulus amplitude is increased to the point where the reflex is inhibited in normal subjects [62]. There are relatively preserved F-waves (as compared with M-waves) in the human extensor digitorum brevis after Bt injection. Both these observations are consistent with decreased Renshaw inhibition [63].

Intramuscular injections of Bt into an agonist muscle increase presynaptic inhibition of the agonist even though Ia reciprocal inhibition at rest seems unchanged [64,65]. This suggests a central effect of Bt on presynaptic inhibitory interneurones rather than a peripheral effect of reduction of spindle activity, since the experiments were performed at rest, i.e. in the absence of gamma motoneuronal activity or significant ongoing stretch [65]. Compelling transcranial magnetic stimulation studies report increased central conduction time to the injected muscle 2 weeks postinjection (but not to its antagonist or to the same muscle contralaterally), consistent with altered responsiveness of spinal motor neurones to descending corticospinal tract impulses [66,67]. Furthermore, the recent finding of decreased F-waves in segments remote from the injection site suggests reduced motorneurone excitability not only in the motorneurones supplying the injected muscles, but also in distant motorneurones [68].

Central reflex changes were noted after blepharospasm injections in one study [69], but not others [70–73]. These central effects do not seem to include changes in conduction along axons [68,74]. Recent studies have also failed to demonstrate effects on ion channels at the presynaptic membrane (i.e. sodium, fast and slow potassium, calcium) [75].

These multiple central effects may partially explain unexpected findings following arm spasticity treatment in our patients. After Bt injections into a spastic agonist, there was reduced spastic cocontraction in both agonist and antagonist [76]. The decrease in Renshaw inhibition on the injected agonist may reduce cocontraction of the antagonist during movements. Indeed, it releases reciprocal Ia inhibition from the injected agonist to the antagonist during movement (in previous studies, changes in reciprocal Ia inhibition have been measured at rest only) [64,65].

Action on gamma motor neurone endings

Limited animal studies suggest that BtA may affect gamma (γ)- as well as alpha (α)-motorneurone endings and perhaps affect γ at lower doses than α endings [77–79]. Acetylcholine's role as a neurotransmitter in intrafusal muscle fibers [79] makes it possible that Bt also blocks intrafusal function. Most intrafusal fibers are encapsulated in spindles and it is not known how readily the 900 Kd molecule of Bt can penetrate the capsule. Rosales *et al.* showed early atrophy in both extrafusal and intrafusal fibers after injection of BtA in rat muscle [79]. However, this histological observation does not prove that spindle function is blocked after injection, as intrafusal fibre atrophy may also result from muscle disuse because of extrafusal dysfunction.

In spastic patients, measurements of stretch-dependent thixotropy before and after injection were unable to generate findings consistent with a γ effect of Bt (Gracies JM, Wilson L, Gandevia S, Burke D, personal communication). The presence and magnitude of a Bt effect on γ endings in humans might be clinically relevant in treating stretch-sensitive forms of muscle overactivity (in particular spastic cocontraction and spastic dystonia) [4]. If γ endings were more sensitive than α, then Bt might target stretch receptors through a reduction in spindle afferent activity (γ effect) with lower doses than those required to provoke significant weakness (α effect), and thus treat stretch sensitive forms of muscle overactivity without significantly weakening muscle.

Bt action on most active terminals

Bt may preferentially block the most active terminals, offering a rationale for methods to increase the efficacy of injections. Experiments in animals [80] and humans [81,82] report improved uptake of Bt by nerve terminals that are more active, whether this increased activity is induced by nerve stimulation [81] or increased voluntary activity [82]. This effect may focus Bt-induced weakness in those muscle fibers that are pathologically overactive. It is difficult to evaluate the clinical significance of this finding. In hemiparetic patients, Hesse *et al.* enhanced the improvement following Bt injection by performing periodic stimulation of the injected muscle and its antagonist for three 30-minute sessions a day during the three days following injection [83,84]. However, the stimulation program by itself also improved the parameters assessed (tone on Ashworth Scale, functional evaluation) [84], consistent with controlled data on electrical stimulation in spasticity [85,86].

Spread of Bt

In animal models BtA readily spreads across muscle fascia [87,88] to *nearby* muscles. It can also cause weakness and endplate dysfunction in human muscles adjacent to injected muscles [70]. Muscles *remote* from injection sites develop subtle EMG abnormalities in endplate function [57,89–93]. These abnormalities may be due to spread of Bt into the systemic circulation. However, as there is no reduction of maximal compound muscle action potentials in distant muscles after local Bt injection [68], there may be some other general stimulus to terminal sprouting that does not involve significant presynaptic inhibition of acetylcholine release in these remote muscles [91].

F-waves reflect motorneurone excitability, and are more persistent and have a greater amplitude in spastic than in normal muscles [94–99]. After focal Bt injections a widespread decrease in F-waves [68] suggests generalized reduction of motorneurone excitability. This might be particularly useful in spasticity, and might help to reduce synergic contractions in muscles remote from the injected muscles, as occurs in some patients with dystonia [63,71,79,100].

How could Bt improve function in patients with spasticity?

This section reviews the likely effects of Bt on mechanisms of functional impairment in spasticity.

Reduction of spastic cocontraction

Spastic cocontraction is the inappropriate recruitment of a muscle, triggered by willed command to its antagonist. It is sensitive to the degree of stretch of the cocontracting muscle [17,101]. The possibility of antagonist cocontraction during active movement is well established [12,17,101–109]. It is a matter of degree, as some cocontraction, i.e. simultaneous activity in both agonist and antagonist, is common even during normal human movement [111]. It becomes excessive in the upper motorneurone syndrome, as shown by comparing EMG activity in a muscle when acting as antagonist against activity in the same muscle when acting as agonist (cocontraction index) [17,76,109–114]. In hemiplegic patients, inappropriate cocontraction of antagonists (plantar flexors) often limits voluntary ankle dorsiflexion torque beyond 90° of dorsiflexion. Placing the knee in extension aggravates these cocontractions by stretching gastrocnemius [17]. Weak spastic arm muscles show a similar increase in cocontraction compared to normal muscles [76].

Voluntary cocontraction involves decreased reciprocal Ia inhibition [116], increased presynaptic inhibition of Ia afferents [117–119], increased fusimotor drive [119,120] and increased recurrent Renshaw inhibition [121]. The pathophysiology of *spastic* cocontraction is now better understood. Like spastic dystonia, spastic cocontraction appears to be primarily due to an abnormal pattern of supraspinal descending drive [13,14,19]. Both are aggravated by abnormal peripheral reflex reactions, in particular the degree of stretch imposed on the overactive muscle [17]. Changes in the baseline excitability of spinal interneurone pathways, and in their regulation during movements, occur in patients with spasticity and may contribute to spastic cocontraction. The changes demonstrated at rest include increased Renshaw inhibition [122], decreased reciprocal Ia inhibition (converted into facilitation from flexors to extensors in lower limb) [123,124], and decreased presynaptic inhibition on the Ia afferents [124–126]. More importantly, the changes demonstrated during voluntary agonist contraction include the lack of increase in reciprocal Ia inhibition directed to the antagonist, and the lack of increase in presynaptic inhibition on the Ia afferents directed to the antagonist [127]. These deficiencies in reciprocal Ia inhibition and presynaptic inhibition on the Ia fibers directed to the antagonist at the onset of active agonist contraction may be responsible for spastic cocontraction in patients with spasticity [127].

Can intervention to weaken the cocontracting muscle, such as an injection of Bt, reduce cocontraction and improve movement? In animals and humans [59,61–63] there is Bt-induced decrease in Renshaw inhibition on the injected agonist that releases reciprocal Ia inhibition from the agonist to the antagonist during movements, and may thus contribute to the decrease in cocontraction of the antagonist. In cerebral palsy, Bt injection into the gastrocnemius and hamstring muscles reduced cocontraction, and was associated with functional improvements [128]. Our work in the hemiplegic arm shows that Bt injected into biceps reduced its cocontraction, improved maximal extensor torque and increased speed of self-paced elbow extensor and flexor movements, as cocontraction was also reduced in the elbow extensors [76].

Reduction of spastic dystonia

Spastic dystonia is the inappropriate recruitment of a muscle at rest. It is sensitive to the degree of stretch of the muscle [4,16]. The concept of spastic dystonia was recognized by Denny-Brown and supported by other authors [16, 129–133]. Denny-Brown pointed out that in monkeys with certain cortical lesions, dystonic and spastic features were superimposed in the same muscle groups, causing abnormal posturing sensitive to the degree of stretch imposed on the muscles [16]. The combination also occurred in patients with spasticity caused by cerebral or spinal lesions.

The pathophysiology of spastic dystonia is still unclear. Decreased presynaptic inhibition on Ia afferents at rest [124–126] may allow minimal tonic stretch stimulus (for instance the stretch imposed by the weight of the forearm for the elbow flexors) to engender prolonged tonic contractions.

Functionally, spastic dystonia is a major cause of deformities, causing disfigurement and social discomfort. It may be evaluated by measuring the resting position at various joints, in various body positions (i.e. standing, sitting, etc.). Photographs or videos of the patient at rest and before and after treatment may be helpful. Although there are numerous encouraging anecdotal reports, there are no systematic studies of the impact of Bt injections on spastic dystonia.

Lengthening of shortened muscles

The pathophysiology and time course of muscle shortening after damage to the central motor pathways was recently reviewed [4]. Spastic overactivity and muscle contracture aggravate each other. In brief, muscle shortening is an acute phenomenon that begins within hours after the onset of muscle immobilization [134–142], in the acute phase of CNS injury while the patient is still in the acute care unit. There is loss of sarcomeres [5], disorganization in the remaining sarcomeres [136–138,141], loss of protein mass [139,140], and accumulation of connective tissue [6,142]. Muscle shortening is functionally critical as it not only contributes to abnormal posturing and deformities (causing social discomfort and impairment in *passive* function), but also limits active ranges of motion and impairs *active* function.

There is a major theoretical reason why treatment with Bt might be efficient in helping to maintain or restore muscle length: secondary muscle overactivity aggravates muscle shortening. The shortening action of muscle overactivity on muscle was shown in the 1920s [143,144], and was later quantified [145]. Any means of reducing muscle overactivity should thus help prevent contracture. The following studies in animals and in human childhood leg spasticity support this concept.

Cosgrove and Graham showed in a randomized trial in the hereditary spastic mouse that BtA injection into gastrocnemius prevented contracture in this muscle [32]. The same group showed that BtA injections into hamstrings and gastrocnemius in children with cerebral palsy increased the length of these muscles [146,147]. The observations that BtA injection may delay tendon lengthening surgery in cerebral palsy are consistent with these results [148,149]. The functional effects of BtA injection are equivalent or superior to those of continuous stretch in several controlled studies [150–152]. Indirect arguments for muscle lengthening after Bt injections exist in other body areas [153–155].

Beside the potential direct lengthening effect of Bt in the injected muscle, there is an additional indirect action. In temporarily relieving muscle overactivity, Bt injections ease extrinsic passive stretching of the injected muscle, whether through antagonist activity, ground reaction force for the calf muscles, or the use of stretching therapies such as posturing, manual stretch and serial casts.

Correction of antagonist weakness

Reducing cocontraction of the injected muscle should increase the torque developed by the antagonist (see above). However, there is no systematic quantitative study of the change in force developed by the antagonist after Bt injection. Our work in the hemiplegic arm showed that 160 mu BtA (Botox®) injected into biceps reduced its cocontraction, and increased maximal extensor torque by 20%, while elbow flexor torque was reduced by 30% [76]. The agonist weakening was not associated with functional deterioration in the movements generated by agonist contraction, since the preferred speed of both flexor and extensor movements increased, and cocontraction was reduced in both the injected agonists (flexors) and its antagonists (extensors) [76].

Summary

Bt in a spastic muscle should, in theory, affect all primary mechanisms of impairment in patients with spasticity. Bt should be able to reduce cocontraction and spastic dystonia of the injected muscle, and cocontraction of the antagonist muscle. It should help to lengthen the injected muscle and increase antagonist torque. However, in spite of these theoretical expectations, the clinical literature assessing functional changes after Bt treatment has been disappointing. This is discussed further below.

Why does treating muscle overactivity matter?

Spastic muscle overactivity is common and can significantly impair long-term quality of life in stable patients, or recovery of function after new lesions. It can cause secondary problems with spasms, impaired movement, hygiene, self-care, poor self-esteem and body image, and pain (Table 10.1).

Muscle overactivity is not always harmful. For example, patients with a combination of muscle weakness and overactivity may rely on the increased tone to maintain their posture and aid standing or walking. There are patients with mild overactivity who need little or no treatment.

Table 10.1 Harmful effects of muscle overactivity.

Muscle spasms	Difficulty with seating, posture or walking
Abnormal trunk and limb posture	Contractures Pressure sores Deformity and its consequences
Loss of function	Reduced mobility Self-care, hygiene, bladder and bowel management
Poor self-esteem	Cosmetic effects of limb deformity Fatigue
Low mood	Depression due to pain and altered self-image
Poor sexual functioning	Sexuality problems and decreased libido Sexual intercourse difficulties
Poor sleep patterns Increased carer burden Pain	

Table 10.2 Some factors aggravating muscle overactivity.

Noxious intrinsic stimuli	Urinary retention, infection, bladder stones
	Constipation and faecal impaction
	Pressure sores and other tissue viability problems
	Skin irritation, e.g. rashes, ingrowing toenails
	Deep vein thrombosis
	Unsuspected lower limb fractures
External stimuli	Ill-fitting orthotic appliances
	Incorrect positioning in bed or chair
	Tight clothing, wrapped pads and catheter leg bags
Medication	Non-tricyclic antidepressants
	Diuretics
	Analgesics

Management of muscle overactivity

Treatment of muscle overactivity is only one part of the wider rehabilitation plan for patients. Management may be complex and requires a multidisciplinary team including the physician, nurse, physiotherapist and occupational therapist, as well as orthotists and rehabilitation engineers. The carers and patients themselves also play an important role. The basis of management is physical and Bt may help to relieve symptoms, improve function and prevent deterioration. Bt should be used in parallel with appropriate physical therapy.

There is a wide range of 'medical' treatments, which the team may deploy in a personalized mix tailored to the muscle overactivity itself, the patient, circumstances and the availability of care and resources. Most clinicians begin with prevention of provocative factors such as pain, constipation, infection and improper postural management.

Avoid aggravating factors

Because muscle overactivity results in part from abnormal processing of sensory input, nociceptive stimuli such as pain and discomfort will exacerbate it and make it harder to treat. Initially therefore the team should identify and eliminate any remedial factors which may be exacerbating muscle overactivity (Table 10.2).

Physical treatment

Physical management remains the cornerstone of spasticity prevention and treatment, and requires education and considerable staff and carer time. There should be a programme of stretching and physical therapy, and regular changes of position to vary pressure points and muscle stretch, together with splints, casts or orthoses. Nursing skills are vital for the management of spasticity, as nurses and carers are responsible for positioning and handling the patient throughout the 24 h period. Therapists also play a critical role in advising on positioning and providing special seating and postural support systems, etc. When planning the postural management programme, it is important to remember that the body needs to change position. There is not just one correct position, but a range of different positions that act to vary the stretch on different muscles and body parts throughout the day. Careful positioning in bed, supported sitting in the wheelchair, periods in a standing frame and splinting/orthotics may all contribute to the maintenance of muscle length and control of spasticity. In addition, these measures reduce the risk of complications such as pressure sores, which may result from abnormal pressure points and shearing forces. Education and advice are important for good physical management of spasticity; it takes considerable staff time, and should involve the entire caregiver team. The aims are to maintain muscle and soft tissue length, improve the posture and symmetry of the body, and to facilitate function or ease of care.

In theory BtA can help at any point in this range of options. It should not be used in isolation, and optimum results require combination with physiotherapy and splinting. Patients who need intensive physiotherapy to gain significantly from BtA must have access to it arranged before starting the injections. Good use of the window of opportunity starting 1–2 weeks after BtA injections permits more effective physical therapies and retraining, and may lead to longer lasting benefit. Physiotherapists can use this time and the impetus of a new treatment to reinvigorate a stalled patient's progress.

Other medical and surgical treatments

Muscle overactivity is asymmetrically distributed across joints in patients with spasticity, with imbalance between more overactive agonists and less overactive antagonists, hence the rationale for preferring focal interventions over systemic treatments. Focal treatments mainly revolve around medical and surgical techniques for blocking the final common pathway of lower motorneurone activity, and now include Bt.

Destructive lesions such as phenol injections or nerve, root or spinal cord surgery can work well, but their effects are not always predictable, and errors or adverse effects may result in long-term problems. Phenol nerve or motor point injections are relatively time consuming, technically challenging and uncomfortable, although they can be very effective. There is a small but significant risk of painful dysaesthesiae or sensory loss if phenol is used in perineural rather than intramuscular injections. Neurosurgical therapies include spinal cord stimulation, selective rhizotomies or neurotomies. Orthopaedic procedures may rescue deforming limbs and return them to more functional postures.

In cases of severe or very widespread muscle overactivity in which priority goes to comfort and passive function rather than active function, systemic treatments may be used, including benzodiazepines, baclofen, tizanidine, dantrolene, piracetam, etc.

[156]. Unfortunately, it can be difficult to achieve a satisfactory balance between good suppression of the most spastic segments, and weakness or excessive loss of muscle tone elsewhere. If these drugs fail or produce unacceptable drowsiness, weakness or other side-effects, intrathecal therapies (baclofen, clonidine, midazolam, morphine, phenol) are used in some centres [156]. However, such therapies require considerable expertise and backup, and carry a significant risk of complications.

How well does Bt work in spasticity?

When considering the literature on the use of Bt in spasticity since the initial publications in the late 1980s [2,157], two findings are remarkably constant, whether obtained from open or controlled studies. The first, and least surprising, is that resistance to passive movement was invariably reduced in joints serviced by injected muscles, whichever scale was used to measure resistance to passive movement: Oswestry [2,157], Ashworth [158–165], or Modified Ashworth [162,163,166–172]. However, similar results were also obtained in earlier studies of systemic oral and intrathecal antispastic treatments [156]. Unfortunately, resistance to passive movement, a phenomenon measured at rest, does not correlate with active function [96,156,161, 173,174]. Indeed, the second consistent finding has been the difficulty of demonstrating functional improvement from Bt in spasticity [175]. Nevertheless, most experienced investigators have observed true functional improvement following Bt injection, at least anecdotally.

To clarify the discussion on the functional impact of antispasticity treatments for patients, we follow Mayer's concept of passive and active function [176]. *Passive* function represents daily activities that are performed by the caregiver when the patient is unable to accomplish them alone. Passive function mainly requires sufficient flexibility and looseness of the limbs (passive range of motion) for the caregiver to accomplish these activities. *Active* function is what the patient can do alone, i.e. activities where active range of motion, strength, concentration, attention, alertness, and even positive mood are essential to the patient's performance. Demonstrating improvement in active function represents the most difficult challenge in clinical research on Bt and spasticity. Meeting this challenge might set local treatment by Bt apart from the systemic antispastic treatments still used as first line therapy by most clinicians.

Upper limb spasticity

We distinguish three eras in the literature to date on Bt and spasticity, based on the scales and study designs that were used to evaluate functional changes.

1989–1995 First era: global assessments of function in mostly open studies (Table 10.3 [2,157–160,167,177])

Until 1996 most studies of Bt injections into paretic arms in spastic hemiplegia were uncontrolled and had limited outcome measurements, mainly focused on tone reduction [2,157–159,166,177] (Table 10.3). Functional assessments usually did not rate the function of the paretic limb itself, but consisted of global assessment of activities of daily living (ADL), such as Barthel Index [2,157,158,177] or the Functional Independence Measure (FIM) [167]. However, these ADL scales measure overall ability to perform tasks, without necessarily focusing on functions involving the affected arm [178]. Therefore they may rate mainly learned adaptive strategies, including one-handed tasks using only the non-paretic arm, corresponding to 'learned disuse' of the affected arm [179]. Other items in these scales such as mobility and continence are unlikely to be affected by localized treatment of arm spasticity.

The work of Dunne and colleagues [160] presaged the next era, in which small investigator-driven trials focused on assessments of functional impairment rather than tone. Dunne *et al's* study rated impairment using blinded video assessments of motor tasks, and Lindmark's Modified Fugl–Meyer Score [180,181], which involves comprehensive testing of active abilities of the paretic arm. The study was also remarkable for the high dilution of toxin used (20 mu/mL Botox®), and the relatively large patient sample size. The improvement reported appeared greater than that noted in previous trials, but this study was uncontrolled. The other important study in this period is the first double blind placebo-controlled trial in the spastic arm, in which a rigid injection protocol of BtA in the elbow and wrist flexors reduced tone in the injected muscles in a dose-dependent fashion. However, the scales used did not demonstrate functional improvement [167].

1996–1999 Second era: targeted assessments of function in mostly open studies (Table 10.4 [83,161,182–184])

Investigators in this period tried to refine evaluation of changes in arm function in small open label protocols [83,161,182–184], and to define subgroups of hemiplegic patients that might predictably benefit from Bt injections [182]. Reiter and colleagues observed that partially paretic patients whose active movements clinically appeared impaired by antagonist overactivity were more likely to benefit from Bt than patients with severe weakness [182]. Other reports confirmed this differential potential of neuromuscular blocking injections according to patient subgroups [161,185]. Bt treatment in severely paretic patients failed to produce significant subjective improvement [161]. A subsequent single blinded study in children supported the importance of residual motor power in the injected limb as a predictor of improvement in active function following Bt injection [185].

A study by Corry and colleagues in children with cerebral palsy [184] pioneered the

Table 10.3 Principal studies of Bt in arm spasticity containing functional assessments in 1989–1995.

Study	Design	N	Muscles injected	Product, dose dilution	Targeting technique	Functional assessments	Change*
Das & Park, 1989 [2,157]	Open	8	Biceps FDP FCU	BTX-A Porton Down 20 ng 10 ng/mL	Plane of motor points	Barthel Index Patient questionnaire	+ +
Mémin et al., 1992 [177]	Open	8	Biceps, BR FCR, FCU FDS, FDP	BTX-A Porton Down <16 ng 20 ng/mL	No specific targeting	Barthel Index Patient questionnaire	0 +
Hesse et al., 1992 [158]	Open	9	Biceps, BR FCU FDS, FDP	BTX-A Porton Down <40 ng dilution not specified	Two different sites per muscle close to motor point	Barthel Index Rivermead Motor Score Therapist + nurse evaluation	0 0 +
Konstanzer et al., 1993 [159]	Open	11	Biceps, BR FCR, FCU FDS, FDP	BTX-A Porton Down <30 ng dilution not specified	No specific targeting	Hygienic Rating Scale	+
Dunne et al., 1995 [160]	Open	13	Biceps, BR FCR, FCU FDS, FDP	Botox® 70–270 mu 20 mu/mL	Multisite EMG-guided mid-belly	Barthel Index Lindmark's Mod. Fugl–Meyer Blinded video-review Subjective self-rating	+ + + +
Simpson et al., 1996 [167]	DB vs. placebo	39	Biceps FCR, FCU	Botox® Placebo/75/150/300 U 25/50/100 mu/mL	No specific targeting biceps 4 sites, FCR, FCU 1 site each	FIM Caregiver Dependency Scale Fugl–Meyer	0 0 0

0, no change: BR, brachioradialis; brach, brachialis; FCR, flexor carpi radialis; FCU, flexor carpi ulnaris; FDP, flexor digitorum profundis; FDS, flexor digitorum superficialis; FIM, Functional Independence Measure; Mod., modified.

*+, trend of improvement.

use of tests of active functional performance in a double blind placebo-controlled design. However, Corry's results, in terms of change in fine motor function, were mixed [184]. Despite more targeted functional assessments and mostly open label designs, investigators in this period were unable to demonstrate consistent gains in active function following BtA injections (Table 10.4).

2000–2002 Recent era: targeted assessments of function in double blind studies (Table 10.5 [162,168–171,186,187])

Table 10.5 summarizes the studies in the recent era. The most recent literature includes at least six double blind placebo-controlled studies with a larger sample size, and using one of two types of targeted functional assessments.

Subjective reports on patients' daily function at home, made by the patient or caregiver, usually combining information on passive and active function. Most of these studies incorporated such assessments [162,168–171,186], and these were mostly rewarding in that they showed the potential for functional improvement following Bt injection in the spastic arm [162,168,170,186]. One placebo-controlled RCT [187] enrolled 126 subjects and tested Botox® 200–240 mu injected into wrist or finger flexors. There were statistically significant benefits favouring Bt for separate Physician and Patient/Carer Global Assessments, and a Disability Assessment Scale.

Direct clinical assessments of performance of functional tasks, made by the clinician, are ostensibly more objective and permit selective testing of active function. However, these tests alone are not sufficient, and it is important to assess whether the performance achieved in the clinic visit is reproduced once the patient is at home. Tests in this cat-egory include the Frenchay Arm test [161,169], grasp and release and coin transfer scores [184], measurements of upper body dressing time [168], Rivermead motor score for the arm [169,170], nine hole peg test [170], and Quality of Upper Extremity Skills Test in children (QUEST) [186]. Unfortunately, significant gains in active functional tests have been more elusive, with the most promising results obtained through a single blind study in children with cerebral palsy [186].

Lower limb spasticity (Table 10.6 [170,188])

The first uncontrolled report of Bt use in lower limb spasticity in adults suggested that it could be beneficial [157]. This was soon supported by a small, early RCT in adductor spasticity [188], and a number of uncontrolled, or open studies and case series. As more results appeared it seemed that measures of impairment and passive function often improved. For instance, most studies reported improved passive range of movement (ROM). However, as for upper limb spasticity and probably for similar reasons, it has proved more difficult to extract proof of benefit for active functions performed by the patients rather than by caregivers.

Table 10.4 Principal studies of Bt in arm spasticity containing functional assessments in 1996–1999.

Study	Design	N	Muscles injected	Product, dose dilution	Targeting technique	Functional assessments	Change*
Reiter et al.. 1996 [182]	Open SB	17	Biceps. BR FCR. FCU FDS, FDP, FPL	Botox® 100–210 mu 50 mu/mL	Plane of motor points	Frenchay Arm Test FIM NHP (quality of life)	+ + ++
Bhakta et al.. 1996 [183]	Open	17	Biceps FCU FDS, FDP	Dysport® 400–1000 mu 200 mu/mL or Botox® 100–200 mu 40 U/mL	No specific targeting	Goal Attainment Scale	+
Sampaio et al.. 1997 [161]	Open	19	FCR, FCU FDS, FDP, FPL	Botox® <150 mu 50 mu/mL	One site per muscle	Frenchay Arm Test Patient Asessment Scale	++ +
Hesse et al.. 1998 [84]	DB vs. placebo	24	Biceps. brach FCR. FCU FDS.FDP	Dysport® 1000 mu 100 mu/mL	Two sites/muscle close to motor point Rigid protocol†	Palm cleaning. nails. sleeve (rated by patient/caregiver)	0
Corry et al.. 1997 [184]	DB vs. placebo	14	Biceps. brach FCR. FCU. PT FPB. AP FDS, FDP, FPL	Dysport® 8–9 mu/kg 100 mu/mL or Botox® 4–7 mu/kg 100 mu/mL	Mutiple sites per muscle	Grasp-and-Release Score Coin Pick-up Score Subjective Opinion of Parent	+ 0 +

0, no change: AP, adductor pollicis: BR. brachioradialis: brach. brachialis; DB, double blind: FCR. flexor carpi ulnaris; FDP. flexor digitorum profundis: FDS, flexor digitorum superficialis; FIM. Functional Independence Measure; FPB, flexor pollicis brevis; FPL, flexor pollicis longus: NHP, Nottingham Health Profile: PT, pronator teres: SB, single blind.

*+, trend of improvement: ++, significant improvement in open or single blind design ($P < 0.05$).

†Rigid protocol means muscle selection and dose per muscle were imposed on the investigator.

Table 10.5 Principal studies of Bt in arm spasticity containing functional assessments in 2000–2002.

Study	Design	N	Muscles injected	Product, dose dilution	Targeting technique	Functional assessments	Change*
Smith et al., 2000 [168]	DB vs. placebo	21	Elbow, wrist, fingers Rigid protocol	Dysport® multiple doses Flexible protocol‡	Multisite EMG-guided	Frenchay Arm Test	0
						Upper Body Dressing Time	0
						Global Assessment Scale	+++
Bakheit et al., 2000 [169]	DB vs. placebo	82	Biceps FCR, FCU FDS, FDP	Dysport® 500/1000/1500 mu 250/500/750 mu/mL	No specific targeting	Barthel Index	0
						Goal Attainment Scale	+
						Rivermead Motor Score (UL)	0
Richardson et al., 2000 [170]	DB vs. placebo	32	Elbow, wrist, fingers	Botox® 50 mu/mL Flexible protocol‡	Multisite EMG-guided	Subj. rating of pb. (flexible)	++
						Rivermead Motor Score	0
						Mod. Goal Attainment Scale	0
						Nine-hole Peg Test	0
Bhakta et al., 2000 [162]	DB vs. placebo	40	Elbow, wrist, fingers	Dysport® 1000 mu 100 mu/mL Flexible protocol‡	No specific targeting	Disability Scale (8 items)	+++
						Carer burden Scale (4 items)	+++
Fehlings et al., 2000 [186]	SB no placebo	30	Biceps, forearm flex AP	Botox® 2–6 mu/kg Flexible protocol‡	Multisite No EMG used	QUEST	++
						Ped. Eval. of Disab. Inventory	++
Bakheit et al., 2001 [171]	DB vs. placebo	59	Biceps FCR, FCU FDS,FDP	Dysport® 1000 mu 500 mu/mL Rigid protocol‡	Muscle belly No EMG used	Barthel Index	0
						Goal Attainment Scale	0
						Subjective evaluation of benefit	+
Brashear et al., 2002 [187]	DB vs. placebo	126	Wrist flexors Finger flexors	Botox® 200–240 mu ?Flexible protocol‡	Multisite ?EMG used	Physician global assessment	++
						Patient/carer global assessment	+++
						Disability Assessment Scale	++

0, no change; AP, adductor pollicis; DB, double blind; EMG, electromyography; FCR, flexor carpi radialis; FCU, flexor carpi ulnaris; FDP, flexor digitorum profundis; FDS, flexor digitorum superficialis; Ped. Eval. of Disab. Inventory, paediatric evaluation of disability inventory; SB, single blind; Subj. rating of pb. subjective rating of problem; QUEST, quality of upper extremity skills test; UL, upper limb.

*+, trend of improvement; ++, significant improvement in open or single blind design (P <0.05); +++ significant improvement in double blind design (P <0.05).

†Flexible protocol means muscle selection and dose per muscle were left to the investigator's discretion.

‡Rigid protocol means muscle selection and dose per muscle were imposed on the investigator.

Table 10.6 Randomized controlled studies of Bt in leg spasticity.

Study	Design	N	Muscles injected	Product, dose dilution*‡	Targeting technique	Functional assessments	Change‡
Snow et al., 1990 [188]	DB Crossover vs. placebo	9	Adductors	Botox® P. 400 mu Rigid‡	Clinical	Hygiene score Spasticity 'score' Spasm frequency	++ ++ +
Grazko, 1995 [189]	DB Crossover vs. placebo	8	Mixed	Botox® P. 90–250 mu Flexible		(Ashworth)§ Spasm frequency	+++ +++
Burbaud et al., 1996 [190]	DB Crossover vs. placebo	23	Gastrosoleus	Dysport® P. 1000 mu Rigid protocol	Clinical Gait velocity Fugl-Meyer	(Modified Ashworth)§ Aids dependency Gait video score 0 0	+++ +++ +++
Kirazli, 1998 [191]	SB Parallel vs. phenol	20	Gastrosoleus Rigid protocol	Botox® 400 mu Phenol Global score	Clinical EMG control	(Ashworth)§ Ambulation score ROM	0* 0* 0* 0*
Hyman et al. 2000 [192]	DB Parallel vs. placebo	74	Adductors	Dysport® P. 500, 1000, 1500 ny Rigid protocol	Pain Global rating	Passive ROM Muscle tone Hygiene score 0 0	+++ ++ +
Richardson, 2000 [170]	DB Parallel vs. placebo	52	Mixed Arm/leg	Botox® P. variable U Flexible	Clinical EMG control	(Ashworth)§ % passive ROM Subjective problem severity Rivermead lower limb	+++ +++ +++ +++
Pittock et al. per.com.	DB Parallel vs. placebo	234	Gastrosoleus	Dysport® P. 500, 1000, 1500 mu Rigid protocol	Clinical 2 min walk	(Modified Ashworth)§ Pain Global score 0 Need for aids	+++ +++ 0 0

0, no change; DB, double blind.; SB, single blind.
*Bt and phenol were reported as being equally 'effective'; hence no difference between them.
†Rigid means that muscle selection and dose per muscle were imposed on the investigator; flexible means that muscle selection and dose per muscle were left to the investigator's discretion.
‡+, trend of improvement; ++, significant improvement in open or single blind design ($P < 0.05$); +++, significant improvement.
§Note that Ashworth scores are not functional assessments but are included here for convenience, in double blind design ($P < 0.05$).

Between 1996 and 2000, four medium size placebo controlled RCTs in adults explored BtA injections for plantarflexor, hip adductor [192], and mixed [170] muscle overactivity.

Plantar flexors

Perhaps because the biomechanical link between gait and plantarflexor activity appears simple, many investigators have tested BtA in open label exploratory studies of the concept of spasticity treatment, using the muscle complex for proof of concept in patients with stroke. Burbaud *et al.* enrolled 23 subjects into their crossover group RCT and demonstrated improvement in quality of gait and dependency on walking aids. However, the improvement in walking speed (+17%) was not statistically significant. Bt was less effective in patients with a longer duration of spasticity [190].

In a larger parallel group dose-ranging study in 234 patients, Pittock *et al.* (personal communication) compared placebo against 500, 1000 or 1500 mu Dysport®. Compared to placebo, treatment with BtA decreased resistance to passive ankle movements (Modified Ashworth Scores), pain, and reliance on walking aids, although there was no statistically significant advantage in other functional gait parameters measured at 12 weeks, including distance walked in 2 min. The lack of benefit in these measures may have resulted from the wide variation in initial impairments. It is difficult to show statistical significance in such a heterogeneous group, and the walking measure itself was confounded by changes in the pattern of walking and because more patients in the BtA group discarded walking aids. Other possible factors include the fixed dose regime and lack of concomitant physiotherapy. Although the greatest improvements occurred in the 1500 mu dose group, gait deteriorated in one patient, possibly because of excessive weakness. There were clear improvements in the placebo group, a warning against over-interpretation of uncontrolled studies.

Hip adductors

The largest placebo controlled RCT in hip adductor spasticity in multiple sclerosis compared 500, 1000 and 1500 mu Dysport®, and showed improvement in muscle tone and passive hip abduction with trends in hygiene scores, and favouring the larger doses. Pain and muscle spasm scores improved in all groups including the placebo group, with no statistically significant benefit favouring Bt. Time until patients requested retreatment significantly favoured Bt. Because there was more muscle weakness in the 1500 mu group, the authors recommended 1000 mu as the optimum dose [192].

Mixed muscles

A parallel group RCT in 52 patients compared variable doses of Botox® with placebo in upper or lower limb spasticity. Summed scores from four postinjection assessments favoured Bt for Ashworth Scale, percentage of passive ROM, Rivermead lower limb and subjective rating of problem severity. However, at 12 weeks there was no difference in a goal attainment score [170].

It may be that those with the greatest initial impairment show the greatest improvement after treatment [188]. However, this proportional response may depend on the severity of muscle overactivity and appears to be lost if there are significant contractures [191,193].

In summary

The literature suggests that subjective improvement in passive function is possible at home, based on patient or caregiver interviews. It has mostly failed so far to show improvement in active performance as rated during tasks performed in the clinic. Ideally, there is a need for more placebo-controlled studies showing gains in both active and passive function to differentiate Bt from systemic antispastic treatments.

Principles of clinical use

Spasticity service

It has emerged from wide clinical experience (but is not yet proven) that Bt treatment in spasticity should be used in the setting of a multidisciplinary rehabilitation service, with a range of staff and facilities as described above. Bt should be injected by clinicians with appropriate knowledge of functional anatomy, general experience in diagnosis and management of spasticity, and specific training in the use of Bt. Guidelines for the development of a Bt service for spasticity have recently been published [194].

Patient selection

It is preferable to define the principles of selection than to provide a precise menu of indications. The underlying cause of the spasticity is rarely relevant to treatment. Patients should have clinically important muscle overactivity that is causing or is about to cause a problem: the presence of spasticity is not in itself an indication for treatment. The classic 'fixed, severe contracture' is *not* a contraindication to Bt injection; an injection trial might in fact partially release movements and disclose underlying overactivity in a muscle that was apparently only 'shortened and silent'. A priority list of muscles where overactivity appears to be most disabling should be selected for injection, compatible with the ceiling doses of Bt when cumulating the required doses (Fig. 10.1). The clinician must understand the dynamic anatomy of the muscle overactivity and be aware of

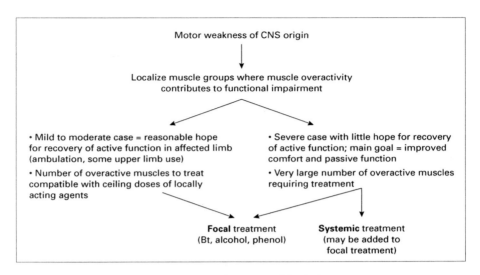

Fig. 10.1 Management strategy depending on the severity of the CNS injury.

the risks of undue weakness of the target or nearby muscles, particularly in distal upper limb injections.

Treatment aims

It is important to define the goals of treatment clearly, and consider how treatment outcomes will be evaluated. Table 10.7 sets out the more common indications for Bt treatment in spasticity. Not all of these have been proven unequivocally in clinical trials. The treatment goals for a patient with spasticity following a single acute insult, such as a mild stroke, may be different from those in a patient with progressive or extensive neurological damage.

In postacute rehabilitation, Bt use may aim to produce long-term gains in active function, although there are no studies proving that this strategy works. Patients may need injections into different muscle groups over several sessions, which may be required within a few weeks of each other, in order to take advantage of the window of opportunity. This should be performed in combination with an intensive stretch schedule to limit and if possible prevent muscle shortening. Under these circumstances, the potential benefits should override the theoretical risk of antibody formation.

In chronic care, particularly in severe cases, the focus may be more on improvement in comfort and passive function, concentrating on pain relief, wearing of splints, prevention of complications (e.g. contractures), easing carer burden and cosmesis.

Table 10.7 Some indications for Bt in spasticity.

Symptom reduction	*Decrease carer burden*
Reduce spasm or pain	Ease dressing and mobility for carers
	Aid hygiene (e.g. perineal, axillary, palmar)
Functional improvement	*Enhance other management strategies*
Improve fit and comfort of orthoses (wrist, ankle)	Optimize physiotherapy
Increase range and control of movement	Reduce need for systemic drugs
Improve mobility: speed, gait quality or range, or wheelchair propulsion	Postpone or avoid orthopaedic surgery
Sexual activity	Predict results of orthopaedic surgery
Improve transfers	Reduce postoperative pain and aid healing
Optimize posture and seating	
Prevention (treatment)	*Cosmetic*
Pressure sores and contractures	More natural arm posture
Injury from involuntary movements	Better fit of clothes

Spasticity syndromes commonly treated with Bt

Spastic upper limb

Common patterns include shoulder adduction, flexion at the elbow, wrist and fingers, pronation of the forearm, thumb in palm and fisting. Occasional variants may occur such as shoulder abduction or wrist supination. All of these can be treated with Bt injections into the appropriate muscles. The total dose required is likely to be up to 1500 mu Dysport®, 400–600 mu Botox®, [194] or equivalent of NeuroBloc®/MYOBLOC™, depending on the number and bulk of muscles needing injection.

Control of muscle spasm and limited ability to reach are common indications for injections around the shoulder, and reducing resistance to passive extension at any level can make dressing easier. Functional improvements can occur, for instance when release of elbow flexion permits a patient to control a wheelchair, or to use the hand to brace an object. In ambulant patients an arm swinging more naturally at the patient's side can help walking, and is a cosmetic bonus, restoring confidence and social activity. It is very difficult to restore fine dexterity, but even fractional release of severe fisting can assist carers in maintaining palmar skin hygiene. The combination of Bt with physiotherapy, regular muscle stretch by the patient and attendants, and progressive splinting, can release flexed postures for longer than the usual duration of Bt-induced weakness.

Spastic lower limb

The simplest situations are dynamic spastic equinus, with or without inversion (tibialis posterior involvement) and toe clawing (toe flexors involvement), and hip adductor overactivity [188,192]. Proximal flexor spasms can arise from hamstrings or hip flexors, and require careful analysis. In practice there can be a mixture, and injections into the hamstrings are technically easier and often work. Psoas, iliacus or rectus femoris injections may be required. We recommend using image guidance with computed tomography (CT) or ultrasound for psoas injections. Other less common injections include Bt into quadriceps to block knee extensor spasms; or toe extensors, especially to suppress an intrusive extensor toe.

Benefits of hip adductor injections include easier perineal hygiene and sexual intercourse, and reduction of gait scissoring. Weakening the hamstrings may block spasms, improve wheelchair posture, and help with walking. Injections into gastrocnemius and soleus may make splints more comfortable to wear.

Situations to avoid

Whether muscle overactivity has primarily a dynamic or a tonic component (spastic dystonia or spastic cocontraction), it may be efficiently relieved by Bt injection. However, patients are less likely to benefit if fixed muscle shortening (contracture) is the predominant problem. We help patients understand this by comparing spastic muscle overactivity with a piece of elastic, a contracture with string. Weakening elastic allows it to stretch, weakening string does not. It is often difficult to know whether a fixed posture is due to contracture only. Assessment during sleep or sedation can help. If the patient is to have surgery for any reason joint ROM may be assessed under anaesthesia. Temporary motor point blocks with lidocaine (lignocaine) may clarify the pattern of muscle involvement, and reveal whether there is severe contracture.

Functional goals must be realistic. There may be little value in abolishing modest overactivity in patients whose main disability is weakness or loss of higher functions such as in sensory inattention. There is unlikely to be much improvement in function, and Bt will only help if the muscle overactivity is causing other problems.

Muscle selection (Table 10.8)

The history may reveal some candidate muscles that appear responsible for spasms, abnormal posturing, or other disability. Examination (including visual inspection and limb palpation) of static posture and the effects of orthoses, and of passive and active movement, muscle hypertrophy and tenderness will be the critical steps to identify the most overactive muscles. It is often not possible to treat all the candidate muscles. Clinicians must judge which would be the most useful ones to weaken within the dose allowed for the injection session.

Distinguish the muscles presenting with spastic dystonia (overactive when examined at rest), and those presenting with spastic cocontraction (overactive when examined during active effort on their antagonist). Treatment of spastic dystonic muscles aims to improve passive function, while treating muscles affected with spastic

Table 10.8 Common patterns of spasticity, muscles involved and treatment benefits.

Pattern	Muscle involved	Benefits
Arm		
Shoulder extension	Latissimus dorsi, long head of triceps, teres major, pectoralis major, scapular adductors (rhomboids, middle trapezius)	Improve reach; Improve balance and symmetry of gait
Shoulder adduction and internal rotation	Pectoralis major, teres major Subscapularis, latissimus dorsi	Sitting posture and ease of dressing Improve balance and symmetry of gait
Elbow flexion	Biceps (attention, also supinator), brachialis, brachioradialis	Improve reach, permit control of an electric wheelchair, improve gait, cosmesis
Pronation of the forearm	Pronator teres, pronator quadratus	Allow supination, improve dexterity
Flexed wrist and clenched hand	Flexor carpi ulnaris and radialis, flexor digitorum superficialis and profundus, flexor pollicis longus	Better dexterity, maintain skin hygiene in palm
Thumb in palm, intrinsic muscle stiffness	Opponens pollicis, adductor pollicis, flexor pollicis brevis, lumbricals, interossei	Improve hand opening, comfort, ease of splinting, function
Leg		
Hip adductor overactivity and spasms	Adductors	Reduce 'scissor gait' Ease perineal hygiene and urinary catheterisation Easier sexual intercourse
Hip and knee flexion or proximal flexor spasms	Psoas major, iliacus, medial hamstring group (gracilis, semitendinosus, semimembranosus), biceps femoris	Improve gait pattern and speed, prevent flexor spasms and improve wheelchair posture
Hamstring overactivity	Semitendinosus, semimembranosus, biceps femoris	Improve late swing phase of gait; allow heel strike
Knee extensor spasms	Quadriceps group	Pain reduction, prevent extension spasms
Ankle plantar flexed and inverted clonus	Gastrocnemius, soleus, tibialis posterior	Correct excessive plantar-flexion, allow heel strike and correct foot inversion, ease of donning orthoses
Toe clawing, turning under	Flexor hallucis longus, flexor digitorum longus, flexor digitorum brevis, palmar interossei	Prevent toe clawing, improve gait
Extensor toe	Extensor hallucis longus	Allows footwear comfort

cocontraction may improve active function. Muscles may display both spastic dystonia and spastic cocontraction. A lidocaine test may clarify the significance of overactivity in muscles that are difficult to see or palpate, such as shoulder extensors, or in obesity. Clear improvement in movement or posture after lidocaine injection in the suspected muscles demonstrates that overactivity in these muscles is disabling. It is usually not necessary in adults to resort to laboratory evaluation with tests such as gait analysis or EMG.

Injection technique

Standard EMG guidebooks can be helpful in locating muscles and injecting safely, but are not written with Bt therapy in mind. Their aim is usually reliable insertion of a diagnostic electrode into an informative site, and this determines the menu of muscles described and the injection points selected. However, these are often different from those needed for Bt injection. A particular problem is the inability of many patients with spastic deformities to achieve the recommended anatomical posture for optimal electrode placement, and this often requires imaginative solutions from clinicians with a good understanding of the dynamic anatomy. It is likely that dedicated books will appear. One current solution is the compact disc guide published by the Movement Disorders Society, which describes techniques for many muscles commonly injected with Bt. A soon-to-be-released DVD published by Comed Communications will provide video demonstrations for the injection of the most commonly injected muscles in spasticity.

Some authors use a simple clinical technique to assist targeting in some large superficial muscles. If the needle is placed in the belly of the muscle and the muscle then gently activated or stretched passively, the differential movement of muscle and skin tilts the needle and syringe and confirms its position inside the muscle fascia [195]. This is helpful in some long limb muscles such as hamstrings or gastrocnemius.

Exploratory stimulation and EMG techniques

We recommend using the *exploratory stimulation technique* when targeting muscles with Bt. This is the most accurate way to distinguish a muscle among its synergic neighbours, and is also the only technique that permits intramuscular localization, for example when injecting around motor points in an attempt to reach areas dense in endplates.

The technique of intramuscular injection must meet two requirements to treat focal muscle overactivity effectively. Bt must be injected into muscular tissue, and not into neighbouring tissues (e.g. blood vessels, subcutaneous tissue, fat, fascia). The needle tip should lie within the muscle responsible for the patient's symptoms, and not in neighbouring muscles. This is particularly challenging when targeting trunk or small limb or neck muscles [196].

In the two commonly used intramuscular injection techniques, the physician inserts the needle at a skin site estimated from surface landmarks. The techniques differ in the method of verification of the position of the needle-tip. In the classical 'passive' EMG technique, the injection needle is used as an exploring electrode to detect motor unit activity occurring spontaneously, on voluntary command, or after reflex activation by selective passive muscle stretch. In the stimulation technique, the injection needle delivers repetitive monopolar cathodal stimulation to the targeted area. The anode is a surface plate electrode taped over the opposite side of the limb in order to avoid confusing contractions due to anodal stimulation. Ideally, the anode should be placed over an antagonist of the target muscle. When a minimal stimulation voltage elicits contraction of the target muscle and no other neighbouring muscle, as confirmed by visual observation or tendon palpation, the needle tip is located inside that muscle and no other.

The classical 'passive' EMG technique has been used more often to date [62,153,160,166]. However, while both techniques ensure that the needle lies in muscle, the stimulation technique verifies more reliably that the needle lies in a specific muscle. A randomized study by Ashby and colleagues indicated that stimulation was superior to passive EMG in the targeting of a single muscle [197]. Detailed guidelines are available for some complex muscles such as flexor digitorum superficialis (FDS), created from a cadaver study, with surface landmarks to localize the skin site corresponding to each finger fascicle in the forearm [198]. The stimulation technique is indispensable when giving injections under anaesthetic, when passive techniques are ineffective. Chapter 4 discusses this point further.

Endplate targeting

The best sites for injection are theoretically the end-plate zones deep in the muscle bulk. Animal studies have shown that intramuscular Bt block is maximal when Bt is injected close to motor endplates [178,199]. The endplate generally lies near the midpoint of any given muscle fibre, and motor endplates classically cluster at characteristic areas (innervation bands) within most skeletal muscles [200]. However, there are exceptions to this rule, such as the sartorius, gracilis and gastrocnemius muscles in humans, where innervation bands are numerous and scattered throughout the muscle [201,202].

Since there is no clinical method to localize endplates reliably, DeLateur proposed an EMG technique to inject as close as possible to endplate areas [203]. It uses a hollow Teflon-coated injection needle as an EMG exploring electrode to find the characteristic endplate potentials in the resting muscle. These include 'endplate ripple' (or 'endplate noise'), and monophasic spike discharges [204–206]. Endplate ripple is a low voltage increase in irregularity of the baseline of about $10–40\,\mu V$ [204]. Monophasic spikes appear when the concentric needle is displaced slightly from the area of endplate ripple. They are almost entirely negative in sign (they may be diphasic with negative onset) and have a random pattern of discharge, as opposed to fibrillation potentials, which are more regular [204]. Movements of the exploring electrode should be slow and smooth, as contact of the needle with endplate zones may be painful. For muscles with a known endplate distribution, there are predetermined skin insertion areas over which skin wheals of xylocaine may be applied. However, this EMG technique is often painful for the patient, and cumbersome for the injector.

It has not yet been demonstrated whether targeting motor endplates inside a muscle improves the clinical efficacy of Bt injection. A controlled study is currently addressing this question in human biceps brachii, for which a cadaver study by Sanders *et al.* has helped define useful surface landmarks to target the endplate zone [202].

Motor points

Since surface landmarks for endplate areas are poorly defined for most human muscles other than biceps brachii, some investigators have tried to target 'motor points' in arm muscles [2,157,158]. These are the points at which the motor nerve penetrates the muscle [207] and are targets for some phenol injections. They are defined physiologically as the sites of lowest percutaneous stimulation threshold evoking a muscle response. However, endplates in long muscles may not be close to the motor point, since axonal branching can occur up to several centimeters before motor nerve endings and neuromuscular junctions arise [208].

The patterns of end-plate zones are not clearly mapped, and it may not always be practical to make multiple passes with an EMG/injection needle looking for their subtle but characteristic electrical signature. Fortunately, small and moderate size muscles will usually respond to Bt injected simply into the belly of the muscle.

Single or multiple injections

Although there is some diffusion through muscle fascia [87], muscles with well-delineated separate components such as quadriceps will need separate injections for each major section. Some authorities recommend multiple scattered smaller injections to spread the toxin. The clinician should consider the discomfort of multiple injections, and consider that patients may let an unpleasant experience persuade them not to undergo repeat injections. The psychology can be important, especially in frail or confused patients, and trying to get a slight extra benefit may be counterproductive in the long run.

Doses

DOSES: A HEALTH WARNING

Please read the warning on p. 35 about doses of Bt. There are three preparations available. *Dysport®* and *Botox®* are type A toxins (BtA), *NeuroBloc®/MYOBLOC™* is type B (BtB). Even though the doses for each are quoted in mouse units (mu), the three preparations have different dose schedules: one mu of *Dysport®* is **not** the same as one mu of *Botox®*, and neither is equivalent to one mu of *NeuroBloc®/MYOBLOC™*.

In most patients with spasticity it is worth giving a full dose of Bt and then reducing it if there are problems. This is appropriate when a rapid response is needed and where undue collateral weakness is unlikely to matter, as commonly occurs in a limb unlikely to be functionally useful even if the muscle overactivity is abolished. Recommended doses for particular muscles are given at the end of this book (Appendix, p. 438), culled from clinical trials and various other sources including We Move Consensus Guidelines, 2002 [194] and the WeMove website (www.wemove.org).

BtA

While there are proposed guidelines based on clinical experience [194], BtA dosages for each muscle are not accurately established and may vary depending upon the size of the muscle injected, the severity of muscle overactivity and the body weight of the patient. Most clinicians stay within a ceiling total dose per injection session or per 2-month period, currently estimated for Botox® as 400–600 mu in adults, and 12–15 mu/kg in children [194]. Equivalent Dysport® doses are 1000–1500 mu and 30–35 mu/kg, respectively. This constraint should not influence the dose used in one particular muscle, which should remain compatible with clinical efficacy. However, the ceiling dose often limits the number of muscles that can be injected in one session.

Botulinum toxin B

Provisional doses of the recently introduced botulinum toxin B (BtB) (MYOBLOC™, NeuroBloc®, Elan®) are available on the WeMove website (www.wemove.org) for spasticity treatment, based on open label studies and investigator reports. Preclinical acute toxicity studies of BtB in monkeys indicated no systemic muscle weakness detected in doses up to 960 mu/kg [209]. It appears safe to use doses at or below 200 mu/kg (15 000 mu in a 70 kg patient) in initial human investigations. There has been no report of systemic muscle weakness with 10 000 mu BtB injected in one session for cervical dystonia [210]. Despite reports of dry mouth following neck injections [210], doses of up to 15 000 mu MYOBLOC™ appear safe and well-tolerated in open label clinical trials in adults with arm spasticity following brain damage [211–214] (Brashear A, personal communication).

Dilution

For large muscles, such as most lower limb muscles and those above the elbow, we recommend using high dilutions for BtA (e.g. Botox® 20 mu/mL), especially when the primary goal is to improve passive function. Studies in animals and in humans (targeting small muscles in healthy volunteers) show that more dilute BtA is more effective [215,216]. In the spasticity literature, dilutions of Bt have varied considerably in the arm and the leg. With Botox®, the dilutions used include 100 mu/mL [66,76,

188,217–220], 50 mu/mL [161,170,182,221–223], 40 mu/mL [183], 25 mu/mL [167,224] and 20 mu/mL [63,96,160,225]. Dysport® dilutions included 800 mu/mL [177], 750 mu/mL [169], 500 mu/mL [169,171], 400 mu/mL [157], 250 mu/mL [83,169], 200 mu/mL [2,84,148,190,226], and 100 mu/mL [162]. We are currently performing a double blind trial in spastic hemiparetic patients, comparing the efficacy of two dilutions of Botox®, 100 mu/mL and 20 mu/mL in biceps brachii [76].

BtB (NeuroBloc®) is supplied at a standard dilution of 5000 mu/mL, and in spasticity treatment there is no published advantage to any different dilution.

Aftercare

Ensure that the team members involved in postinjection management are consulted or aware of preinjection assessment and goal setting. It is important to have clear goals for the injection and for subsequent therapy and to explain that the outcome is a result of combined efforts. The degree and duration of benefit differ between patients, so monitor the evolving effects of the toxin, preferably using standardized assessment and evaluation.

Therapists

Once muscle weakening is apparent (range 1–10 days postinjection), assess the need for splinting and provide new splints if necessary. Splinting is only an adjunct to physical therapy and should not be used in isolation. It must be carried out by trained staff with knowledge of how to position and align a limb, an understanding of muscle tone, and an ability to apply casts.

Splinting aims to correct or prevent flexion contractures and should provide prolonged stretch to the treated muscle. There is little reliable evidence regarding splinting [14], but clinical judgement suggests that splints should be applied 1–14 days postinjection. The optimal duration of splinting is unclear. There is some evidence that splints should be worn daily for at least 6 h and they should be reviewed and revised regularly [227] as toxin-induced weakness and joint ranges of movement evolve.

Educate patients and carers about stretching regimes, and give guidance on activity levels. Grade the intensity of the stretches over time to prevent intramuscular haematomas due to tearing of stiffened muscle fibres. When possible, arrange therapy to facilitate activity and increase the strength of the opposing muscle groups.

Medical follow-up

We recommend medical review at 4–6 weeks postinjection to determine whether or not the treatment goals have been achieved, and at 3–4 months to consider further injections as the previous toxin is wearing off. Documentation for all injections should include a clear statement of treatment aims and appropriate baseline outcome measures;

Bt agent, dose, dilution and muscles injected; follow-up treatment plan; evaluation of outcome and repeat measures; plans for future management.

Evaluating effectiveness in individual patients

Most studies have examined technical features and impairment, i.e. spasticity scales, spasm scores, adductor tone and range of joint motion. Global functional measures such as the Barthel or FIM have rarely been sensitive to this Bt treatment. Measurement methods include the following.

Physical measures (section to join with impairment scales down below)

Impairment measures include goniometry or spasm frequency counts. Functional benefit is unlikely if there is no change in impairment.

Techniques to quantify individual symptoms

It is helpful to record a Visual Analogue Scale (VAS) score before and after treatment, except inpatients with brain injuries who may have visuo-spatial problems, making the VAS less reliable. Some patients may find it easier to complete a verbal questionnaire or Lickert Scale (e.g. major deterioration . . . no change . . . major improvement). These provide fewer possibilities and are less sensitive, but may sometimes be more reliable.

Measure goal attainment

Document clear treatment goals in the medical records. Suitable goals may reflect impairment, disability or handicap.

Formal scales

Standardized scales also allow comparison between individuals and groups. The choice of scale will depend on the goals for treatment.

Impairment scales

Video recordings before and after Bt injection can be helpful in monitoring the overall affect of Bt and for measurement through a variety of scales and scoring systems.

The Ashworth Scale is a widely used measure of resistance to passive movement. Its validity and sensitivity are poor, but it can be a useful baseline indicator of severity. Table 10.6 sets out specific measures. There are at least four levels of quantitative assessment for each joint movement: (i) passive range of motion (PROM)—i.e. the angle of movement arrest at slow speed of stretch; (ii) spasticity angle (Tardieu Scale [14])—given by the subtraction of the angle of catch-and-release at fast speed from the angle of movement arrest at slow speed; (iii) active range of motion (AROM); (iv) performance on rapid alternating movements. This is particularly helpful in patients with mild syndromes in whom AROM may be normal or subnormal, and in whom the impairment of motor function is detected with greater sensitivity by tests of rapid alternating movements.

Focal measures of disability (active function)

Focal measures help in limbs with residual function, but where the quality or speed of movement is affected by increased tone. The Frenchay arm test is useful in the arm, and a 10 m walking time or a 2 min walking distance in the leg.

Global functional ratings

Rarely, reduction of muscle overactivity may provide critical benefits which change the global picture of disability. The Barthel Index [228] and the FIM Motor Scale [229] are well validated and widely used measures of independence. They are divided into sub-scales and in some circumstances it may be appropriate to record the relevant subscale rather than the whole instrument.

Dependency and care needs assessment

For severely dependent patients, the assistance of two or more people may be needed for hygiene and handling tasks. These may take much longer then usual because of the need to undertake spasm-reducing manoeuvres prior to moving the patient. Bt may occasionally make a critical difference to the number of people or the time taken to perform care tasks, and may be cost-effective.

The FIM and Barthel correlate with care needs, but cannot measure them directly since they discount the number of people and the time taken to complete a task. The Northwick Park Dependency Score [229] and Care Needs Assessment can predict reduced care needs and community savings from reduced dependency.

Handicap (participation)

While health professionals may focus on impairment and disability as direct indicators of successful treatment, patients and their families are more interested in handicap and quality of life. Because of the wide range of different goals and outcomes for Bt injection, there are currently no suitable validated scales. However, quality-of-life measures may reflect treatment outcome satisfaction.

Multi-level instruments

Some authors have developed standard scales, which reflect outcome at the level of impairment, disability and handicap for the targeted problem. For example, Snow *et al.* [188] used a standardized measure of focal tone, spasm frequency and ease of hygiene in their double blind trial of Bt for adductor spasticity. Such instruments should be validated before use, but may be appropriate in the future.

Reinjection

The general principles set out in Chapter 3 apply in spasticity, with several additional points. Especially in early mild spasticity, a single injection cycle is occasionally sufficient and frees movement enough for physiotherapy and splinting to take over. If it were possible to weaken all the relevant muscles in the initial treatment session, it may be appropriate simply to reinject some or all of the same muscles. However, in some patients clinicians can inject only a selection of many large affected muscles. At each visit, assess the residual pattern of muscle overactivity and decide the most useful combination of muscles requiring reinjection, bearing in mind that earlier injections may still be wearing off. It is important to realize that antibodies to Bt do not cause significant resistance to Bt injections in spasticity, despite the relatively large doses used [230].

Complications

Patients with spasticity are often on anticoagulants, mandating caution in injecting deep muscles, but this is not an absolute contraindication to Bt therapy. Other problems are those of Bt injections in general (see Chapter 3).

How can trials demonstrate functional gains?

RCTs have so far failed to demonstrate improvements in 'active' function in spasticity, perhaps due to inadequate trial methods [231]. These could include inadequate statistical power, inappropriate patient selection, injection protocols or outcome measures, and general problems of study design. Below are some principles that we suggest should be applied in future clinical trials aiming to evaluate the impact of BT on active function.

Individualized injection protocols (muscle selection, doses, dilution)

Bt should not be tested in clinical trials as if it were an oral medication. Bt is an injectable drug designed for focal treatment and administered muscle by muscle. It permits *flexibility* and the ability to individualize the muscles selected, doses and the techniques of injection. This potentially decisive advantage over 'rigid' treatments such as oral therapy or intrathecal infusions has often been ignored in controlled trials that imposed rigid injection protocols [84,167–169] with the assumption that they would be more rigorous or more easily controlled. Only one of these studies reported subjective improvement in home function in a Patient-Reported Global Assessment Scale [168]. Other placebo-controlled designs left the choice of target muscles and doses to the investigator's discretion [162,170,186], and showed subjective improvement in home function, with one also suggesting improvement in active functional performance [186].

Doses

While it is necessary to remain within a ceiling total dose of Bt (see above), we recommend leaving the choice of dose per muscle to the investigator's discretion when designing studies aimed at showing functional improvement with Bt. This permits individualization and optimization of the injection regimen for each patient, and is also realistic as it reflects common clinical practice.

Injection technique — use exploratory stimulation

We recommend using the *exploratory stimulation technique* in trials with Bt. As discussed above, it is the most accurate technique to distinguish a muscle among its synergic neighbours, and is also the only technique that permits intramuscular localization, for example when injecting around motor points in an attempt to reach areas dense in endplates.

Include the shoulder muscles among target arm muscles

The shoulder is the most important arm joint functionally for *reaching* movements, which represent the majority of common arm movements. Surprisingly, the shoulder has consistently been overlooked in studies of Bt and upper limb spasticity [2,84,157–172,177,182–186,232]. Cocontraction in shoulder extensors contributes to the impediment of active shoulder flexion in most spastic patients. Important muscles include latissimus dorsi, teres major, posterior deltoid, long head of triceps, the scapular adductors, rhomboids, middle and lower trapezius (for shoulder flexion over 60°), and pectoralis major (for shoulder flexion over 90°) [233]. Baseline preinjection active shoulder flexion greater than 45° may predict greater potential for recovery of active function and reaching movements in arm spasticity patients after Bt injection [76].

Individualized outcome measures

Tests of active performance at the clinic

Use a combination of two types of functional tests. There should be a subjective rating of the limb function at home, by the patient or the caregiver, and an objective rating of patient performance on active tasks, preferentially using video-assessments by blinded investigators.

Individualization of subjective ratings of function at home

Functional impairment in arm spasticity varies between patients. Individualize assessments and treatment goals. There are two strategies to achieve this end.
• Use a global subjective self-assessment of the targeted limb by the patient or carer, such as the one shown in Appendix 1 of this chapter. Question 2 relates more to passive function and question 3 to active function. The patient may then express his/her own particular problem in this global opinion.
• Ask the subject to choose priority goals in a list of preselected common problems (i.e. a goal attainment scale) [171]. Outcomes might include the ability to put the affected arm through a sleeve, to open the affected hand to clean the palm, cut the fingernails, etc. The patient then rates the change in these priority areas after treatment.

Blinded assessments of active performance at the clinic

Such tests help to identify changes in active function more objectively, as opposed to subjective impressions or changes limited to passive function. Impairment evaluations such as the Fugl–Meyer Score [160,180,181] are time-consuming and do not necessarily relate well to daily functioning. Among assessments of arm function, the Frenchay Arm Test [161,169,178] contains arm tasks that are relevant for daily living. It takes only a few minutes, and is likely to be more sensitive to changes after arm treatment with Bt than global assessments by interview such as the Barthel Scale or the FIM. However, the Frenchay Arm Test gives ordinal scores, which permit only non-parametric tests. An alternative is the Modified Frenchay Assessment (Appendix 2), which uses blinded video-assessments and contains more bimanual activities. It more closely reflects the way a hemiplegic patient should function in real life. The clinician rates each of the 10 tasks on a 10-point analogue scale, from 'not done' to 'normal'. This test permits parametric analysis. When used by blinded physical therapists, intra-and inter-rater reliability of this Modified Frenchay Assessment was good to excellent as measured by Intra Class Correlation Coefficients (ICC) [234], inter-rater reliability ICC $(2,1)=0.77$–0.81, and intrarater reliability ICC $(2,1)=0.83$–0.98 (Gracies, Dean, Gandevia, Burke, unpublished).

Controlled evaluation of methods to enhance the effects of Bt injection: stretch in the injected muscle; training of the antagonist; electrical stimulation

Muscle stretch

Muscle stretch is the cornerstone of physical treatment of spastic muscle overactivity

[4]. Muscle overactivity is a factor in muscle shortening [141,143,145]. Muscle shortening in turn increases spindle sensitivity [19–21], so that muscle contracture and stretch-sensitive muscle overactivity are intertwined [16]. Thus, lengthening muscles also helps to treat stretch-sensitive muscle overactivity and its functional consequences. Indeed, there is now considerable evidence that chronic stretch is useful in spasticity [4].

Stretch is often performed during physiotherapy sessions, and commonly involves passive range of motion exercises or short posturing sessions. However, to prevent the development of contractures, muscle stretch is probably most efficient when applied continuously for several hours each day [227]. Hence, rigid or semirigid devices have been used, including rigid splints, serial casting and dynamic splints [14,235,236]. However, an intensive home stretching program may be the most satisfactory strategy in selected subjects. Rodriquez and colleagues instructed subjects in a home stretching program of the long finger flexors after finger flexion injection, and obtained good results in an open study focusing on hand opening [163]. No sham-controlled study has yet systematically measured the effect of prolonged daily stretch combined with Bt injections in the arm.

Training of the antagonist

Motor skill training in brain-injured individuals can drive plastic brain reorganization and optimize functional performance [237–239]. Recent changes in training interventions in spasticity include increasing emphasis on active exercise and task-specific training, and active and passive methods of preserving muscle extensibility [240,241]. Therapists rely increasingly on circuit training and group exercise and on technological advances such as interactive computerized systems and treadmills, which all increase time spent in active practice [240].

The muscle relaxation afforded by Bt treatment provides significant opportunities for strengthening the weak antagonist muscle and functional retraining [242]. In the open study discussed above, Rodriquez *et al.* instructed subjects in an exercise program to improve finger extension control after finger flexor Bt injection, and obtained improvement in active finger extension [163]. Again, there is no published sham-controlled study assessing the effect of the combination of antagonist training and agonist Bt injection on active function in the spastic arm.

Electrical stimulation

The promising studies by Hesse *et al.* in hemiparetic patients suggested that a program of periodic stimulation of the injected muscle and its antagonist for three 30 min sessions a day during the three days following injection may improve the outcome following Bt injection [83,84]. A recent study in the lower limb tested a program of stimulation of the injected muscle only and did not confirm these results [243]. Sham-controlled studies (e.g. with stimulation below and above sensory or motor threshold) are required to establish the advantage of combining Bt injections with a stimulation program in patients with spasticity.

Controlled comparisons of Bt with other muscle blocking agents

Local treatments with alcohol compounds (alcohol, phenol)

Potential advantages of alcohol and phenol over Bt include low cost, better stability, and the absence of antibodies. Their disadvantages are tissue destruction, lack of selectivity on motor function, and adverse effects including chronic painful dysaesthesia, muscle induration and vascular reactions [244,245]. Some rehabilitation teams have combined local treatments. Conventionally, alcohol or phenol has been used for perineural injections to block large proximal muscles for which the Bt ceiling dose would be rapidly reached. Bt can then be reserved for intramuscular injection into smaller and more distal muscles that can be selectively targeted.

The patient's prognosis and overall disability are also relevant. Because of the potential for chronic adverse effects and for destruction of muscle and sensory fibers, alcohol or phenol may be more appropriate than Bt in severe cases in which passive function and comfort are more important than active function. Conversely, the absence of tissue destruction after repeated Bt injections, and the specific action on efferent fibers might render Bt preferable where there is reasonable hope for recovery of active function. Differences in cost should further encourage properly controlled comparisons.

Kirazli *et al.* compared BtA injected intramuscularly and 5% phenol injected perineurally to treat overactive calf muscles in chronic stroke patients [191]. Intramuscular BtA was safer than perineural phenol, as complications such as common peroneal nerve palsy occurred with perineural phenol only. The two techniques appeared equally effective. However, alcohol injections can be limited to muscle motor points, which reduces the risk of dysaesthesia. There has not been a comparison of these two agents using a similar intramuscular technique.

Systemic treatments (oral antispastic agents)

Clinicians usually prescribe oral antispasticity agents before considering local injection treatments. Since the safety and efficacy of local treatments, in particular Bt, are becoming increasingly apparent, it is appropriate to question whether systemic drugs are appropriate first line treatments. A recent extensive review of the 29 available oral or intrathecal systemic antispasticity treatments drew the following conclusions [156]:
• Apart from piracetam, all systemic antispastic agents have been approved by regulatory agencies, or accepted by the community, based only on their capacity to reduce stretch responses, much like the data generated in the first era of Bt studies.
• Agents that reduce spasticity (response to muscle stretch) are non-selective and

often depress other CNS responses. Systemic administration of these agents also causes numerous central effects on higher functions, such as sedation, drowsiness, hypotension, bradycardia, depression, cognitive impairment, tolerance.

• Most systemic agents that reduce spasticity improve patient comfort, which may lead to positive subjective patient assessments. Some improve *passive* function in controlled studies. No antispastic systemic agent has improved *active* function in controlled studies, except piracetam (one study); some may actually impair active function.

Oral agents appear acceptable when passive function and comfort are priorities. However, no study has yet compared systemic and local treatments in these situations. When active function is the priority, systemic treatments may be deleterious because of the lack of selectivity of their CNS action. A controlled comparative study of systemic and local Bt treatment would clarify and differentiate their respective effects. Such a protocol is under development.

How many injection cycles do muscles need? Is Bt a life-long treatment?

Retrospective long-term studies suggest that Bt continues to work even after multiple large dose injections [163,172]. Equally, some patients can eventually discontinue Bt injections in specific muscles when they are sufficiently relaxed and lengthened for long-term exercise and use of the antagonist to maintain the improvement. This is easier with appropriate programs of stretch and training, particularly with patient compliance to these regimens. This concept of limited duration of treatment with Bt in spasticity remains to be demonstrated in a prospective study.

Conclusions

Local treatment with Bt may become a first-line therapy for patients with spasticity, and may be preferable to systemic (oral or intrathecal agents) or to local alcohol treatments, especially in patients who have the potential to recover active function. Unfortunately, most protocols to date have emphasized changes in resistance to passive movement as a primary outcome measure (e.g. Ashworth Scale, etc.). However, although it does respond to treatments such as Bt, oral agents and alcohol compounds, resistance to passive movement does not correlate with active function. Trials have shown a variety of improvements in passive function and ease of caring but have mostly been unable to demonstrate active functional gain.

It is important to develop efficient trial designs that apply some of the following principles:

1 *Flexibility* of the injection regimens, permitting *individualization* of target muscles and of the doses injected.

2 *Inclusion* of the shoulder muscles among the arm muscles targeted for Bt injection.

3 *Improved injection techniques*, including increased dilution in large muscles and muscle targeting using the stimulation technique.

4 *Individualization* of subjective functional assessments, in particular of patient ratings of home function (goal attainment scales).

5 *Blinded video-assessments* of active functional performance at the clinic.

It will also be useful to prove, using sham-controlled protocols, that (i) stretch in the injected muscle; (ii) motor training of the antagonist; (iii) electrical stimulation in both injected muscle and its antagonist, may enhance the effects of Bt injection. If proven, systematic combination of these enhancing techniques with Bt injections should improve functional outcome.

References

1 Das TK, Park DM. Effect of treatment with botulinum toxin on spasticity. *Postgrad Med J* 1989; **65**: 208–10.

2 Gracies JM, Simpson D. Therapy with Botulinum toxin. *Neurologist* 2000; **6**: 98–115.

3 Brown P. Pathophysiology of spasticity. *J Neurol, Neurosurg Psychiatry* 1994; **57**: 773–7.

4 Gracies JM. Pathophysiology of impairment in spasticity: stretch as a treatment of spastic hypertonia. *Phys Med Rehabil Clin N Am* 2001; **12**: 747–68.

5 Tabary JC, Tabary C, Tardieu C, Tardieu G, Goldspink G. Physiological and structural changes in cat's soleus muscle due to immobilization at different lengths by plaster casts. *J Physiol* 1972; **224**: 231–44.

6 Tardieu C, Tardieu G, Colbeau-Justin P, Huet de la Tour E, Lespargot A. Trophic muscle regulation in children with congenital cerebral lesions. *J Neurol Sci* 1979; **42**: 357–64.

7 Krenz NR, Weaver LC. Sprouting of primary afferent fibers after spinal cord transection in the rat. *Neuroscience* 1998; **85**: 443–58.

8 Hall M. *On the Diseases and Derangements of the Nervous System.* London: Baillière, 1841.

9 Little WJ. Course of lectures on the deformities of the human frame. *Lancet* 1843; **1**: 350–4.

10 Charcot JM. Histologie de la sclérose en plaques. *Gaz Hop (Paris)* 1868; **41**: 554–5.

11 Farmer SF, Harrison LM, Ingram DA, Stephens JA. Plasticity of central motor pathways in children with hemiplegic cerebral palsy. *Neurology* 1991; **41**: 1505–10.

12 Dewald JP, Pope PS, Given JD, Buchanan TS, Rymer WZ. Abnormal muscle coactivation patterns during isometric torque generation at the elbow and shoulder in hemiparetic subjects. *Brain* 1995; **118**: 495–510.

13 Reddy H, De Stefano N, Mortilla M, Federico A, Matthews PM. Functional reorganization of motor cortex increases with greater axonal injury from CADASIL. *Stroke* 2002; **33**: 502–8.

14 Gracies JM, Marosszeky JE, Renton R, Sandanam J, Gandevia SC, Burke D. Short-term effects of dynamic lycra splints on upper limb in hemiplegic patients. *Arch Phys Med Rehabil* 2000; **81**: 1547–55.

15 Lance JW. Symposium synopsis. In: Feldman, RG, Young, RR, Koella, WP, eds. *Spasticity, Disordered Motor Control.* Chicago: Yearbook Medical, 1980: 485–94.

16 Denny-Brown D. *The Cerebral Control of Movement.* Liverpool: Liverpool University Press, 1966: 124–143, 171–84.

17 Gracies JM, Wilson L, Gandevia SC, Burke D. Stretched position of spastic muscles aggravates their cocontraction in hemiplegic patients. *Ann Neurol* 1997; **42**: 438–9.

18 Ashworth B. Preliminary trial of carisoprodol in multiple sclerosis. *Practitioner* 1964; **192**: 540–2.

19 Maier A, Eldred E, Edgerton VR. The effects on spindles of muscle atrophy and hypertrophy. *Exp Neurol* 1972; **37**: 100–23.

20 Williams RG. Sensitivity changes shown by spindle receptors in chronically immobilized skeletal muscle. *J Physiol* 1980; **306**: 26P–7P.

21 Gioux M, Petit J. Effects of immobilising the cat peroneus longus muscle on the activity of its own spindles. *J Appl Physiol* 1993; **75**: 2629–35.

22 Kernell D, Eerbeek O, Verhey BA, Donselaar Y. Effects of physiological amounts of high- and low-rate chronic stimulation on fast-twitch muscle of the cat hindlimb. I. Speed and force related properties. *J Neurophysiol* 1987; **58**: 598–613.

23 Edström L. Selective changes in the sizes of red and white muscle fibres in upper motor lesions and Parkinsonism. *Neurol Sci* 1970; **11**: 537–50.

24 Williams PE, Goldspink G. Changes in sarcomere length and physiological properties in immobilised muscle. *J Anat* 1978; **127**: 459–68.

25 Dietz V, Berger W. Normal and impaired regulation of muscle stiffness in gait: a new hypothesis about muscle hypertonia. *Exp Neurol* 1983; **79**: 680–7.

26 Tonge DA. Chronic effects of botulinum toxin on neuromuscular transmission and sensitivity to acetyl-choline in slow and fast skeletal muscles of the mouse. *J Physiol* 1974; **241**: 127–39.

27 Sellin LC, Thesleff S, Dasgupta BR. Different effects of types A and B botulinum toxin on transmitter release at the rat neuromuscular junction. *Acta Physiol Scand* 1983; **119**: 127–33.

28 Hallett M, Glocker FX, Deuschl G. Mechanism of action of botulinum toxin. *Ann Neurol* 1994; **36**: 449–50.

29 Coffield JA, Bakry N, Zhang RD, Carlson J, Gomella LG, Simpson LL. *In vitro* characterization of botulinum toxin types A, C and D action on human tissues: combined electrophysiologic, pharmacologic and molecular biologic approaches. *J Pharmacol Exp Ther* 1997; **280**: 1489–98.

30 Sanchez-Prieto J, Sihra TS, Evans D, Ashton A, Dolly JO, Nicholls DG. Botulinum toxin A blocks glutamate exocytosis from guinea-pig cerebral cortical synaptosomes. *Eur J Biochem* 1987; **165**: 675–81.

31 Kauffman JA, Way JF Jr, Siegel LS, Sellin LC. Comparison of the action of types A and F botulinum toxin at the rat neuromuscular junction. *Toxicol Appl Pharmacol* 1985; **79**: 211–17.

32 Cosgrove AP, Graham HK. Botulinum toxin A prevents the development of contractures in the hereditary spastic mouse. *Dev Med Child Neurol* 1994; **36**: 379–85.

33 Callaway JE, Arezzo JC, Grethlein AJ. Botulinum toxin type B, an overview of its biochemistry and preclinical pharmacology. *Semin Cutan Med Surg* 2001; **20**: 127–36.

34 Black JD, Dolly JO. Interaction of 125I-labeled botulinum neurotoxins with nerve terminals. I. Ultrastructural autoradiographic localization and quantitation of distinct membrane acceptors for types A and B on motor nerves. *J Cell Biol* 1986; **103**: 521–34.

35 Black JD, Dolly JO. Interaction of [125I]-labeled botulinum neurotoxins with nerve terminals. II. Autoradiographic evidence for its uptake into motor nerves by acceptor-mediated endocytosis. *J Cell Biol* 1986; **103**: 535–44.

36 Molgo J, Siegel LS, Tabti N, Thesleff S. A study of synchronization of quantal transmitter release from mammalian motor endings by the use of botulinal toxins type A and D. *J Physiol* 1989; **411**: 195–205.

37 Maselli RA, Burnett ME, Tonsgard JH. *In vitro* microelectrode study of neuromuscular transmission in a case of botulism. *Muscle Nerve* 1992; **15**: 273–6.

38 Boroff DA, Chen GS. On the question of permeability of the blood–brain barrier to botulinum toxin. *Int Arch Allergy Appl Immunol* 1975; **48**: 495–504.

39 Habermann E, Heller I. Direct evidence for the specific fixation of Cl. botulinum A neurotoxin to brain matter. *Naunyn Schmiedebergs Arch Pharmacol* 1975; **287**: 97–106.

40 Black JD, Dolly JO. Selective location of acceptors for botulinum neurotoxin A in the central and peripheral nervous systems. *Neuroscience* 1987; **23**: 767–79.

41 Tonello F, Morante S, Rossetto O, Schiavo G, Montecucco C. Tetanus and botulism neurotoxins: a novel group of zinc endopeptidases. *Adv Exp Med Biol* 1996; **389**: 251–60.

42 Ogasawara J, Kamata Y, Sakaguchi G, Kozaki S. Properties of a protease-sensitive acceptor compo-

nent in mouse brain synaptosomes for clostridium botulinum type B neurotoxin. *FEMS Microbiol Lett* 1991; **63**: 351–5.

43 Yokosawa N, Tsuzuki K, Syuto B, Fujii N, Kimura K, Oguma K. Binding of botulinum type Cl, D and E neurotoxins to neuronal cell lines and synaptosomes. *Toxicon* 1991; **29**: 261–4.

44 Herreros J, Marti E, Ruiz-Montasell B, Casanova A, Niemann H, Blasi J. Localization of putative receptors for tetanus toxin and botulinum neurotoxin type A in rat central nervous system. *Eur J Neurosci* 1997; **9**: 2677–86.

45 Agui T, Syuto B, Oguma K, Iida H, Kubo S. Binding of *Clostridium botulinum* type C neurotoxin to rat brain synaptosomes. *J Biochem (Tokyo)* 1983; **94**: 521–7.

46 Murayama S, Syuto B, Oguma K, Iida H, Kubo S. Comparison of *Clostridium botulinum* toxins type D and C1 in molecular property, antigenicity and binding ability to rat-brain synaptosomes. *Eur J Biochem* 1984; **142**: 487–92.

47 Kozaki S. Interaction of botulinum type A, B and E derivative toxins with synaptosomes of rat brain. *Naunyn Schmiedebergs Arch Pharmacol* 1979; **308**: 67–70.

48 Dolly JO, Williams RS, Black JD, Tse CK, Hambleton P, Melling J. Localization of sites for ^{125}I-labelled botulinum neurotoxin at murine neuromuscular junction and its binding to rat brain synaptosomes. *Toxicon* 1982; **20**: 141–8.

49 Wiegand H, Erdmann G, Wellhoner HH. ^{125}I-labeled botulinum A neurotoxin: pharmacokinetics in cats after neuromuscular injection. *Naunyn Schmiedebergs Arch Pharmacol* 1976; **292**: 161–5.

50 Habermann E, Erdmann G. Pharmacokinetic and histoautoradiographic evidence for the intraaxonal movement of toxin in the pathogenesis of tetanus. *Toxicon* 1978; **16**: 611–23.

51 Mikhailov VV, Denisova DA. Role of axoplasm synthesis disorders in the nerve cell in lesions of the peripheral neuromuscular apparatus induced by botulinum toxin [Article in Russian]. *Biull Eksp Biol Medical* 1966; **31**: 44–7.

51 Kristensson K, Olsson T. Uptake and retrograde axonal transport of horseradish peroxidase in botulinum-intoxicated mice. *Brain Res* 1978; **155**: 118–23.

53 Enerback L, Kristensson K, Olsson T. Cytophotometric quantification of retrograde axonal transport of a fluorescent tracer (primuline) in mouse facial neurons. *Brain Res* 1980; **186**: 21–32.

54 Mikhailov VV, Barashkov GN. Mechanism of disorders of inhibition of electrogenesis in spinal alpha-motor neurons in experimental local botulin poisoning [Article in Russian]. *Biull Eksp Biol Medical* 1977; **83**: 651–4.

55 Moreno-Lopez B, Pastor AM, de la Cruz RR, Delgado-Garcia JM. Dose-dependent, central effects of botulinum neurotoxin type A. A pilot study in the alert behaving cat. *Neurology* 1997; **48**: 456–64.

56 Pastor AM, Moreno-Lopez B, De La Cruz RR, Delgado-Garcia JM. Effects of botulinum neurotoxin type A on abducens motoneurons in the cat: ultrastructural and synaptic alterations. *Neuroscience* 1997; **81**: 457–78.

57 Wiegand H, Wellhoner HH. Proceedings: type A botulinum toxin in cats, neural ascent and action on spinal cord reflexes. *Naunyn Schmiedebergs Arch Pharmacol* 1974; **282**: R106.

58 Wiegand H, Wellhöner HH. The action of botulinum A neurotoxin on the inhibition by antidromic stimulation of the lumbar monosynaptic reflex. *Naunyn Schmiedebergs Arch Pharmacol* 1977; **298**: 235–8.

59 Hagenah R, Benecke R, Wiegand H. Effects of type A botulinum toxin on the cholinergic transmission at spinal Renshaw cells and on the inhibitory action at Ia inhibitory interneurones. *Naunyn Schmiedebergs Arch Pharmacol* 1977; **299**: 267–72.

60 Mikhailov VV. Electrophysiological analysis of disturnaces in reflex activity of the spinal cord in experimental botulism. *Bull Exp Biol Med* 1958; **46**: 1188–92.

61 Hagenah R. Neuropharmacologic and neurotoxic studies on the Renshaw mechanism [Article in German] *Fortschr Medical* 1979; **97**: 1840–4.

62 Tyler HR. Physiological observations in human botulism. *Arch Neurol* 1963; 9: 661–70.

63 Hamjian JA, Walker FO. Serial neurophysiological studies of intramuscular botulinum-A toxin in humans. *Muscle Nerve* 1994; **17**: 1385–92.

64 Priori A, Berardelli A, Mercuri B, Manfredi M. Physiological effects produced by botulinum toxin treatment of upper limb dystonia. Changes in reciprocal inhibition between forearm muscles. *Brain* 1995; **118**: 801–7.

65 Modugno N, Priori A, Berardelli A, Vacca L, Mercuri B, Manfredi M. Botulinum toxin restores presynaptic inhibition of group Ia afferents in patients with essential tremor. *Muscle Nerve* 1998; **21**: 1701–5.

66 Pauri F, Boffa L, Cassetta E, Pasqualetti P, Rossini PM. Botulinum toxin type-A treatment in spasticity increases the central conduction time to brain stimulation. *Electroencephalogr Clin Neurophysiol* 1999; **51**: 250–9.

67 Pauri F, Boffa L, Cassetta E, Pasqualetti P, Rossini PM. Botulinum toxin type-A treatment in spastic paraparesis: a neurophysiological study. *J Neurol Sci* 2000; **181**: 89–97.

68 Wohlfarth K, Schubert M, Rothe B, Elek J, Dengler R. Remote F-wave changes after local botulinum toxin application. *Clin Neurophysiol* 2001; **112**: 636–40.

69 Behari M, Raju GB. Electrophysiological studies in patients with blepharospasm before and after botulinum toxin A therapy. *J Neurol Sci* 1996; **135**: 74–7.

70 Girlanda P, Quartarone A, Sinicropi S, Nicolosi C, Messina C. Unilateral injection of botulinum toxin in blepharospasm: single fiber electromyography and blink reflex study. *Mov Disord* 1996; **11**: 27–31.

71 Valls-Sole J, Tolosa ES, Ribera G. Neurophysiological observations on the effects of botulinum toxin treatment in patients with dystonic blepharospasm. *J Neurol Neurosurg Psychiatry* 1991; **54**: 310–13.

72 Valls-Sole J, Tolosa ES, Marti MJ, Allam N. Treatment with botulinum toxin injections does not change brainstem interneuronal excitability in patients with cervical dystonia. *Clin Neuropharmacol* 1994; **17**: 229–35.

73 Grandas F, Traba A, Alonso F, Esteban A. Blink reflex recovery cycle in patients with blepharospasm unilaterally treated with botulinum toxin. *Clin Neuropharmacol* 1998; **21**: 307–11.

74 Guyton AC, McDonald MA. Physiology of Botulinus toxin. *Arch Neurol Psychiatry (Chicago)* 1947; **57**: 578–92.

75 Mallart A, Molgo J, Angaut-Petit D, Thesleff S. Is the internal calcium regulation altered in type A botulinum toxin-poisoned motor endings? *Brain Res* 1989; **479**: 167–71.

76 Gracies JM, Weisz DJ, Yang BY, Flanagan S, Simpson D. Evidence for increased antagonist strength and movement speed following botulinum toxin injections in spasticity. *Neurology* 2001; **56**: A3.

77 Manni E, Bagolini B, Pettorossi VE, Errico P. Effect of botulinum toxin on extraocular muscle proprioception. *Doc Ophtalmol* 1989; **72**: 189–98.

78 Filippi GM, Errico P, Santarelli R, Bagolini B, Manni E. Botulinum A toxin effects on rat jaw muscle spindles. *Acta Otolaryngol* 1993; **113**: 400–4.

79 Rosales RL, Arimura K, Takenaga S, Osame M. Extrafusal and intrafusal muscle effects in experimental botulinum toxin-A injection. *Muscle Nerve* 1996; **19**: 488–96.

80 Hughes R, Whaler BC. Influence of nerve ending activity and of drugs on the rate of paralysis of rat diaphragm preparations by clostridium botulinum type A toxin. *J Physiol* 1962; **160**: 221–3.

81 Eleopra R, Tugnoli V, De Grandis D. The variability in the clinical effect induced by botulinum toxin type A. the role of muscle activity in humans. *Mov Disord* 1997; **12**: 89–94.

82 Chen R, Karp BI, Goldstein SR, Bara-Jimenez W, Yaseen Z, Hallett M. Effect of muscle activity immediately after botulinum toxin injection for writer's cramp. *Mov Disord* 1999; **14**: 307–12.

83 Hesse S, Jahnke MT, Luecke D, Mauritz KH. Short-term electrical stimulation enhances the effectiveness of botulinum toxin in the treatment of lower limb spasticity in hemiparetic patients. *Neurosci Lett* 1995; **201**: 37–40.

84 Hesse S, Reiter F, Konrad M, Jahnke MT. Botulinum toxin type A and short-term electrical stimulation in the treatment of upper limb flexor spasticity after stroke: a randomized, double blind, placebo-controlled trial. *Clin Rehabil* 1998; **12**: 381–8.

85 Pandyan AD, Granat MH, Stott DJ. Effects of electrical stimulation on flexion contractures in the hemiplegic wrist. *Clin Rehab* 1997; **11**: 123–30.

86 Chae J, Bethous F, Bohinc T, Dobos L, Davis T, Friedl A. Neuromuscular stimulation for upper extremity motor and functional recovery in acute hemiplegia. *Stroke* 1998; **29**: 975–9.

87 Shaari CM, George E, Wu BL, Biller HF, Sanders I. Quantifying the spread of botulinum toxin through muscle fascia. *Laryngoscope* 1991; **101**: 960–4.

88 George EF, Zimbler M, Wu BL, Biller HF, Sanders I. Quantitative mapping of the effect of botulinum toxin injections in the thyroarytenoid muscle. *Ann Otol Rhinol Laryngol* 1992; **101**: 888–92.

89 Sanders DB, Massey EW, Buckley EG. Botulinum toxin for blepharospasm: single fiber EMG studies. *Neurology* 1986; **36**: 545–7.

90 Lange DJ, Brin MF, Warner CL, Fahn S, Lovelace RE. Distant effects of local injection of botulinum toxin. *Muscle Nerve.* 1987; **10**: 552–5. Erratum. *Muscle Nerve.* 1988; 11: 520.

91 Olney RK, Aminoff MJ, Gelb DJ, Lowenstein DH. Neuromuscular effects distant from the site of botulinum neurotoxin injection. *Neurology* 1988; **38**: 1780–3.

92 Lange DJ, Rubin M, Greene PE *et al.* Distant effects of locally injected botulinum toxin: a double blind study of single fiber EMG changes. *Muscle Nerve* 1991; **41**: 672–5. Comment: *Muscle Nerve* 1993; **16**: 677.

93 Girlanda P, Vita G, Nicolosi C, Milone S, Messina C. Botulinum toxin therapy. distant effects on neuromuscular transmission and autonomic nervous system. *J Neurol Neurosurg Psychiatry* 1992; **55**: 844–5.

94 Bischoff C, Schoenle PW, Conrad B. Increased F-wave duration in patients with spasticity. *Electromyogr Clin Neurophysiol* 1992; **32**: 449–53.

95 Drory VE, Neufeld MY, Korczyn AD. F-wave characteristics following acute and chronic upper motor neuron lesions. *Electromyogr Clin Neurophysiol* 1993; **33**: 441–6.

96 Fisher MA. Are H reflexes and F responses equally sensitive to changes in motoneuronal excitability? *Muscle Nerve* 1996; **19**: 1345–6.

97 Hultborn H, Nielsen JB. H-reflexes and F-responses are not equally sensitive to changes in motoneuronal excitability. *Muscle Nerve* 1995; **18**: 1471–4.

98 Hultborn H, Nielsen JB. Comments. methodological problems of comparing F responses and H reflexes. *Muscle Nerve* 1996; **19**: 1347–8.

99 Leis AA, Stetkarova I, Beric A, Stokic DS. The relative sensitivity of F wave and H reflex to changes in motoneuronal excitability. *Muscle Nerve* 1996; **19**: 1342–4.

100 Gelb DJ, Yoshimura DM, Olney RK, Lowenstein DH, Aminoff MJ. Change in pattern of muscle activity following botulinum toxin injections for torticollis. *Ann Neurol* 1991; **29**: 370–6.

101 Tardieu G, Tardieu C, Hariga J. Infiltrations par l'alcool à 45° des points moteurs, des racines par voie épidurale, ou du nerf tibial postérieur. Leurs indications et contre-indications dans les divers modes de 'spasticité' (experience de dix ans). *Rev Neurol (Paris)* 1971; **125**: 63–8.

102 Tardieu G. Troubles du maintien postural des membres supérieurs. In: Tardieu G, ed. *Les Feuillets de l'Infirmité Motrice Cérébrale.* Paris: Association Nationale des IMC, 1972: 1–10.

103 Tardieu G, Tardieu C, Hariga J. Selective partial denervation by alcohol injections and their results in spasticity. *Reconstr Surg Traumat* 1972; **13**: 18–36.

104 McLellan DL. Co-contraction and stretch reflexes in spasticity during treatment with baclofen. *J Neurol Neurosurg Psychiat* 1977; **40**: 30–8.

105 Knutsson E, Richards C. Different types of disturbed motor control in gait of hemiparetic patients. *Brain* 1979; **102**: 405–30.

106 Knutsson E, Martensson A. Dynamic motor capacity in spastic paresis and its relation to prime mover dysfunction. spastic reflexes and antagonist coactivation. *Scand J Rehab Med* 1980; **12**: 93–106.

107 Hammond MC, Fitts SS, Kraft GH, Nutter PB, Trotter MJ, Robinson LM. Cocontraction in the hemiparetic forearm: quantitative EMG evaluation. *Arch Phys Med Rehabil* 1988; **69**: 348–51.

108 Wing AM, Lough S, Turton A, Fraser C, Jenner JR. Recovery of elbow function in voluntary positioning of the hand following hemiplegia due to stroke. *J Neurol Neurosurg Psychiatry* 1990; **53**: 126–34.

109 Levin MF, Hui-Chan C. Ankle spasticity is inversely correlated with antagonist voluntary contraction in hemiparetic subjects. *Electromyogr Clin Neurophysiol* 1994; **34**: 415–25.

110 Levin MF. Interjoint coordination during pointing movements is disrupted in spastic hemiparesis. *Brain* 1996; **119**: 281–93.

111 Levin MF, Dimov M. Spatial zones for muscle coactivation and the control of postural stability. *Brain Res* 1997; **757**: 43–59.

112 Levin MF, Selles RW, Verheul MH, Meijer OG. Deficits in the coordination of agonist and antagonist muscles in stroke patients: implications for normal motor control. *Brain Res* 2000; **853**: 352–69.

113 Unnithan VB, Dowling JJ, Frost G, Volpe Ayub B, Bar-Or O. Cocontraction and phasic activity during GAIT in children with cerebral palsy. *Electromyogr Clin Neurophysiol* 1996; **36**: 487–94.

114 Unnithan VB, Dowling JJ, Frost G, Bar-Or O. Role of cocontraction in the O_2 cost of walking in children with cerebral palsy. *Med Sci Sports Exerc* 1996; **28**: 1498–504.

115 Gracies JM. Evaluation de la spasticité. Apport de l'Echelle de Tardieu. *Motricité Cérébrale* 2001; 22: 1–16.

116 Nielsen J, Kagamihara Y. The regulation of disynaptic reciprocal Ia inhibition during cocontraction of antagonistic muscles in man. *J Physiol* 1992; **456**: 373–91.

117 Nielsen J, Kagamihara Y. The regulation of presynaptic inhibition during co-contraction of antagonistic muscles in man. *J Physiol* 1993; **464**: 575–93.

118 Nielsen J, Sinkjaer T, Toft E, Kagamihara Y. Segmental reflexes and ankle joint stiffness during co-contraction of antagonistic ankle muscles in man. *Exp Brain Res* 1994; **102**: 350–8.

119 Llewellyn M, Yang JF, Prochazka A. Human H-reflexes are smaller in difficult beam walking than in normal treadmill walking. *Exp Brain Res* 1990; **83**: 22–8.

120 Nielsen J, Nagaoka M, Kagamihara Y, Kakuda N, Tanaka R. Discharge of muscle afferents during voluntary co-contraction of antagonistic ankle muscles in man. *Neurosci Lett* 1994; **170**: 277–80.

121 Nielsen J, Pierrot-Deseilligny E. Evidence of facilitation of soleus-coupled Renshaw cells during voluntary co-contraction of antagonistic ankle muscles in man. *J Physiol* 1996; **493**: 603–11.

122 Katz R, Pierrot-Deseilligny E. Recurrent inhibition of alpha-motoneurons in patients with upper motor neuron lesions. *Brain* 1982; **105**: 103–24.

123 Crone C, Nielsen J, Petersen N, Ballegaard M, Hultborn H. Disynaptic reciprocal inhibition of ankle extensors in spastic patients. *Brain* 1994; **117**: 1161–8.

124 Nakashima K, Rothwell JC, Day BL, Thompson PD, Shannon K, Marsden CD. Reciprocal inhibition between forearm muscles in patients with writer's cramp and other occupational cramps, symptomatic hemidystonia and hemiparesis due to stroke. *Brain* 1989; **112**: 681–97.

125 Faist M, Mazevet D, Dietz V, Pierrot-Deseilligny E. A quantitative assessment of presynaptic inhibition of Ia afferents in spastics. Differences in hemiplegics and paraplegics. *Brain* 1994; **117**: 1449–55.

126 Nielsen J, Petersen N, Crone C. Changes in transmission across synapses of Ia afferents in spastic patients. *Brain* 1995; **118**: 995–1004.

127 Morita H, Crone C, Christenhuis D, Petersen NT, Nielsen JB. Modulation of presynaptic inhibition and disynaptic reciprocal Ia inhibition during voluntary movement in spasticity. *Brain* 2001; **124**: 826–37.

128 Hesse S, Brandl-Hesse B, Seidel U, Doll B, Gregoric M. Lower limb muscle activity in ambulatory children with cerebral palsy before and after the treatment with Botulinum toxin A. *Restor Neurol Neurosci* 2000; **17**: 1–8.

129 Tardieu G. Description classique et étude critique des cinq formes d'infirmité motrice cerébrale internationalement retenues. Classifications diverses. In: Tardieu G, ed. *Les Feuillets de l'Infirmité Motrice Cérébrale*. Paris: Association Nationale des IMC, 1969: 1–8.

130 Lance JW, McLeod JG. *A Physiological Approach to Clinical Neurology*, 3rd edn. London: Butterworths, 1981: 145.

131 Burke D. An approach to the treatment of spasticity. *Drugs* 1975; **10**: 112–20.

132 Burke D. Spasticity as an adaptation to pyramidal tract injury. *Adv Neurol*, **47**. Waxman SG, ed. *Functional Recovery in Neurological Disease*. New York: Raven Press, 1988: 401–23.

133 Young RR. Spasticity: A review. *Neurology* 1994; **44**: S12–S20.

134 Baker JH, Hall-Craggs EC. Changes in length of sarcomeres following tenotomy of the rat soleus muscle. *Anat Rec* 1978; **192**: 55–8.

135 Baker JH, Hall-Craggs EC. Changes in sarcomere length following tenotomy in the rat. *Muscle Nerve* 1980; **3**: 413–16.

136 McLachlan EM. Rapid atrophy of mouse soleus muscles after tenotomy depends on an intact innervation. *Neurosci Lett* 1981; **25**: 269–74.

137 McLachlan EM, Chua M. Rapid adjustment of sarcomere length in tenotomized muscles depends on an intact innervation. *Neurosci Lett* 1983; **35**: 127–33.

138 McLachlan EM. Atrophic effects of proximal tendon transection with and without denervation on mouse soleus muscles. *Exp Neurol* 1983; **81**: 651–68.

139 Booth FW, Seider MJ. Early change in skeletal muscle protein synthesis after limb immobilization of rats. *J Appl Physiol* 1979; **47**: 974–7.

140 Booth FW. Effect of limb immobilization on skeletal muscle. *J Appl Physiol* 1982; **52**: 1113–18.

141 McLachlan EM. Modification of the atrophic effects of tenotomy on mouse soleus muscles by various hind limb nerve lesions and different levels of voluntary motor activity. *Exp Neurol* 1983; **81**: 669–82.

142 Williams PE, Goldspink G. Connective tissue changes in immobilised muscle. *J Anat* 1984; **138**: 343–50.

143 Ranson SW, Dixon HH. Elasticity and ductility of muscle in myostatic contracture caused by tetanus toxin. *Am J Physiol* 1928; **86**: 312–19.

144 Pollock LJ, Davis L. Studies in decerebration. VI. The effect of deafferentation upon decerebrate rigidity. *Am J Physiol* 1930; **98**: 47–9.

145 Huet de la Tour E, Tardieu C, Tabary JC, Tabary C. Decrease of muscle extensibility and reduction of sarcomere number in soleus muscle following a local injection of tetanus toxin. *J Neurol Sci* 1979; **40**: 123–31.

146 Thompson NS, Baker RJ, Cosgrove AP, Corry IS, Graham HK. Musculoskeletal modelling in determining the effect of botulinum toxin on the hamstrings of patients with crouch gait. *Dev Med Child Neurol* 1998; **40**: 622–5.

147 Eames NW, Baker R, Hill N, Graham K, Taylor T, Cosgrove A. The effect of botulinum toxin A on gastrocnemius length: magnitude and duration of response. *Dev Med Child Neurol* 1999; **41**: 226–32.

148 Cosgrove AP, Corry IS, Graham HK. Botulinum toxin in the management of the lower limb in cerebral palsy. *Dev Med Child Neurol* 1994; **36**: 386–96.

149 Koman LA, Mooney JF III, Smith BP, Walker F, Leon JM. Botulinum toxin type A neuromuscular blockade in the treatment of lower extremity spasticity in cerebral palsy: a randomized, double blind, placebo-controlled trial. Botox® Study Group. *J Pediatr Orthop* 2000; **20**: 108–15.

150 Corry IS, Cosgrove AP, Duffy CM, McNeill S, Taylor TC, Graham HK. Botulinum toxin A compared with stretching casts in the treatment of spastic equinus: a randomized prospective trial. *J Pediatr Orthop* 1998; **18**: 304–11.

151 Reiter F, Danni M, Lagalla G, Ceravolo G, Provinciali L. Low-dose botulinum toxin with ankle taping for the treatment of spastic equinovarus foot after stroke. *Arch Phys Med Rehabil* 1998; **79**: 532–5.

152 Flett PJ, Stern LM, Waddy H, Connell TM, Seeger JD, Gibson SK. Botulinum toxin A versus fixed cast stretching for dynamic calf tightness in cerebral palsy. *J Paediatr Child Health* 1999; **35**: 71–7.

153 Scott AB. Injection treatment of endocrine orbital myopathy. *Doc Ophthalmol* 1984; **58**: 141–5.

154 Scott AB, Kraft SP. Botulinum toxin injection in the management of lateral rectus paresis. *Ophthalmology* 1985; **92**: 676–83.

155 Scott AB. Change of eye muscle sarcomeres according to eye position. *J Pediatr Ophthalmol Strabismus* 1994; **31**: 85–8.

156 Gracies JM, Elovic E, McGuire J, Simpson D. Traditional pharmacologic treatments of spasticity. Part II Systemic Treatments. In: Mayer NH, Simpson DM, eds. *Spasticity: Etiology, Evaluation, Management, and the role of Botulinum Toxin.* New York: WEMOVE; 2002: 65–93.

157 Das TK, Park DM. Botulinum toxin in treating spasticity. *Br J Clin Prac* 1989; **43**: 401–3.

158 Hesse S, Friedrich H, Domasch C, Mauritz KH. Botulinum toxin therapy for upper limb flexor spasticity: preliminary results. *J Rehab Sci* 1992; **5**: 98–101.

159 Konstanzer A, Ceballos-Baumann AO, Dressnandt J, Conrad B. Lokale Injektionsbehandlung mit Botulinum-Toxin A bei schwerer Arm- und Beinspastik. (Local injection treatment with botulinum toxin A in severe arm and leg spasticity). *Nervenarzt* 1993; **64**: 517–23.

160 Dunne JW, Heye N, Dunne S. Treatment of chronic limb spasticity with botulinum toxin A. *J Neurol Neurosurg Psychiatry* 1995; **58**: 232–5.

161 Sampaio C, Ferreira JJ, Pinto AA, Crespo M, Ferro JM, Castro-Caldas A. Botulinum toxin type A for the treatment of arm and hand spasticity in stroke patients. *Clin Rehabil* 1997; **11**: 3–7.

162 Bhakta BB, Cozens JA, Chamberlain MA, Bamford JM. Impact of botulinum toxin type A on disability and carer burden due to arm spasticity after stroke: a randomized double blind placebo controlled trial. *J Neurol Neurosurg Psychiatry* 2000; **69**: 217–21.

163 Rodriquez AA, McGinn M, Chappell R. Botulinum toxin injection of spastic finger flexors in hemiplegic patients. *Am J Phys Med Rehabil* 2000; **79**: 44–7.

164 Friedman A, Diamond M, Johnston MV, Daffner C. Effects of botulinum toxin A on upper limb spasticity in children with cerebral palsy. *Am J Phys Med Rehabil.* 2000; **79**: 53–9, 75–6.

165 Hurvitz EA, Conti GE, Flansburg EL, Brown SH. Motor control testing of upper limb function after botulinum toxin injection: a case study. *Arch Phys Med Rehabil* 2000; **81**: 1408–15.

166 Yablon SA, Agana BT, Ivanhoe CB, Boake C. Botulinum toxin in severe upper extremity spasticity among patients with traumatic brain injury: an open labeled trial. *Neurology* 1996; **47**: 939–44.

167 Simpson D, Alexander DN, O'Brien CF *et al.* Botulinum toxin type A in the treatment of upper extremity spasticity: a randomized, double blind, placebo-controlled trial. *Neurology* 1996; **46**: 1306–10.

168 Smith SJ, Ellis E, White S, Moore AP. A double blind placebo-controlled study of botulinum toxin in upper limb spasticity after stroke or head injury. *Clin Rehabil* 2000; **14**: 5–13.

169 Bakheit AM, Thilmann AF, Ward AB *et al.* A randomized, double blind, placebo-controlled, dose-ranging study to compare the efficacy and safety of three doses of botulinum toxin type A (Dysport®) with placebo in upper limb spasticity after stroke. *Stroke* 2000; **31**: 2402–6.

170 Richardson D, Sheean G, Werring D *et al.* Evaluating the role of botulinum toxin in the management of focal hypertonia in adults. *J Neurol Neurosurg Psychiatry* 2000; **69**: 499–506.

171 Bakheit AM, Pittock S, Moore AP *et al.* A randomized, double blind, placebo-controlled study of the efficacy and safety of botulinum toxin type A in upper limb spasticity in patients with stroke. *Eur J Neurol* 2001; **8**: 559–65.

172 Lagalla G, Danni M, Reiter F, Ceravolo MG, Provinciali L. Poststroke spasticity management with repeated botulinum toxin injections in the upper limb. *Am J Phys Medical Rehabil* 2000; **79**: 377–84, 391–4.

173 Sahrmann SA, Norton BJ. The relationship of voluntary movement to spasticity in the upper motor neuron syndrome. *Ann Neurol* 1977; **2**: 460–5.

174 Norton BJ, Bomze HA, Sahrmann SA, Eliasson SG. Correlation between gait speed and spasticity at the knee. *Phys Ther* 1975; **55**: 355–9.

175 Sheean GL. Botulinum treatment of spasticity: why is it so difficult to show a functional benefit? *Curr Opin Neurol* 2001; **14**: 771–6.

176 Mayer NH, Esquenazi A, Keenan MA. Patterns of upper motoneuron dysfunction in the lower limb. *Adv Neurol* 2001; **87**: 311–19.

177 Mémin B, Pollak P, Hommel M, Perret J. Traitement de la spasticité par la toxine botulique. *Rev Neurol (Paris)* 1992; **148**: 212–14.

178 Wade DT, Langton-Hewer R, Wood VA, Skilbeck CE, Ismail HM. The hemiplegic arm after stroke, measurement and recovery. *J Neurol Neurosurg Psychiatry* 1983; **46**: 521–4.

179 Taub E, Uswatte G, Pidikiti R. Constraint-Induced Movement Therapy, a new family of techniques with broad application to physical rehabilitation. A clinical review. *J Rehabil Res Dev* 1999; **36**: 237–51.

180 Fugl-Meyer AR, Jaasko L, Leyman I, Olsson S, Steglind S. The poststroke hemiplegic patient. 1. A method for evaluation of physical performance. *Scand J Rehab Med* 1975; **7**: 13–31.

181 Lindmark B, Hamrin E. Evaluation of functional capacity after stroke as a basis for active intervention. Validation of a modified chart for motor capacity assessment. *Scand J Rehabil Med* 1988; **20**: 111–15.

182 Reiter F, Danni M, Ceravolo MG, Provinciali L. Disability changes after treatment of upper limb spasticity with botulinum toxin. *J Neuro Rehab* 1996; **10**: 47–52.

183 Bhakta BB, Cozens JA, Bamford JM, Chamberlain MA. Use of botulinum toxin in stroke patients with severe upper limb spasticity. *J Neurol Neurosurg Psychiatry* 1996; **61**: 30–5.

184 Corry IS, Cosgrove AP, Walsh EG, McClean D, Graham HK. Botulinum toxin A in the hemiplegic upper limb: a double blind trial. *Dev Med Child Neurol* 1997; **39**: 185–93.

185 Fehlings D, Rang M, Glazier J, Steele C. Botulinum toxin type A injections in the spastic upper extremity of children with hemiplegia: child characteristics that predict a positive outcome. *Eur J Neurol* 2001; **8**: 145–9.

186 Fehlings D, Rang M, Glazier J, Steele C. An evaluation of botulinum-A toxin injections to improve upper extremity function in children with hemiplegic cerebral palsy. *J Pediatr* 2000; **137**: 331–7.

187 Brashear A, Gordon M, Elovic E *et al.* A multicenter, double blind, randomized, placebo-controlled, parallel study of the safety and efficacy of Botox® (botulinum toxin type A) purified neurotoxin in the treatment of focal upper limb spasticity poststroke. *Neurology* 2001; **56**: A78.

188 Snow BJ, Tsui JKC, Bhatt MH, Varelas M, Hashimoto SA, Calne DB. Treatment of spasticity with botulinum toxin: a double blind study. *Ann Neurol* 1990; **28**: 512–15.

189 Grazko MA, Polo KB, Jabbari B. Botulinum toxin A for spasticity, muscle spasms and rigidity. *Neurology* 1995; **45** (4): 712–17.

190 Burbaud P, Wiart L, Dubos JL *et al.* A randomized, double blind, placebo controlled trial of botulinum toxin in the treatment of spastic foot in hemiparetic patients. *J Neurol Neurosurg Psychiatry* 1996; **61**: 265–9.

191 Kirazli Y, On AY, Kismali B, Aksit R. Comparison of phenol block and botulinum toxin type A in the treatment of spastic foot after stroke: a randomised, double blind trial. *Am J Phys Med Rehabil* 1998; **77** (6): 510–15.

192 Hyman N, Barnes M, Bhakta B *et al.* Botulinum toxin (Dysport®) treatment of hip adductor spasticity in multiple sclerosis: a prospective, randomized, double blind, placebo-controlled, dose-ranging study. *J Neurol Neurosurg Psychiatry* 2000; **68**: 707–12.

193 Molteni F. Botulinum toxin and rehabilitation programs in lower limb spasticity. *Eur J Neurol* 1995; **2**: 61–7.

194 The Wemove Spasticity Study Group. Dosing, administration and a treatment algorithm for use of botulinum toxin type A for adult-onset muscle overactivity in patients with on . . . motorneuron lesion. In: Mayer N, Sunpson D, eds. *Spasticity: Etiology, Evaluation, Management and the Role of Botulinum Toxin* 2002, 154–66.

195 Cosgrove AP, Graham HK. Cerebral palsy. In: Moore P, ed. *Handbook of Botulinum Toxin Treatment.* Oxford: Blackwell Scientific, 1995: 222–47.

196 Comella CL, Buchman AS, Tanner CM, Brown-Toms NC, Goetz CG. Botulinum toxin injection for spasmodic torticollis, increased magnitude of benefit with electromyographic assistance. *Neurology* 1992; **42**: 878–82.

197 Geenen C, Consky E, Ashby P. Localizing muscles for botulinum toxin treatment of focal hand dystonia. *Can J Neurol Sci* 1996; **23**: 194–7.

198 Bickerton LE, Agur AM, Ashby P. Flexor digitorum superficialis. locations of individual muscle bellies for botulinum toxin injections. *Muscle Nerve* 1997; **20**: 1041–3.

199 Childers MK, Kornegay JN, Aoki R, Otaviani L, Bogan DJ, Petroski G. Evaluating motor end-plate-targeted injections of botulinum toxin type A in a canine model. *Muscle Nerve* 1998; **21**: 653–5.

200 Zack SI. *The Motor Endplate*. Philadelphia: WB Saunders, 1971.

201 Aquilonius SM, Askmark H, Gillberg PG, Nandedkar S, Olsson Y, Stalberg E. Topographical localization of motor endplates in cryosections of whole human muscles. *Muscle Nerve* 1984; **7**: 287–93.

202 Sanders I, Mu L, Amirali A *et al*. Motor endplate mapping of the human biceps brachii muscle. Abstract. *Ann Neurol* 1998; **44**: 501.

203 DeLateur BJ. A new technique of intramuscular phenol neurolysis. *Arch Phys Med Rehabil* 1972; **53**: 179–81.

204 Buchthal F, Rosenfalck P. Spontaneous electrical activity of human muscle. *Electroencephalogr Clin Neurophysiol* 1966; **20**: 321–36.

205 Jones RV Jr, Lambert EH, Sayre GP. Source of type of insertion activity in electromyography with evaluation of histologic method of localization. *Arch Phys Med* 1955; **36**: 301–10.

206 Wiederholt WC. 'End-plate noise' in electromyography. *Neurology* 1970; **20**: 214–24.

207 Del Toro DR, Park TA. Abductor hallucis false motor points. electrophysiologic mapping and cadaveric dissection. *Muscle Nerve* 1996; **19**: 1138–43.

208 Kadrie HA, Yates SK, Milner-Brown HS, Brown WF. Multiple point electrical stimulation of ulnar and median nerves. *J Neurol Neurosurg Psychiatry* 1976; **39**: 973–85.

209 Arezzo JC, Litwak M, Caputo FA *et al*. Botulinum toxin type B (BoNT-B): Safety studies in adult and juvenile cynomolgus monkeys. Neurology 2001 (Supple 3); **56** (8): A387.

210 Lew MF, Brashear A, Factor S. The safety and efficacy of botulinum toxin type B in the treatment of patients with cervical dystonia: summary of three controlled clinical trials. *Neurology* 2000; **55**: S29–S35.

211 Cullis PA. Safety and efficacy of botulinum toxin type B. an open label, dose escalation study. *J Neurol Sci* 2001 (Suppl 1); **187**: ••.

212 McAfee A, Kuhn ER, Ambrosius WT, Brashear A. An open label trial of botulinum toxin type B in upper limb spasticity. *Arch Phys Medical Rehabil* 2002; (In press).

213 O'Brien C, Mancini F. Botulinum toxin type B for limb spasticity. *Arch Phys Medical Rehabil* 2002; (In press).

214 NeuroBloc® SPC, (European Package Insert). Elan, 2002.

215 Shaari CM, Sanders I. Quantifying how location and dose of botulinum toxin injections affect muscle paralysis. *Muscle Nerve* 1993; **16**: 964–9.

216 Bigalke H, Wohlfarth K, Irmer A, Dengler R. Botulinum A toxin. Dysport® improvement of biological availability. *Exp Neurol* 2001; **168**: 162–70.

217 Hesse S, Lücke D, Malezic M *et al*. Botulinum toxin treatment for lower limb extensor spasticity in chronic hemiparetic patients. *J Neurol Neurosurg Psychiatry* 1994; **57**: 1321–4.

218 Hesse S, Krajnik J, Luecke PT, Jahnke MT, Gregoric M, Mauritz KH. Ankle muscle activity before and after botulinum toxin therapy for lower limb extensor spasticity in chronic hemiparetic patients. *Stroke* 1996; **27**: 455–60.

219 Corry IS, Cosgrove AP, Walsh EG, McClean D, Graham HK. Botulinum toxin A in the hemiplegic upper limb: a double blind trial. *Dev Med Child Neurol* 1997; **39**: 185–93.

220 Childers MK, Stacy M, Cooke DL, Stonnington HH. Comparison of two injection techniques using botulinum toxin in spastic hemiplegia. *Am J Phys Med Rehabil* 1996; **75**: 462–9.

221 Borg-Stein J, Pine ZM, Miller JR, Brin MF. Botulinum toxin for the treatment of spasticity in multiple sclerosis. New observations. *Am J Phys Med Rehabil* 1993; **72**: 364–8.

222 Kirazli Y, On AY, Kismali B, Aksit R. Comparison of phenol block and botulinus toxin type A in the treatment of spastic foot after stroke: a randomized, double blind trial. *Am J Phys Med Rehabil* 1998; **77**: 510–15.

223 Sloop RR, Escutin RO, Matus JA, Cole BA, Peterson GW. Dose–response curve of human extensor digitorum brevis muscle function to intramuscularly injected botulinum toxin type A. *Neurology* 1996; **46**: 1382–6.

224 Girlanda P, Quartarone A, Sinicropi S *et al*. Botulinum toxin in upper limb spasticity: study of reciprocal inhibition between forearm muscles. *Neuroreport* 1997; **8**: 3039–44.

225 Arens LJ, Leary PM, Goldschmidt RB. Experience with botulinum toxin in the treatment of cerebral palsy. *S Afr Med J* 1997; **87**: 1001–3.

226 Dengler R, Neyer U, Wohlfahrt K, Bettig U, Janzik HH. Local botulinum toxin in the treatment of spastic drop foot. *J Neurol* 1992; **239**: 375–8.

227 Tardieu C, Lespargot A, Tabary C, Bret MD. For how long must the soleus be stretched each day to prevent contracture. *Dev Med Child Neurol* 1998; **30**: 3–10.

228 Wade DT. *Neurological rehabilitation*. London: Churchill Livingstone, 1990.

229 Turner Stokes L, Ward A. On behalf of the working party on botulinum toxin in spasticity. *Guidelines for the use of botulinum toxin (BTX) in the management of spasticity in adults*. London: Royal College Physicians, 2002.

230 Turkel CC, Dru RM, Daffe HS, Brin M. Neutralizing antibody formation is . . . following repeated injections of a low protein formulation of botulinum toxin type A (BTX-A) in patients with poststroke spasticity. *Neurology* 2002, **58** (Suppl 7): A316.

231 Sheean G. Botulinum treatment of spasticity: why is it so difficult to show a functional benefit? *Curr Opin Neurol* 2001; **14**: 771–5.

232 Panizza M, Castagna M, di Summa A, Saibene L, Grioni G, Nilsson J. Functional and clinical changes in upper limb spastic patients treated with botulinum toxin (BTX). *Funct Neurol* 2000; **15**: 147–55.

233 Hislop HJ, Montgomery J. Techniques of manual examination. In: Hislop HJ, Montgomery J, eds. *Daniel's and Woringham's Muscle Testing*, 6th edn. Philadelphia: WB Saunders, 1995: 69–80, 83–8.

234 Fleiss JL. *The Design and Analysis of Clinical Experiments*. New York: John Wiley and Sons, 1986.

235 Gracies JM, Fitzpatrick R, Wilson L, Burke D, Gandevia SC. Lycra garments designed for patients with upper limb spasticity: mechanical effects in normal subjects. *Arch Phys Med Rehab* 1997; **78**: 1066–71.

236 Feldman PA. Upper extremity casting and splinting. In: Glenn MB, Whyte J, eds. *The Practical Management of Spasticity in Children and Adults*. London: Lea & Febiger, 1990, pp. 149–66.

237 Nudo RJ, Wise BM, SiFuentes F, Milliken GW. Neural substrates for the effects of rehabilitative training on motor recovery after ischemic infarct. *Science* 1996; **272**: 1791–4.

238 Xerri C, Merzenich MM, Peterson BE, Jenkins W. Plasticity of primary somatosensory cortex paralleling sensorimotor skill recovery from stroke in adult monkeys. *J Neurophysiol* 1998; **79**: 2119–48.

239 Butefisch CM, Davis BC, Sawaki L *et al*. Modulation of use-dependent plasticity by d-amphetamine. *Ann Neurol* 2002; **51**: 59–68.

240 Shepherd RB. Exercise and training to optimize functional motor performance in stroke: driving neural reorganization? *Neural Plast* 2001; **8**: 121–9.

241 Dean CM, Shepherd RB. Task-related training improves performance of seated reaching tasks after stroke. A randomized controlled trial. *Stroke* 1997; **28**: 722–8.

242 Leach J. Children undergoing treatment with botulinum toxin. the role of the physical therapist. *Muscle Nerve*. 1997; **6**: S194–207.

243 Detrembleur C, Lejeune TM, Renders A, Van Den Bergh PY. Botulinum toxin and short-term electrical stimulation in the treatment of equinus in cerebral palsy. *Mov Disord* 2002; **17**: 162–9.

244 Gracies JM, Elovic E, McGuire J, Simpson D. Traditional pharmacologic treatments of spasticity. Part I. Local treatments. *Muscle Nerve*, 1997; **20**: S61–91.

245 Gracies JM, Simpson D. Neuromuscular blockers. *Phys Med Rehabil Clin N Am* 1999; **10**: 357–83, viii.

Patient self-assessment

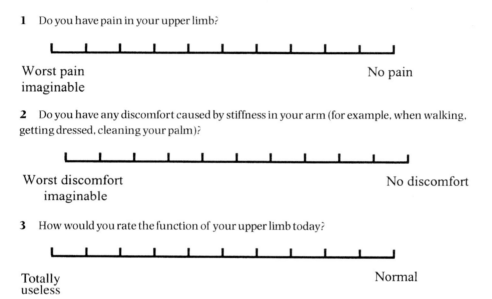

1 Do you have pain in your upper limb?

Worst pain imaginable   No pain

2 Do you have any discomfort caused by stiffness in your arm (for example, when walking, getting dressed, cleaning your palm)?

Worst discomfort imaginable   No discomfort

3 How would you rate the function of your upper limb today?

Totally useless   Normal

Modified Frenchay Scale

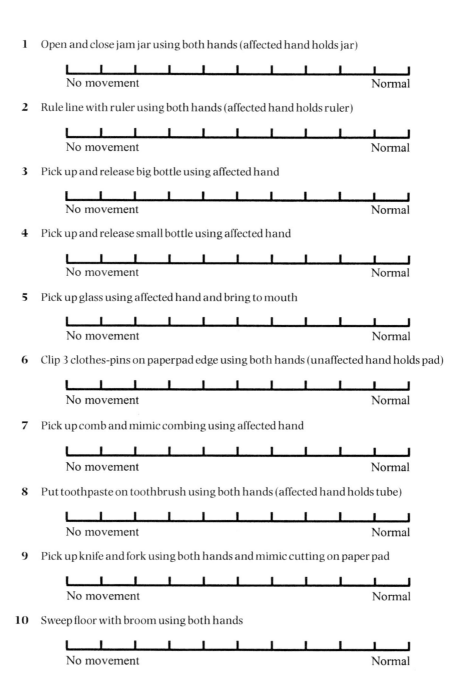

1   Open and close jam jar using both hands (affected hand holds jar)

No movement   Normal

2   Rule line with ruler using both hands (affected hand holds ruler)

No movement   Normal

3   Pick up and release big bottle using affected hand

No movement   Normal

4   Pick up and release small bottle using affected hand

No movement   Normal

5   Pick up glass using affected hand and bring to mouth

No movement   Normal

6   Clip 3 clothes-pins on paperpad edge using both hands (unaffected hand holds pad)

No movement   Normal

7   Pick up comb and mimic combing using affected hand

No movement   Normal

8   Put toothpaste on toothbrush using both hands (affected hand holds tube)

No movement   Normal

9   Pick up knife and fork using both hands and mimic cutting on paper pad

No movement   Normal

10 Sweep floor with broom using both hands

No movement   Normal

CHAPTER 11

Spasticity in children

STEFFEN BERWECK, H KERR GRAHAM & FLORIAN HEINEN

A word of caution

The registration of botulinum toxin A (BtA) preparations Botox® and Dysport® varies from country to country. For example, as of April 2001, BtA registration in Germany and Australia only covered the treatment of spastic equinus in children with cerebral palsy from 2 years of age, and at a maximum dose of 4 mu Botox® per kg body weight. NeuroBloc®/MYOBLOC™ (botulinum toxin B [BtB]) does not yet hold any licences for paediatric use. In most cases this means that the parent or guardian must understand and accept that the proposed treatment is effectively 'off-label'. Some countries require institutional ethical approval and written consent for each individual case before starting treatment with botulinum toxin (Bt).

Physicians administering BtA must have adequate training and experience in general paediatrics, orthopaedics and rehabilitation, with specific additional training in when and how to use BtA.

Introduction

Clinical experience with BtA in the treatment of spasticity in children goes back to the early 1990s with the first trials reported from the US by Koman and coworkers [1] and from the UK by Graham and coworkers [2]. Several open label and placebo-controlled studies have documented efficacy, safety and side-effects [3]. The therapeutic principle is disarmingly simple. BtA injections result in a localized, temporary chemodenervation of affected muscles, which in turn can lead to functional gains. However the heterogeneity and complexity of spastic motor disorders in children ensure that the application of this principle is challenging even for the most experienced clinician.

Therapeutic principle and limitations

• The treatment converts paresis with muscular *hyper*activity to paresis with muscular *hypo*activity.
• A *focal* therapy is applied to a *non-focal* motor disorder.
• A *chronic* disorder is treated with an agent that has a relatively *short duration* of activity.

Mode of action

BtA is well known as a cause of food poisoning and infant botulism. It is a potent neurotoxin produced by the bacterium *Clostridium botulinum* under anaerobic conditions.
It binds to cholinergic nerve endings and inhibits release of the neurotransmitter
acetylcholine by blocking the binding of acetylcholine vesicles to the interior of
the motor endplate plasma membrane. The sprouting of new nerve endings restores
neurotransmission. It takes about 3 months for the original nerve endings to be restored
while the 'new' nerve endings are concurrently being eliminated. The effect of BtA
is pharmacologically as well as clinically completely reversible [4]. There is no evidence
for central nervous system (CNS) effects of the toxin after intramuscular injection
[5] or for accumulation or persistence in the central or peripheral nervous systems.
However, BtA therapy has some effect on the activity of the spinal motorneurone since
both extrafusal and intrafusal neuromuscular junctions are affected. Furthermore,
there is some evidence that BtA therapy might have an effect on sensorimotor system
organization [6]. Pauri *et al.* observed prolonged motor evoked potential latencies
and prolonged central conduction time after BtA injections in patients with spastic
paraparesis [7].

Spastic motor disorders

The expression 'spastic motor disorder' is used as an umbrella term. It is purely descriptive and does not imply any particular aetiology or pathology. It refers to complex disorders involving cortical, spinal and musculoskeletal systems and feedback mechanisms.
The common denominator is 'early onset' of the disorder in childhood and the most
common clinical syndrome is cerebral palsy.

Classification

Motor disorders in children can be classified according to the aetiology and CNS lesion,
the type of movement disorder, the topographical distribution and functional status.
Population-based studies are clarifying their aetiology [8]. Advances in neuroimaging
are also helping to define the patterns, sites and extent of the CNS lesions associated
with the cerebral palsies. Movement disorders in children are primarily spastic or
mixed but dyskinetic syndromes also occur. The most common topographical distribu-
tions are hemiplegia, diplegia and quadriplegia. Monoplegia and triplegia are rare (Fig.
11.1 [10]). Functional classifications, such as the Gross Motor Function Classification
System (GMFCS), are important in describing affected populations and defining indications for intervention (Table 11.1 [9]). More detailed functional classifications can make
useful outcome measures, e.g. the Gillette Functional Assessment Questionnaire
(Fig. 11.1 [10]).

Table 11.1 Degree of functional disability in spastic motor disorders: Levels 1–5 for 2 and 3 year olds defined according to the Gross Motor Function Classification System (GMFCS). The complete classification system encompasses the age groups <2 years, 2 and 3 years, 4 and 5 years, and 6–12 years (see also Outcome evaluation section) (adapted from Palisano [9]).

Level I

Sits unaided, arms free

Movements in and out of floor sitting and standing without adult assistance

Free walking (without support/aids)

Level II

Sits unaided, but some difficulties to hold balance when arms are free; can attain standing from a firm base

Crawls reciprocally

Cruises holding onto furniture, walking with support or aids

Level III

The only attainable free sitting position is w-sitting (some assistance may be required)

Creeping in prone position or crawling (often not reciprocally)

Attains standing from a firm base; may walks indoors short distances using aids and requiring assistance from caregiver

Level IV

Requires assistance to attain sitting on the floor, only able to sit with arms propping

Requires frequently adaptive equipment for sitting and standing

Moves short distances (indoors) by rolling, creeping or crawling non-reciprocally

Level V

Unable to hold head and trunk upright when sitting, or up when in prone position

All motor functions impaired, unable to move along unaided, some mobility may be possible using a power wheel-chair

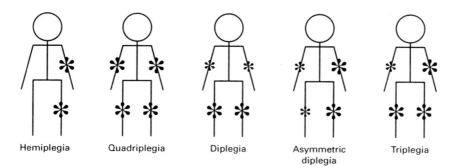

| Hemiplegia | Quadriplegia | Diplegia | Asymmetric diplegia | Triplegia |

Fig. 11.1 Classification of infantile cerebral palsy according to localization and ranking of neurological findings (adapted from Michaelis [10]).

Suitability of local therapy

Spasticity is only one component of the upper motorneurone syndrome and it is frequently not the most important factor in determining function. When considering treatment with BtA, remember that muscle hyperactivity may not be the sole cause of impaired motor function in children with spasticity. Indeed, in some patients it may play no part at all. In others it combines with weakness, impaired motor control, poor balance, sensory and intellectual deficits. The hyperactivity is sometimes helpful, as when quadriceps maintains a 'spastic prop' that prevents the knee from giving way. Whatever the underlying cause, local administration of BtA may temporarily reduce muscular hyperactivity.

General guidelines

Indications for treatment with BtA rest on the following principles.
• The disability is focal, i.e. only a few muscles are affected.
• The disability is dynamic, i.e. due to muscular hyperactivity.
• It is possible to identify individual therapy goals that would benefit the patient's daily routine.

Patient selection

Irrespective of the aetiology, the specific type or severity of the spastic motor disorder, it may be worth treating children of any age if they meet the above criteria. The results of treatment depend on the combination of the local effects with other factors, such as adjuvant treatments, motivation, ability to learn, psychosocial integration and expectations, and concomitant disorders such as epilepsy.

Timing of treatment

In childhood, normal motor development is a dynamic process leading to mature walking by the age of 7 years [11]. Children with motor disorders may acquire motor skills late, but their early natural history is nonetheless one of continuously improving motor skills. Thus we can only judge the functional benefits of BtA therapy with reference to a control group (Fig. 11.2 [12]).

Early or late treatment?

For spasticity associated with *cerebral palsy*, 'early treatment' means to begin treating at the age of 1–4 years. For spasticity following *traumatic brain injury*, it means to begin treating with BtA at the first signs of spasticity.

Early treatment of spasticity may be indicated when:

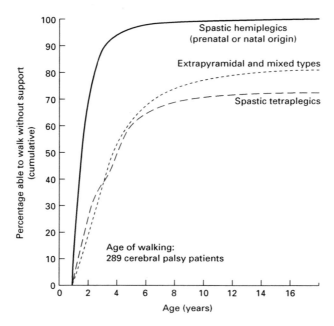

Fig. 11.2 Percentage of cerebral palsy patients able to walk at different ages. Up to about 7 years, an increasing proportion of patients learn to walk. Thereafter, the proportions of patients able to walk level off in all three groups (from Bleck [12] with permission, redrawn from Crothers and Paine [11]).

- intervention may help achieve a developmentally appropriate goal;
- associated interventions, such as casting, will not disrupt developmental progress;
- musculoskeletal pathology has not progressed to fixed contracture or bony torsion.
  Indications for *late* treatment are:
- easier care;
- pain relief;
- maintaining function;
- postoperative care.

Interdisciplinary treatment—combination therapy

It is rarely appropriate to manage spasticity with BtA alone. Although BtA has a predictable local *biological* effect when injected into large muscle groups, the *functional* outcome is less predictable and it is unusual to achieve sustained functional gains without a coordinated, well planned approach.

Responsibility for the care of children with motor disorders varies within and between countries and medical systems. Paediatric orthopaedic surgeons ran early trials of BtA in cerebral palsy but many surgeons are not involved nor are they interested in wider spasticity management. In some areas, paediatricians or neurologists coordinate spasticity management for children who have cerebral palsy. Paediatric rehabilitation specialists in Europe and physiatrist in the US are taking an increasing lead in co-ordinating spasticity management in children. Whatever local arrangements exist, it is clear that close cooperation between neuropaediatricians, orthopaedic surgeons and physiotherapists is essential to maximize benefit for the individual patient.

Physiotherapy

The physiotherapist is central to the multidisciplinary spasticity team, with responsibilities and expertise in:
- developmental assessment;
- establishing appropriate functional goals;
- identifying and selecting target muscles for injection;
- adjunctive therapy such as casting;
- postural management;
- strengthening programmes;
- educating parents and carers;
- continuity of care and communication.

Orthoses

Orthoses and treatment with BtA are complementary and frequently synergistic. The most common and best example is management of dynamic equinus secondary to calf spasticity. Such children will typically present with toe walking and tripping. Spasticity is the positive feature of the upper motorneurone syndrome. The negative feature is loss of selective motor control, which is seen clinically as inability to dorsiflex the ankle with the knee extended. During the stance phase of gait, the children stand on their toes. During the swing phase, they catch their toes and trip. Calf spasticity can often be managed very effectively by intramuscular injection of BtA, and an ankle-foot orthosis (AFO) compensates for inability to achieve dorsiflexion during the swing phase of gait. BtA makes it easier to wear orthoses and may make it possible to wear them for the first time. Other combinations of BtA therapy and orthotic management include:
- hamstring injection plus three-point splints for crouch gait;
- adductor injections and hip abduction bracing for scissoring gait and hip migration;
- injection of the thumb adductor plus abduction splinting for 'thumb-in-palm' deformity in the hemiplegic upper limb.

Casting

There is good evidence from animal experiments and some clinical evidence to show that serial casting can correct minor degrees of muscle shortening, by stimulating the addition of sarcomeres and functionally lengthening the muscle belly [13]. However, one study using sonography suggested that it is contraction of the aponeurosis that causes fixed shortening of the gastrocnemius muscle in diplegia, and that contracture is not due to decreased fibre length [14]. Given that BtA acts mainly on muscle tone or stiffness, and casting on muscle length, there are many clinical indications to use combinations of BtA and casting. Despite the fact that most centres routinely use these treatments sequentially, there are no systematic trials investigating the best way to combine injection and casting. In many centres, BtA injection is performed first and a decision on casting is deferred until 2–3 weeks after injection. By this stage, it is felt that casting is more effective and better tolerated. Casting without preinjection with BtA typically requires 4–6 weeks. After BtA injection, 1–3 weeks is usually enough. We need clinical trials in this area as soon as possible.

Intrathecal baclofen

BtA is not effective as the sole treatment in severe, generalized spasticity in older children and adolescents, and large doses may be dangerous. Clinicians are making increasing use of continuous intrathecal infusion of baclofen by an implanted pump. The legs and the trunk benefit most, and additional focal management of arm spasticity with intramuscular BtA is often very effective. We have used BtA arm injections in several adolescents who have intrathecal baclofen pumps in place, helping them to realize specific goals such as reaching and activating wheelchair control switches. This may increase their independence in the community.

Orthopaedic surgery

Most children with spasticity develop fixed musculoskeletal deformities as they grow, because muscle growth lags behind bone growth. Corrective orthopaedic surgery for fixed deformities is used in older children, when BtA therapy is ineffective. Although most children with spasticity eventually still need orthopaedic surgery, the sequential use of BtA and surgery offers many advantages. Children are older at first surgery, there is less need for repeat surgery and surgery is less radical and more successful after appropriate use of BtA. BtA can bridge the gap for many years until the optimum age and time for surgery. In some instances, BtA injections can simulate the effects of surgery and help surgeons to plan complex multilevel operations and predict the outcome. Perioperative BtA can relieve painful postoperative spasms, which facilitates postural correction and enhances functional outcomes [15]. Many children have a mixture of dynamic and fixed contractures which respond to creative combinations of BtA injections and soft tissue surgery.

Evidence for BtA efficacy

There are now many published short-term open and uncontrolled studies. They generally report good results and have supplied an impressive weight of evidence of important benefits from using BtA in paediatric spasticity. BtA appears to improve posture, spasms, function and ease of care, and may reduce the need for other treatments. Adverse events are transient and minor. However, it is difficult to draw secure conclusions from these open studies because of the wide variety of indications, doses and techniques examined, and because it is clear that children in placebo groups in controlled studies do improve, as one would expect, as they grow. Purchasers of health care have increasingly been demanding higher quality evidence before agreeing to fund BtA treatment.

It is more difficult to generate this evidence in part because of the sheer variety of problems arising from spasticity. Available outcome measures are often insufficiently sensitive when applied to a group average, or are unlikely to show major improvement over the 3-month period of typical randomized controlled trials (RCTs) in this field. Some research programmes have chosen to test BtA in highly circumscribed situations to produce statistically significant results from reasonably small numbers of patients. The hope is that these indications will be accepted as exemplars of benefit in the wider field of paediatric spasticity, but this approach has led to relatively restricted licences to use BtA. Trials of treatment as used by experienced centres in service clinics would enroll children with more heterogeneous types of spasticity, and become unwieldy.

Leg spasticity

In the last few years several RCTs of BtA for spastic equinus have been completed, using Botox® [3,16] and Dysport® [17; Botulinum toxin study group, DYSP/040, unpublished data]. Although they were still short-term, single injection cycle studies and numbers remain small (total 259 children randomized) a Cochrane systematic review was able to perform meta-analysis on some of the outcomes measured [18]. There were statistically significant benefits favouring BtA for some outcomes, but not for others (Table 11.2).

These results show that short-term clinical benefits are measurable and probably

Table 11.2 Meta-analysis of RCTs of BtA in paediatric spastic equinus. Outcomes favouring BtA over placebo [18].

	Peak effect (4–8 weeks)	End effect (12–16 weeks)
Video gait analysis	$P < 0.0001$	$P < 0.0001$
Dynamic spasticity	$P < 0.0005$	$P < 0.0001$
Parental opinion	$P < 0.01$	NS
GMFM overall change	$P < 0.06$	NS
GMFM walking change	NS	NS

GMFM, Gross Motor Function Measure; NS, not significant.

worthwhile for spastic equinus. The persistence of measurable benefit at 12–16 weeks supports the suggestion that there may be benefit outlasting the simple weakening effect of BtA. Side-effects were temporary and acceptable. There were no economic data presented, and there is still no long-term controlled information. Extrapolation from the literature suggests that BtA injections continue to produce a detectable effect after multiple treatment cycles. Table 11.3 [3,15,17,21] summarizes the outcomes following treatment with BtA classified on the basis of the AACPDM model for coding dimensions of disablement.

Two RCTs compared BtA against casting for dynamic equinus and found that the two treatments were equally effective in the short term, but that BtA was better tolerated and the benefits lasted longer [19,20]. Many centres combine the two.

Arm spasticity

Anecdotal reports suggest that it is relatively easy to use BtA to relieve pain and spasm in the arms, and to release fisting or shoulder adduction to facilitate palmar or axillary hygiene. BtA can relax elbow flexion to a more natural and cosmetically acceptable posture. This more normal elbow posture indirectly improves gait. It may allow children to reach out and to use the hand, for instance to control a wheelchair or to brace objects, even if the hand itself remains clumsy. Wrist and finger flexor injections can improve hand posture especially if combined with good physiotherapy and regularly adjusted splinting. It is more difficult to increase dexterity as other motor control and sensory deficits may swamp the benefits of muscle relaxation.

Thus many experts believe that BtA is indeed helpful for arm spasticity, but available controlled data come from only two small studies [22,23] (Table 11.4 [22,23]), and it is not possible to combine them in a meta-analysis. Both examined the effects of a single injection cycle of BtA into clinically selected spastic arm muscles, with follow-up of 3 [22] and 6 [23] months. *Blinded* outcomes showed significant benefits at peak effect, with improved Ashworth scores and active ranges of motion [22]. These benefits were lost in the later follow-up visits. Assessment of function showed improvement in one study, using the Quality of Upper Extremity Skills Test [23], but not the other, which used a coin-transfer test [22]. *Unblinded* evaluation of wider outcomes with the Pediatric Evaluation of Disability Inventory (PEDI) in one study showed improvement 1, 3 and 6 months after the first injection [23].

Thus the evidence for benefit in arm spasticity is as yet inconclusive, and more trials are needed. Unfortunately several factors make it difficult to conduct RCTs. Whilst there are common patterns of spasticity in the arm, there is a great deal of variability. Some patterns are straightforward and easy to analyse and treat with BtA, but many are highly complex and require detailed knowledge of functional anatomy, realistic assessment of the potential benefits, and the technical skills to inject BtA into these small muscles. The heterogeneous problems and technical factors require large trials to generate convincing evidence.

Table 11.3 Efficacy of BtA in the treatment of calf spasticity [3,17,21] and in the preoperative treatment of adductor spasm [15] as assessed in randomized, double blind, placebo-controlled studies. The table summarizes the various methods used for assessment and the results obtained.

Study	Method	Results*
Pathophysiology		
Koman *et al.* 2000 [3] n=114	M-response on stimulation of peroneal nerve	Treatment with BtA results in significant partial denervation of the muscle (M-response reduced by 20%)
Sutherland *et al.* 1999 [21] n=20	EMG of tibialis anterior, gastrocnemius, and soleus muscles during walking	No significant changes in the activation patterns of ankle joint agonists and antagonists during gait cycle
Koman *et al.* 2000 [3] n=114	Determination of antibodies to BtA before and 12 weeks after treatment	None of the patients had any detectable levels of antibodies to BtA
Impairment		
Sutherland *et al.* 1999 [21] n=20	Three-dimensional gait analysis before and 8 weeks after treatment	Significantly increased dorsal flexion of ankle joint during various phases of the gait cycle. Length of step and walking speed not significantly changed
Koman *et al.* 2000 [3], Ubhi *et al.* 2000 [17] n=154	Joint angle on passive dorsiflexion of ankle joint	Not significantly changed
Koman *et al.* 2000 [3] n=114	Joint angle on active dorsiflexion of ankle joint	Significantly increased
Ubhi *et al.* 2000 [17] n=40	Physiological Cost Index (change of heart rate while walking a distance of 6 m, and time required)	Not significantly changed
Barwood *et al.* 2000 [15] n=16	Standardized assessment of postoperative pain and recording of postoperative requirements for analgesics	Preoperative treatment before adductor tenotomy reduced postoperative pain highly significantly and lowered postoperative requirements for analgesics
Functional limitation/activity		
Ubhi *et al.* 2000 [17] n=40	Gross Motor Function Measure	The GMFM dimension, 'walking, running and jumping' improved significantly; changes of the GMFM Total Score were not significant
Koman *et al.* 2000 [3], Sutherland *et al.* 1999 [21], Ubhi *et al.* 2000 [17] n=174	Blinded evaluation of a randomized sequence of Video records of the patient's gait pattern (e.g. the Physicians Rating Scale)	Significantly improved gait patterns as assessed according to the Physicians Rating Scale
Disability/participation		
Barwood *et al.* 2000 [15] n=16	Length of postoperative hospitalization	Significantly reduced stay in hospital

n, the number of children studied.
*statistically significant, $P < 0.05$.

Table 11.4 Efficacy of BtA in treating arm spasticity. The table summarizes the results from a randomized, double blind, placebo-controlled [22], and a randomized, single blind study (ergotherapy vs. ergotherapy plus BtA) [23].

Study	Method	Results*
Impairment		
Corry *et al.* 1997 [22], Fehlings *et al.* 2000 [23] *n* = 43	Ashworth scale to assess muscle tonus (thumb, carpal joint, supination/pronation, elbow)	Significant improvements in carpal and elbow joints after 2 weeks, in carpal joints also after 4 weeks [22]. Other improvements were either statistically not significant or absent [22,23]
Corry *et al.* 1997 [22] *n* = 14	Mobility range in active abduction of the thumb, extension of the thumb, extension of the metacarpophalangeal, carpal, and elbow joints; Grasp-and-release Score	Significant improvements in active extension of elbow joint and base joint of the thumb for simple grasping tasks and opening of the hand in test situations
Fehlings *et al.* 2000 [23] *n* = 29	Passive joint angle for extension of elbow and carpal joints, basal joint of the thumb, and pronation/supination	No significant changes. But this was to be expected because only patients who did not show any structural contraction of the muscle/tendon apparatus were included in the study
Fehlings *et al.* 2000 [23] *n* = 29	Quality of Upper Extremity Skills Test (QUEST)	Compared to placebo, QUEST scores for the BtA group improved significantly after 1 month, but not after 3 and 6 month of treatment (although the BtA group tended to score more favourably)
Fehlings *et al.* 2000 [23] *n* = 29	Grip strength	No significant increase
Functional Limitation/activity		
Corry *et al.* 1997 [22] *n* = 14	Number of coins transferred per minute	Not significantly improved
Fehlings *et al.* 2000 [23] *n* = 29	Pediatric Evaluation of Disability Inventory (PEDI)	Compared to placebo, PEDI scores for the BtA group improved significantly after 1, 3 and 6 months of treatment
Disability/participation		
Corry *et al.* 1997 [22] *n* = 14	Cosmetic effects on the upper extremities after BtA injection as judged by patient and/or parents	Patients and parents emphasized the aesthetic gain due to the reduced involuntary flexion of the elbow joint
Fehlings *et al.* 2000 [23] *n* = 29	Pediatric Evaluation of Disability Inventory (PEDI)	Compared to placebo, PEDI scores for the BtA group improved significantly after 1, 3 and 6 months of treatment

n, the number of children studied.
*statistically significant, $P < 0.05$.

Dosage

General dose guidelines

DOSES: A HEALTH WARNING

Please read the warning on p. 35 about doses of Bt. There are three preparations available. *Dysport®* and *Botox®* are type A toxins (BtA), *NeuroBloc®/MYOBLOC™* is type B (BtB). Even though the doses for each are quoted in mouse units (mu), the three preparations have different dose schedules: one mu of *Dysport®* is **not** the same as one mu of *Botox®*, and neither is equivalent to one mu of *NeuroBloc®/MYOBLOC™*.

Accordingly, always calculate doses for the specific commercial preparation to be used.
    Remember the following key points:
- Dose per muscle—should be distributed between several injection sites. This is increasingly important with higher doses and larger muscles.
- Dose per patient—as much as is necessary, as little as possible.
- Reinjection intervals—as long as possible, and never less than 3 months.

Dose per muscle

Table 11.5 provides some guidance with regard to children older than 2 years (or with a body weight between 10 and 30 kg). Consider the size of individual muscles and other dose modifiers (Table 11.6). There are limits to the amount of BtA that individual muscles can take up. There is no further muscle relaxation or functional gain if the BtA dose exceeds the 'saturation capacity' of a specific muscle, and systemic side-effects become more likely. The dose should not exceed 50 mu Botox® or 250 mu Dysport® *per injection site*, and 100 mu Botox® or 500 mu Dysport® *per muscle*.

Reinjection intervals

Avoid reinjections within less than 12 weeks. There are two reasons for this, based on neurological experience with adults. First, more frequent injections or boosters are

Table 11.5 Dose per patient (total dose per kg body weight).*

Clinically tested dose range for Botox®	*Clinically tested dose range for Dysport®*
Up to 12 mu per kg body weight	Up to 30 mu per kg body weight

*Children should not receive more than 400 mu Botox® or 1000 mu Dysport® in total per injection session. Inexperienced clinicians should avoid higher doses as serious systemic side-effects can occur. However, higher total doses may be beneficial and can be safe in experienced hands.

Table 11.6 Dose ranges for therapy with BtA. The doses printed in boldface are recommended as upper limits per muscle. To ensure safe treatment, it is important that the *total dose per kg body weight* administered to the patient at a single session does not exceed the safe upper limits. For details please refer to the text.

Target muscle	Botox® dose (mu)		Dysport® dose (mu)	
	Per target muscle (kg body weight)	Total per muscle	Per target muscle (kg body weight)	Total per muscle
Small muscles Adductor pollicis brevis Hand and finger flexors Brachialis Brachioradialis	1–3	10–**50**	5–10	50–**150**
Large muscles Gastrocnemius Soleus Tibialis posterior Adductor muscles Gracilis Hamstrings Rectus femoris Iliopsoas Biceps brachii	3–6	30–**100**	10–30	100–**500**

more likely to give rise to antibodies and thus might increase the number of secondary non-responders. Second, a *non-linear* dose–response relationship is likely with shorter injection intervals.

Specific indications

Calf spasticity

The most common deformity in cerebral palsy is spastic equinus and the most frequent indication for the use of BtA is dynamic equinus. Equinus often appears in younger children with spastic hemiplegia or diplegia when they begin to pull to stand and walk with assistance. The equinus posture may make it difficult to walk independently, and early intervention with BtA injections may accelerate progress in motor skills. A plantigrade foot position during stance can usually be achieved by injection of BtA and maintained using an AFO. The duration of response to calf injection for dynamic equinus is variable. There are so-called 'golden responders', children who after only a few injections are permanently relieved from the burden of equinus (about 5%). More typically, dynamic equinus is managed by injections every 4–9 months until definitive surgical correction at the age of 6–12 years.

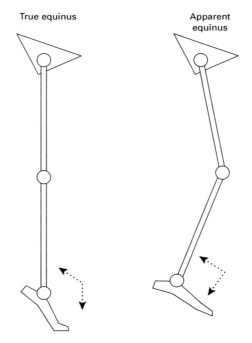

Fig. 11.3 'True equinus': plantar flexion of the ankle due to calf spasticity. 'Apparent equinus': the child is walking on tiptoe but the posture is imposed because of excessive hip and knee flexion. The problem is primarily in the hip flexors and hamstrings and not the calf muscles.

Management of dynamic equinus is complicated by the fact that not every child who walks on tiptoe has a true equinus gait. 'True equinus' refers to plantarflexion of the ankle because of calf spasticity or shortening and is usual in spastic *hemi*plegia. In spastic *di*plegia, true equinus in the younger child often gives way gradually to 'apparent equinus'. The biomechanics of this gait pattern are commonly misunderstood. The child is walking on tiptoe but the posture is imposed by excessive hip and knee flexion. The problem is primarily in the hip flexors and hamstrings and not the calf muscles (Fig. 11.3). Injection of the calf muscles in children with 'apparent equinus' usually results in crouch gait, i.e. increased hip and knee flexion. The child is then worse off and the overall gait disturbance is more difficult to manage. We frequently see children mismanaged in this way. The correct strategy is to inject the hamstring and iliopsoas muscles and to provide ground reaction AFOs.

Individual therapy goals

The goals of managing spastic equinus vary from facilitating independent walking to better tolerance of an AFO. Start treatment as early as possible while the children are learning to stand and walk, i.e. in the 2nd–4th year of life. In children who are already walking independently, BtA may improve both the appearance and efficiency of gait. Note that injection of the spastic gastrocsoleus can paradoxically increase power generation, as measured by forceplate during instrumented gait analysis [24].

Type and extent of spastic equinus

When measuring maximum joint ranges of movement and muscle lengths, stretch muscles slowly enough to avoid triggering stretch reflexes that might restrict the movement and invalidate the measurement. Slow stretch gives a range close to that found under anaesthesia, and measures true maximum muscle length or contracture. Because the measurement is performed slowly, and with the patient on an examination couch, we refer to the maximum length as the 'static muscle length' or R2.

Measure dynamic joint range of motion by performing the same type of examination much more quickly. The aim is to deliberately provoke a stretch reflex, if it is present. Typically this first catch or R1 appears at a repeatable joint angular position. This is usually 20–50° prior to R2, the static muscle length [25]. The difference between R1 and R2 represents the part of the deformity that is dynamic, as opposed to fixed. R2 approximates to the degree of 'myostatic contracture' or fixed shortening, and R1 the limit of spasticity or dynamic shortening. Perform these simple clinical tests of R1 and R2, representing static and dynamic muscle length, to assess the length of the adductors of the hip, the hamstrings, quadriceps and the calf muscles, some of the most important lower limb muscle groups to be affected by spasticity (Fig. 11.4) [26].

Measurements of R2 and R1 are of great practical relevance in the management of spasticity because they help to:
- distinguish between spasticity and contracture;
- quantify the degree of spasticity present;
- select which muscles might respond to spasticity management;
- monitor the response to spasticity management.

R2 measures the static muscle length or contracture, which may require tendon lengthening. R1 reflects the degree of spasticity or dynamic shortening, which may respond to spasticity management.

EXAMPLE 1

A 3-year-old child with spastic diplegia has an equinus gait affecting both lower limbs equally.

R1: negative 35° (35° of equinus).

R2: positive 5° (5° of dorsiflexion).

R2 minus R1 = 40°.

Spasticity management will probably help because there are 40° of dynamic shortening to be exploited by spasticity management. Surgical lengthening of the heel cord is contraindicated because the degree of fixed contracture is so small.

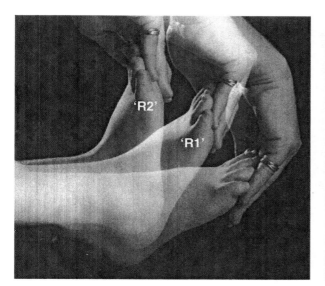 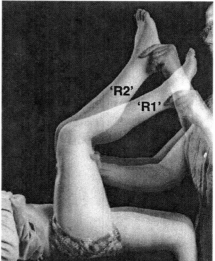

Fig. 11.4 Assessment of dynamic range of motion R1 of ankle and knee using the authors' modification of the Tardieu scale. R2 is the slow passive range of motion (conducted at Tardieu velocity V1). R1 is the point of 'catch' in the range of motion during fast movement of the ankle through the full available range of motion (Tardieu velocity V3). The angle at which the muscle reaction ('catch' or R1) occurs is best measured by goniometry. (a) The Tardieu measure is performed at the ankle to test the gastrocnemius with the knee extended. (b) The Tardieu measure is performed for the hamstring muscles with the hip flexed to 90° and the opposite hip extended (from Boyd [26] with permission.)

EXAMPLE 2

A 10-year-old boy with hemiplegia walks with an equinus gait on the affected side.

R1: negative 30° (30° of equinus).

R2: negative 20° (20° of equinus).

R2 minus R1 = 10°.

Surgical lengthening of the Achilles tendon is indicated because R2 minus R1 = 10°. This is not enough dynamic shortening for spasticity management and there would be too much residual contracture.

Equinovarus and equinovalgus

Equino*varus* posturing and deformity are very common in spastic hemiplegia and less common in spastic diplegia. They are usually caused by calf spasticity together with spasticity of the tibialis posterior. Combined calf and tibialis posterior injections can be very helpful. Manual palpation of tibialis posterior is unreliable. Identify it by muscle stimulation or visualize it by sonography before injection.

Equino*valgus* is very common in spastic diplegia and spastic quadriplegia. There is calf spasticity but there is rarely spasticity in the peroneal muscles. The valgus is a passive biomechanical phenomenon, secondary to dynamic or fixed calf shortening. It is usually managed by an orthosis or surgical stabilization of the foot, only rarely by injecting the peronei with BtA.

Combining BtA with other treatments

The transition from dynamic spasticity to fixed contracture is gradual. Most children have a mixed picture, part dynamic and part fixed. In our experience, a combination of BtA injection with a short period of casting can be very effective. An appropriate AFO can often maintain the correction following cast removal.

Injection sites and dose

• Medial and lateral bellies of gastrocnemius, one or two injection sites each (Fig. 11.5).
• Soleus, one or two injection sites (Fig. 11.6).
• Tibialis posterior, one to two injection sites (Fig. 11.7).
The clinically tested maximum dose per patient is 12 mu Botox® or 30 mu Dysport® per kg body weight.

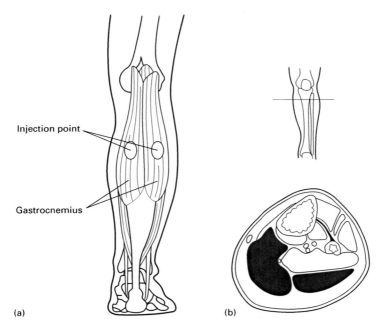

Fig. 11.5 Injection sites for treatment of spastic equinus: *gastrocnemius* muscle. (a) Posterior view and (b) cross-section (proximal third of the calf; gastrocnemius shaded black). If using two injection sites per muscle, place injections 5–10 cm apart.

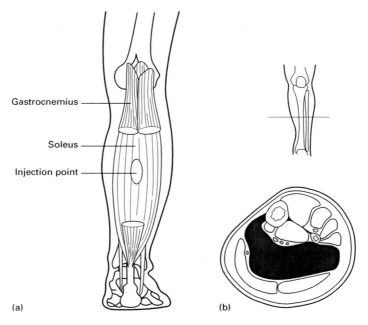

Fig. 11.6 Injection sites for treatment of spastic equinus: *soleus* muscle. (a) Posterior view and (b) cross-section view (middle of the calf; soleus shaded black). If using two injection sites per muscle, place injections 5–10 cm apart.

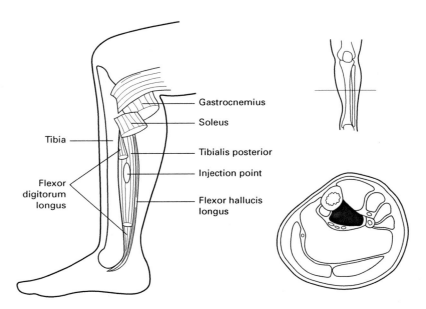

Fig. 11.7 (a).(b) Injection sites for treatment of spastic equinus: *tibialis posterior* muscle. (a) Medial view and (b) cross-section (middle of the calf; tibialis posterior shaded black). If using two injection sites per muscle, place injections 5–10 cm apart.

In all cases of unilateral injection we advise that operators label the extremity selected for treatment clearly during the clinical examination. This safeguards against a possible mix-up of sides when the patient is later put in prone position for the injection procedure.

Hamstring spasticity

Hamstring spasticity is common in spastic diplegia and in some types of spastic hemiplegia. Children may have difficulty in long sitting and may stand and walk in 'apparent equinus' or in crouch gait. We inject the hamstrings in combination with calf injections in most children with spastic diplegia, and in Winters and Gage type 3 and 4 hemiplegia. The response to hamstring injection is variable. After injection, some children walk with increased knee extension, increased speed and decreased energy cost [27]. Others gain little or no benefit. The indications and adjunctive therapies need to be refined. Some centres combine hamstring injection with injection of the iliopsoas and other muscle groups in a multilevel treatment strategy, similar to the strategy of multilevel surgery [28]. Such a sophisticated approach depends on instrumented gait analysis to choose target muscles and evaluate the outcome after injection.

When surgical lengthening of the hamstrings is required, many children with diplegia benefit from concomitant transfer of the rectus femoris muscle. This addresses the phenomenon of rectus-hamstrings 'cospasticity' which results in a characteristic stiff knee gait. Given that this is spasticity rather than a contracture, on theoretical grounds it should respond to BtA injections. We have tried to alleviate stiff knee gait using combined BtA injections to the medial hamstrings and rectus femoris, but the results obtained so far are rarely convincing.

Children with spastic quadriplegia may benefit from combined hamstring/adductor injections to improve seating, comfort and ease of care (Fig. 11.8).

Adductor spasticity

This is the second most frequent indication for BtA in children and adolescents. Adductor spasm produces scissor-like positioning of the legs that affects gait and sitting. In severely affected cases, hyperactivity of adductors and hamstrings often leads to substantial difficulties in patient care and to progressive subluxation of hip joints that can be painful. Randomized controlled studies are in progress in several countries.

Individual therapy goals

The priorities for patients with spastic quadriplegia are comfort and ease of care. Any gains in motor function should primarily reduce or eliminate hip pain, ease the task of moving the patient around or improve the patient's sitting posture, the ability to crawl reciprocally or even to walk. Several open studies have investigated the therapeutic effi-

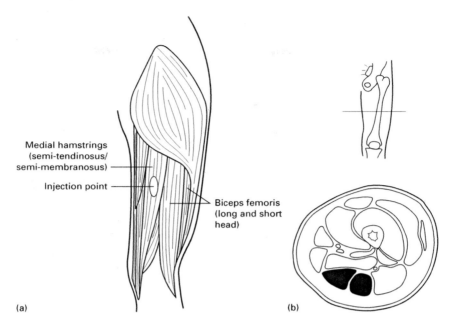

Medial hamstrings
(semi-tendinosus/
semi-membranosus)

Injection point

Biceps femoris
(long and short
head)

(a)   (b)

Fig. 11.8 Injection sites for treatment of the medial hamstring muscles. (a) Posterior view, and (b) cross-sectional view (middle of thigh; medial hamstrings shaded black). If using two injection sites per muscle, place injections 5–10 cm apart.

cacy of BtA in achieving these goals [29–31]. Placebo-controlled studies are currently testing whether regular treatment of the adductors with BtA can prevent progression of hip displacement.

Sitting may not stretch the adductors efficiently in nonambulant children, and BtA injections may need to be combined with a hip abduction orthosis. We use BtA injections to the hip adductors and medial hamstrings in children with scissoring postures, difficulties in sitting and radiological evidence of 'hips at risk'. Monitor hip migration radiologically by obtaining an anteroposterior X-ray of the hips every 6 months and measuring the migration percentage of Reimers [32] (Fig. 11.9). We usually manage hip migration with BtA and bracing when the migration percentage is below 40%. Intervene surgically when the migration percentage exceeds 40%.

Age of patients

The potentially favourable influence on hip development and the patient's ability to sit up suggest that treatment of adductor spasm should begin early in life. Thus, treatment may be indicated from the 2nd year on, depending on the child's specific motor problem and the condition of the hip joints. Both younger and older children (>10 years) may benefit from pain relief and improved ease of care.

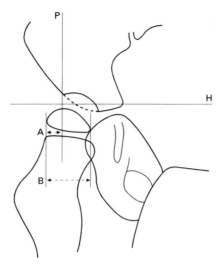

Fig. 11.9 Migration percentage (MP) is the percentage of the femoral head that is lateral to Perkins' line on a frontal view. MP = A/B × 100%. H, Hilgenreiner line; P, Perkins line.

Type and extent of adductor spasm

Fixed contractures of the adductors are less frequent than with the other muscles. However, any already established luxation or subluxation of the hip with osseous restriction of movement could also reduce the local efficacy of BtA. Note that adduction of the hip joint is mediated not only by the true adductors (adductor longus, brevis, magnus) but also involves gracilis and the hamstrings. In selected patients, treatment may be extended to psoas.

Combination with other methods of treatment

In addition to ensuring physiotherapy and the supply of aids, the physician must decide on the regular use of abduction splints during the night or of abduction wedges to facilitate sitting and lying. Preoperative use of BtA in children who undergo adductor-release surgery decreases the time that children spend in hospital, lessens postoperative pain and thus the need for analgesics, and lowers the need for repeated stationary treatment [15].

Injection sites and doses

- Adductor group (longus/magnus/brevis), one or two injection sites (Fig. 11.10).
- Medial hamstrings, one or two injection sites (Fig. 11.8).
- Gracilis, one or two injection sites (Fig. 11.11).

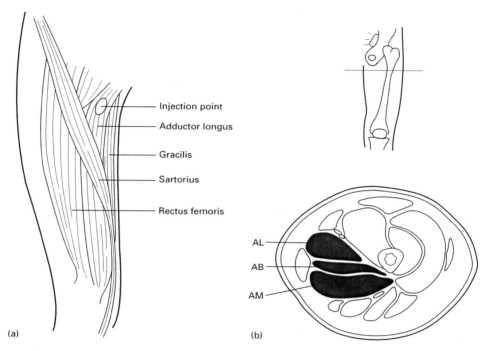

Fig. 11.10 Injection sites for treatment of adductor spasm: *adductor longus* (AL), *magnus* (AM), and *brevis* (AB) muscles. (a) Anteromedial view and (b) cross-sectional view (proximal third of thigh, adductor muscles shaded black). If using two injection sites per muscle, place injections 5–10 cm apart.

The clinically tested maximum total dose per patient is 12 mu of Botox® or 30 mu of Dysport® per kg body weight. How the dose should be distributed will depend on whether the planned injections are unilateral or bilateral, symmetric or asymmetric, and whether they include the hamstrings.

Arm spasticity

Several studies have shown that BtA can effectively reduce the muscle hyertonus in arm flexion spasm [22,23,33]. However, treatment is not so easy to plan and implement since the muscles that move the hands and fingers are complex. The clinician must be able to analyse the dynamic anatomy producing deformity or dysfunction, be able to select the most important muscles for injection, and divide the dose of BtA according to the size and contribution of individual muscles. Identification and precise injection of the forearm muscles in children use techniques similar to those for adults but are much trickier because of their smaller size and the limited ability of children to cooperate.

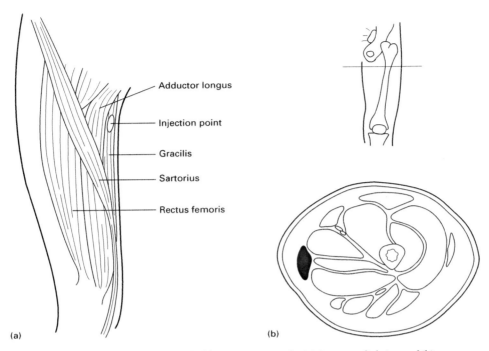

Fig. 11.11 Injection sites for treatment of adductor spasm: *gracilis*. (a) Anteromedial view and (b) cross-sectional view (proximal third of thigh; gracilis shaded black). If using two injection sites per muscle, place injections 5–10 cm apart.

Individual therapy goals

The most frequent indications are to improve passive spontaneous posture of the upper limbs, enable easier dressing and general caring for the patient, easier opening of the hand and care of the palm when there is maceration of the palmar skin, and cosmetic correction of abnormal posture. Children and teenagers perceive elbow flexion as disfiguring and may gain confidence in social affairs when the arm hangs more naturally after elbow flexor injections. BtA may improve posture in clinically relevant malpositions of the thoracic girdle, the elbow, wrist or hand. It is more difficult to improve function because of the many other problems associated with spasticity. Although BtA usually produces a convincing effect, gains in function are less clear cut and remain controversial. For instance, the 'reward' for finger flexor injections may be a flaccid paresis but with impaired prehensile function that hampers satisfactory functional gain. On the other hand, blocking elbow flexion spasms may permit the hand to reach down to control a wheelchair or to stabilize a cup or piece of paper.

Muscle selection and doses

Treatment of spasticity in the upper limbs is complex in both adults and children because each movement involves so many muscles. In elbow flexion spasticity, biceps brachii, brachialis and brachioradialis may all be active. Pronator teres and pronator quadratus both contribute to wrist pronation. The muscles that are of biomechanical importance in hand and finger flexion spasticity include flexor carpi ulnaris, flexor carpi radialis, flexor digitorum profundus and superficialis, flexor pollicis brevis, opponens pollicis and adductor pollicis. The various muscles involved and respective therapeutic goals vary widely between patients. This makes it impossible to provide specific dose recommendations here and treating physicians are referred to the General dose guidelines section (see p. 283).

Combination with other methods of treatment

BtA-induced weakness provides a window of opportunity for physiotherapists, carers and cooperative children to stretch muscles more easily and frequently to deal with incipient contracture. However, the weakness also makes it easier to overstretch muscles inadvertently and cause sprains. Wherever practical, it is worth using extension or other appropriate splinting to maintain the muscles' stretched position for as much of the time as possible. Experienced clinical centres use BtA as an aid for planning and to complement hand surgery [34].

Other indications

Focal motor problems due to spasticity can occur in any part of the body. Apply the principles outlined above. Assess the type and extent of the problem, decide on individual therapy goals and develop a suitable interdisciplinary approach. Worth mentioning are retro- and laterocollis (splenius muscle, sternocleidomastoid muscle, trapezius muscle), malposition of the shoulder joint (pectoralis muscle, teres major muscle), scoliosis (paravertebral musculature), hip flexion contracture (iliopsoas muscle, two injection sites (Fig. 11.12) and stiff gait pattern (rectus femoris muscle).

Adverse side-effects

Local side-effects

Any intramuscular injection can cause a local haematoma. In patients with dynamic equinus who have been able to walk, a transiently unsteady gait may be observed (for about 10 days) if treatment caused excessive local paresis. However, as the peak induced paresis tails off slightly, or once the patient has adapted to the new freedom of movement, this is usually soon superseded by a significantly improved gait.

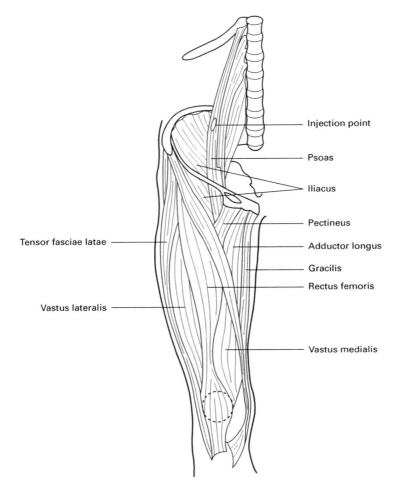

Fig. 11.12 Injection site for treatment of hip flexion contracture: *psoas.* Anterior view. If using two injection sites per muscle, place injections 5–10 cm apart.

Systemic side-effects [35]

Distant and thus systemic adverse side-effects may occur with doses that exceed the maximum recommended dose per kg body weight, and occasionally with lesser doses. Temporary double vision, dysphagia, general weakness of muscles, feeling tired, and impaired bladder function have been described in adults and occasionally in children, especially where the muscles are already compromised. For instance in children with pre-existing dysphagia, further deterioration of swallowing can lead to aspiration and consequently to aspiration pneumonia. Monitor patients carefully whenever aspiration is suspected. Children who have had a squint or squint surgery may experience temporary reactivation of the squint. Recently acquired or precarious sphincter control may lapse briefly. These possibilities should be expressly pointed out to parents or guardians and caregivers. Tell them that most side-effects are not dangerous, will resolve spontaneously and do not need investigation.

Provided physicians adhere strictly to clinically proven dose ranges and reinjection intervals, adverse side-effects should occur only rarely, and those that do should be mild and reversible.

Long-term effects

Adverse effects

We do not know for certain whether there will be any late sequelae of treatment of spasticity with BtA. However, significant circumstantial evidence suggests that adverse long-term effects are unlikely. Most importantly, there are no reports of permanent adverse effects of BtA in adults after long-term treatment of focal dystonic motor disorders over more than 15 years. In infant botulism, the prognosis is for full and complete recovery. After accidental intoxication through food contaminated with Bt, neuromuscular transmission is restored, although some adults have reported chronic weakness and fatigue as sequelae [36]. The amounts of BtA ingested were many times greater than any BtA dose conceivably used for therapy.

Neutralizing antibodies are not in themselves dangerous, but may cause BtA to become ineffective. Available retrospective data suggest that the incidence of antibodies to BtA and of secondary non-responders in adults is in the range of 2–15% [37,38]. Strategies for avoiding the development of neutralizing antibodies are discussed in Chapter 3.

Benefits

Many centres base their policy of repeating injections on personal and anecdotal experience, and suggest that multiple injection cycles continue to work. However, all the available randomized controlled data in children pertain to single injection cycles with 3–6 month follow-up, so we do not yet know whether the strategy of repeated BtA treatments produces long-term benefit. Early animal experiments on the hereditary spastic mouse suggested that pretreatment with BtA, before the onset of spasticity, could prevent the biomechanical changes of muscle contracture [39]. One study examined whether treatment with BtA can prevent contractures in children, or achieve permanent lengthening of muscles [40]. Although some patients showed a response at 1 year, the cohort as a whole did not show long-term lengthening. First published results of a randomized controlled dose-ranging study included only the data from the 4-week follow-up [41]. After 10 years of treatment with BtA it seems reasonable that treatment with BtA may have a role in delaying the need for surgery in young children.

Clinical procedure

Analgesia and sedation

General anaesthesia is not routinely required [42]. Pain arises on penetration of skin and muscle fascia with the needle, but mainly when the injected volume distends the surrounding muscle. In children younger than 10 years, combined analgesia and sedation with amnesic effect, such as rectal administration of midazolam and pethidine, helps the patient to accept needles and makes the injection procedure easier. Some centres use oral or intranasal midazolam. In addition, or as an alternative, injection sites can be anaesthetized with a surface anaesthetic such as chlorethane spray or lidocaine cream. It is worth discussing options with parents and older children. Bear in mind that an unpleasant experience for either party may compromise future willingness to have injections. Occasional children will not tolerate BtA injections and require an anaesthetic. If a child is due to have an anaesthetic for any other reason it may be possible to inject BtA during the procedure, with the added advantage of an opportunity to measure contracture definitively. Some injections may be technically more difficult under anaesthesia as the target muscle's relaxation makes it harder to palpate and to activate using reflex stimuli.

Injection

We recommend dissolving the contents of one vial of BtA (100 mu Botox® or 500 mu Dysport®) in 2 mL of 0.9% NaCl. One millilitre tuberculin syringes with 27-gauge needle are often suitable. Obese children may need larger needles. Hold the muscle belly between index and middle finger of the palpating hand ('billiard position'), fingers spread so as to compress the fatty tissue layer beneath. Use the other hand to insert the needle, aspirate to ensure it is not in a blood vessel, and then inject. Inject the BtA solution slowly. Special situations, such as injection of forearm muscles or tibialis posterior, may require electromyography (EMG) with special Teflon®-coated needles that allow injection and simultaneous recording of the muscle potentials. EMG-guided injections do take longer, and this can be a major drawback in very young or handicapped children with limited ability to cooperate. We prefer to use high-resolution ultrasonography to identify muscles and control injections—it is fast, painless and reliable (Fig. 11.13, Fig. 11.14).

If neither EMG nor sonography is available, check visually whether the needle is in the 'correct' muscle by observing movement of the detached needle on passive stretching of the target muscle.

Outcome evaluation

Reliable evaluation of the therapeutic outcome is essential, especially because treatment with BtA is a relatively new treatment. A selection of evaluation methods appears below.

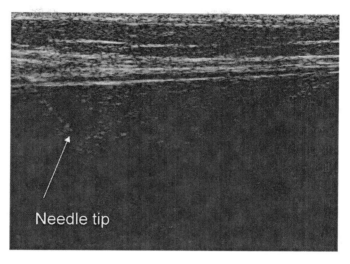

Fig. 11.13 Ultrasound visualization of the 27-gauge needle inserted into gastrocnemius: longitudinal-section view.

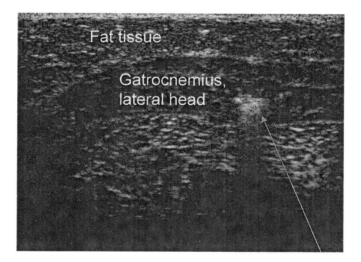

Fig. 11.14 Intramuscular cloud-like echogenic appearance immediately after injection of BtA solution.

Gross Motor Function Classification System [9]

GMFCS is a validated and reliable method that classifies the severity of functional impairment in children with cerebral palsy. It grades motor function in accordance with the patient's age using a five-step scale. The greatest possible independent motor ability is classified as grade I, a complete lack of independent mobility as grade V. Classification with the GMFCS also helps to predict the child's motor function development [43]. Table 11.1 shows the scoring system for the age-band 2–3 years.

Joint range of motion [26,44]

Assess the range of motion of individual joints to detect fixed musculoskeletal contractures as well as to evaluate the effects of treatment. As explained above, measure the joint range of motion on slow (R2) as well as on fast (R1) passive movement. The same person should examine the child before and after treatment.

Ashworth Scale [45–47]

Use the modified Ashworth Scale to record baseline and changes in muscle tone.

Goal attainment scaling [48]

Goal attainment scaling provides a means to establish therapy goals and grade the therapeutic results attained in a standardized fashion. It is a simple and reliable method that can greatly assist in the overall evaluation of therapeutic outcome. It helps to avoid misunderstandings between patients, physiotherapists and physicians about the therapy goals, promotes compliance and makes it easier to determine indications for treatment. The initial situation of the child before treatment is given the score '-2'. Assign the score '0' to any realistically achievable therapy goal, and define it precisely. Therapeutic results that fall short of the defined goal are scored from '–2' (no change) to '–1' (below the established goal), those that do exceed the defined goal are scored from '+1' (a little more than the established goal) to '+2' (markedly above the established goal) (Table 11.7).

Video documentation

Standardized video documentation of the patient's condition before and during the course of treatment allows comparative evaluation of therapeutic outcome, provided this is used together with a standardized rating scale, such as the Physician Rating Scale [16,49].

Table 11.7 Goal Attainment Scale. A means to establish therapy goals and grade the therapeutic results attained in a standardized fashion. For details please refer to the text.

−2	No change of the child's initial condition
−1	Slight improvement but below the defined therapeutic goal
0	Attains the defined therapeutic goal
+1	Improvement slightly exceeds the defined therapeutic goal
+2	Improvement clearly exceeds the defined therapeutic goal

Gross Motor Function Measure [50]

Gross Motor Function Measure (GMFM) is a reliable and valid measure specifically designed for the quantitative evaluation of change in motor function in children with spasticity. On one hand this method can be highly recommended and there is really no good alternative to it, but on the other hand it has some serious drawbacks. First, the required procedure is too involved for routine use and, second, this method is primarily suited to detect changes that can be achieved in children with spasticity of intermediate severity [31]. The 'functionally very good' and 'functionally very poor' do not show any change in the GMFM after BtA therapy. The authors who developed the GMFM were able to show that GMFM scores closely correlated with the 'overall gain' reported by caregivers [51].

Other evaluation methods [52]

Methods designed to assess local changes as well as gains in the patient's daily routine and general quality of life are still undergoing clinical evaluation or have been used only rarely. They involve tools such as standardized interviews and questionnaires for parents and physiotherapists, such as the Pediatric Evaluation of Disability Inventory (PEDI) [53].

Three-dimensional gait analysis is the most comprehensive investigation for a systematic record of normal and pathological gait patterns [54]. It includes kinetic and kinematic data in combination with EMG to analyse forces, joint movements and pathological cocontraction during the gait cycle. The results allow a detailed planning of the conservative or operative management of the patient. Gait analysis has been used in BtA therapy as an evaluation instrument [21,24,55]. Its broader use is limited by the high expenditure of manpower and time to run a gait laboratory.

Most families can fill in a chart using a weekly visual analogue scale for factors selected and defined individually for each child. Such charts give an immediate graphical representation of the perceived benefits or adverse effects, and an excellent idea of the timing of effect onset, the plateau phase and gradual wearing off. The comparative benefits of consecutive injection cycles are easy to compare (a typical scale is given in Chapter 3).

Setting up a paediatric BtA service

BtA treatment should be given as part of a wider spasticity or disability service and should not be used in isolation. The best results will arise where there is good paediatric diagnosis, assessment and monitoring and ready access to physiotherapy, splinting and orthoses, as well as paediatric orthopaedic and sometimes neurosurgery links. Staff require specific training to use BtA to its full advantage.

We do not know the community prevalence of children who might benefit from

BtA treament, nor do we know how long treatment should continue. It is therefore difficult to predict the optimum capacity of BtA clinics, and there is great debate about the distribution of services. Should only major centres give BtA or should it be devolved to smaller units? Funding issues are important and units intending to use BtA should budget for the staff and other support costs as well as the toxin supplies. BtA clinics do not get smaller! As yet there are no reliable economic data to support the reasonable notion that effective use of BtA ultimately reduces health and community care costs.

A 10-point checklist

1 *Aetiology and phenomenology*
  Established aetiology.
  Type, topographical distribution and functional status (e.g. GMFCS) of spastic motor disorder.
2 *Information to parents*
  Individual informed consent.
3 *Goal of therapy*
  Focal motor problem (due to muscular hyperactivity).
  Relevance for daily routine.
4 *Initial dose and reinjection*
  Dose per target muscle.
  Number of injection sites.
  Dose per kg body weight.
  Reinjection interval.
5 *Limitations*
  There are limitations as to how many muscles may be injected in one treatment period.
  Non-focal disorder—focal therapy.
  Chronic disorder—temporary treatment.
6 *Procedure*
  27-gauge injection needle, 1 mL tuberculin syringe.
  Analgesia and sedation (pethidine/midazolam) if required.
  Local anaesthetic (lidocaine [lignocaine] cream, chlorethane spray) if required.
7 *Evaluation*
  Local therapeutic result (joint range of motion measured on fast passive movement).
  Functional therapeutic result (GMFM, video records, Physician Rating Scale).
  Overall evaluation (e.g. 6–12 month after initiating treatment).
8 *Criteria for discontinuation*
  Cost–benefit ratio.
  Adverse side-effects.

9   *Interdisciplinary approach*

Develop an overall therapy concept (goals, methods, time schedule) coordinated between neuropaediatricians, orthopaedic surgeons, physiotherapists and family members or guardians.

10   *Combination therapy*

Physiotherapy.

Orthoses.

Casting.

Orthopaedic surgical care.

Baclofen.

References

1   Koman LA, Mooney JF, Smith B, Goodman A, Mulvaney T. Management of cerebral palsy with botulinum-A toxin: preliminary investigation. *J Pediatr Orthop* 1993; **13**: 489–95.

2   Cosgrove AP, Corry IS, Graham HK. Botulinum toxin in the management of the lower limb in cerebral palsy. *Dev Med Child Neurol* 1994; **36**: 386–96.

3   Koman LA, Mooney JF, Smith BP, Walker F, Leon JM. Botulinum toxin type A neuromuscular blockade in the treatment of lower extremity spasticity in cerebral palsy: a randomized, double blind, placebo-controlled trial. Botox® Study Group. *J Pediatr Orthop* 2000; **20**: 108–15.

4   de Paiva A, Meunier FA, Molgo J, Aoki KR, Dolly JO. Functional repair of motor endplates after botulinum neurotoxin type A poisoning: biphasic switch of synaptic activity between nerve sprouts and their parent terminals. *Proc Natl Acad Sci U S A* 1999; **96**: 3200–5.

5   Hagenah R, Benecke R, Wiegand H. Effects of type A botulinum toxin on the cholinergic transmission at spinal Renshaw cells and on the inhibitory action at Ia inhibitory interneurones. *Naunyn Schmiedebergs Arch Pharmacol* 1977; **299**: 267–72.

6   Hallett M. How does botulinum toxin work? *Ann Neurol* 2000; **48**: 7–8.

7   Pauri F, Boffa L, Cassetta E, Pasqualetti P, Rossini PM. Botulinum toxin type-A treatment in spastic paraparesis: a neurophysiological study. *J Neurol Sci* 2000; **181**: 89–97.

8   Krageloh-Mann I, Hagberg G, Meisner C *et al*. Bilateral spastic cerebral palsy: a comparative study between south-west Germany and western Sweden. I. Clinical patterns and disabilities. *Dev Med Neurol* 1993; **35**: 1037–47.

9   Palisano R, Rosenbaum PL, Walter S, Russell D, Wood E. Development and reliability of a system to classify gross motor function in children with cerebral palsy. *Dev Med Child Neurol* 1997; **39**: 214–23.

10   Michaelis R. Die sogenannten Zerebralparesen. In: Michaelis R, Niemann GW, eds. *Entwicklungsneurologie und Neuropädiatrie*. Stuttgart: Thieme Verlag, 1999: 86–101.

11   Crothers B, Paine RS. *Natural History of Cerebral Palsy*. Cambridge MA: Harvard University Press, 1959.

12   Bleck EE. Prognosis and structural changes. In: Bleck EE, ed. *Orthopaedic Management in Cerebral Palsy*. London: McKeith Press, 1987: 121–41.

13   O'Dwyer NJ, Neilson PD, Nash J. Mechanisms of muscle growth related to muscle contracture in cerebral palsy. *Dev Med Child Neurol* 1989; **31**: 543–7.

14   Shortland AP, Harris CA, Gough M, Robinson RO. Is decreased fibre length responsible for contracture of the medial gastrocnemius in spastic diplegia? *Dev Med Child Neurol* 2001; **43**: 4.

15   Barwood S, Baillieu C, Boyd R *et al*. Analgesic effects of botulinum toxin A: a randomized, placebo-controlled clinical trial. *Dev Med Child Neurol* 2000; **42**: 116–21.

16 Koman LA, Mooney JF, Smith BP, Goodman A, Mulvaney T. Management of spasticity in cerebral palsy with botulinum-A toxin: report of a preliminary, randomized, double blind trial. *J Pediatr Orthop* 1994; **14**: 299–303.

17 Ubhi T, Bhakta BB, Ives HL, Allgar V, Roussounis SH. Randomized double blind placebo controlled trial of the effect of botulinum toxin on walking in cerebral palsy. *Arch Dis Child* 2000; **83**: 481–7.

18 Ade-Hall RA, Moore AP. Botulinum toxin type A in the treatment of lower limb spasticity in cerebral palsy (Cochrane Review). In: *The Cochrane Library*, Issue 3. Oxford: Update Software, 2002.

19 Corry IS, Cosgrove AP, Duffy CM, McNeill S, Taylor TC, Graham HK. Botulinum toxin A compared with stretching casts in the treatment of spastic equinus: a randomized prospective trial. *J Pediatr Orthop* 1998; **18**: 304–11.

20 Flett PJ, Stern LM, Waddy H, Connell TM, Seeger JD, Gibson SK. Botulinum toxin A versus fixed cast stretching for dynamic calf tightness in cerebral palsy. *J Paediatr Child Health* 1999; **35**: 71–7.

21 Sutherland DH, Kaufman KR, Wyatt MP, Chambers HG, Mubarak SJ. Double blind study of botulinum A toxin injections into the gastrocnemius muscle in patients with cerebral palsy. *Gait Posture* 1999; **10**: 1–9.

22 Corry IS, Cosgrove AP, Walsh EG, McClean D, Graham HK. Botulinum toxin A in the hemiplegic upper limb: a double blind trial. *Dev Med Child Neurol* 1997; **39**: 185–93.

23 Fehlings D, Rang M, Glazier J, Steele C. An evaluation of botulinum-A toxin injections to improve upper extremity function in children with hemiplegic cerebral palsy. *J Pediatr* 2000; **137**: 331–7.

24 Boyd RN, Pliatsios V, Starr R, Wolfe R, Graham HK. Biomechanical transformation of the gastroc-soleus muscle with botulinum toxin A in children with cerebral palsy. *Dev Med Child Neurol* 2000; **42**: 32–41.

25 Tardieu G, Shentoubs Delarue R. A la recherche d'une technique de mésure de la spasticité: Imprimé avec le periodique. *Revue Neurologique* 1954; **91**: 143–4.

26 Boyd RN, Graham HK. Objective measurement of clinical findings in the use of botulinum toxin type A for the management of children with cerebral palsy. *European J Neurol* 1999; **6**: S23–S35.

27 Corry IS, Cosgrove AP, Duffy CM, Taylor TC, Graham HK. Botulinum toxin A in hamstring spasticity. *Gait Posture* 1999; **10**: 206–10.

28 Molenaers G, Eyssen M, Desloovere K, Jonkers I, De Cock P. A multilevel approach to botulinum toxin type A treatment of the (ilio) psoas in spasticity in cerebral palsy. *Eur J Neurol* 1999; **6**: S59–S62.

29 Heinen F, Wissel J, Philipsen A *et al.* Interventional neuropediatrics: treatment of dystonic and spastic muscular hyperactivity with botulinum toxin A. *Neuropediatrics* 1997; **28**: 307–13.

30 Heinen F, Linder M, Mall V, Kirschner J, Korinthenberg R. Adductor spasticity in children with cerebral palsy and treatment with botulinum toxin type A: the parents' view of functional outcome. *European J Neurol* 1999; **6**: S47–S50.

31 Mall V, Heinen F, Kirschner J *et al.* Evaluation of botulinum toxin A therapy in children with adductor spasm by gross motor function measure. *J Child Neurol* 2000; **15**: 214–17.

32 Reimers J. The stability of the hip in children. A radiological study of the results of muscle surgery in cerebral palsy. *Acta Orthop Scand* 1980; **184**: S1–100.

33 Friedman A, Diamond M, Johnston MV, Daffner C. Effects of botulinum toxin A on upper limb spasticity in children with cerebral palsy. *Am J Phys Med Rehabil* 2000; **79**: 53–9.

34 Autti-Ramo I, Larsen A, Peltonen J, Taimo A, von Wendt L. Botulinum toxin injection as an adjunct when planning hand surgery in children with spastic hemiplegia. *Neuropediatrics* 2000; **31**: 4–8.

35 Mohamed K, Moore AP, Rosenbloom L. Adverse events following repeated injections with botulinum toxin A in children with spasticity. *Dev Med Child Neurol* 2001; **43**: 791–2.

36 Schechter R, Arnon SS. Botulism. In: Behrman RE, Kliegman R, Jenson HB, eds. *Nelson Textbook of Pediatrics*. Philadelphia: WB Saunders Co., 2000: 875–8.

37 Kessler KR, Skutta M, Benecke R. Long-term treatment of cervical dystonia with botulinum toxin A: efficacy, safety, and antibody frequency. German Dystonia Study Group. *J Neurol* 1999; **246**: 265–74.

38 Herrmann J, Mall V, Bigalke H, Geth K, Korinthenberg R, Heinen F. Secondary non-response due to development of neutralising antibodies to Botulinum Toxin A during treatment of children with cerebral palsy. *Neuropediatrics* 2000; **31**: 333–4.

39 Cosgrove A, Graham H. Botulinum toxin A prevents the development of contractures in the hereditary spastic mouse. *Dev Med Child Neurol* 1994; **36**: 379–85.

40 Eames NW, Baker R, Hill N, Graham K, Taylor T, Cosgrove A. The effect of botulinum toxin A on gastrocnemius length: magnitude and duration of response. *Dev Med Child Neurol* 1999; **41**: 226–32.

41 Baker R. Botulinum toxin A for treatment of dynamic equinus spasticity associated with cerebral palsy: results of a double blind placebo-controlled dose-ranging study. *Dev Med Child Neurol* 2000; **42**: S10.

42 Moore A, Ade-Hall R, McDowell M, Rosenbloom L, Mohamed K, Walsh H. Children with cerebral palsy tolerate repeated botulinum toxin injection sessions without general anaesthetic. *Mov Disord* 2001; **16**: 381.

43 Wood E, Rosenbaum P. The gross motor function classification system for cerebral palsy: a study of reliability and stability over time. *Dev Med Child Neurol* 2000; **42**: 292–6.

44 Gajdosik RL, Bohannon RW. Clinical measurement of range of motion. Review of goniometry emphasizing reliability and validity. *Phys Ther* 1987; **67**: 1867–72.

45 Bohannon RW, Smith MB. Inter-rater reliability of a modified Ashworth Scale of muscle spasticity. *Phys Ther* 1987; **67**: 206–7.

46 Allison SC, Abraham LD. Correlation of quantitative measures with the modified Ashworth Scale in the assessment of plantar flexor spasticity in patients with traumatic brain injury. *J Neurol* 1995; **242**: 699–706.

47 Allison SC, Abraham LD, Petersen CL. Reliability of the modified Ashworth Scale in the assessment of plantarflexor muscle spasticity in patients with traumatic brain injury. *Int J Rehabil Res* 1996; **19**: 67–78.

48 Palisano RJ. Validity of goal attainment scaling in infants with motor delays. *Phys Ther* 1993; **73**: 651–8.

49 Graham HK, Aoki KR, Autti-Ramo I *et al*. Recommendations for the use of botulinum toxin type A in the management of cerebral palsy. *Gait Posture* 2000; **11**: 67–79.

50 Russell DJ, Rosenbaum PL, Cadman DT *et al*. The gross motor function measure. A means to evaluate the effects of physical therapy. *Dev Med Child Neurol* 1989; **31**: 341–52.

51 Russell D, Rosenbaum P, Gowland C *et al. Gross Motor Function Measure Manual*, 2nd edn. Hamilton, ON: McMaster University, 1993.

52 Ketelaar M, Vermeer A, Helders P. Functional motor abilities of children with cerebral palsy: a systematic literature review of assessment measures. *Clin Rehabil* 1998; **12**: 369–80.

53 Haley SM, Coster WJ, Faas RM. A content validity study of the Pediatric Evaluation of Disability Inventory. *Pediatric Physical Therapy* 1991; **3**: 177–84.

54 Gage JR. *Gait Analysis in Cerebral Palsy*. New York: MacKeith, 1991.

55 Molenaers G, Desloovere K, Nijs J. The effect of an integrated BTA-A treatment on the gait pattern of children with CP. *Dev Med Child Neurol* 2001; **43**: 4–5.

CHAPTER 12

Tremor

BIMSARA SENANAYAKE & LESLIE J. FINDLEY

Introduction

Symptomatic tremor is the commonest movement disorder in everyday clinical practice and can represent normal or abnormal functioning of the nervous system. There are many underlying pathologies, and tremor mechanisms are not well understood. Our ability to attenuate pathological tremor is poor. Treatment with botulinum toxin type A (BtA) is proving to be a valuable option, but our experience is still limited. Appreciating the possibilities requires an understanding of the different types of tremor, their patho-physiology and available treatments.

The International Tremor Foundation has been established to provide support for patients with tremor of all types. It offers an information service, fund raising and funds for research into all types of tremor and their treatments.

Definition of tremors

Tremor is an involuntary rhythmical oscillation of a body part. By convention, it is pri-marily classified according to the behavioural situation in which it occurs, or to the frequency of oscillation, distribution over the body or underlying disease processes [1]. The Tremor Investigation Group (TRIG) of the International Tremor Foundation recommends the definitions shown in Table 12.1 [2].

The most effective way of establishing the type of tremor and any underlying cause is clinical assessment by history and examination (Table 12.2 [1]). Measurement of tremor frequency may clarify the type of tremor [1]. Always consider drugs in the differ-ential diagnosis as they can act at almost any level of the nervous system to produce tremor as a side-effect (Table 12.3 [2]).

Recently (1998), the Movement Disorders Society issued a consensus statement on tremor in an effort to create a common terminology for tremor disorders [3]. It provides a clinical definition for enhanced physiological tremor and subclassifies essential tremor (ET) and Parkinson's disease (PD) tremor. Dystonic tremor is considered separately. Palatal myoclonus is grouped with tremors. The eponymous term 'Holmes tremor' sub-stitutes for 'rubral' tremor because G. Holmes published one of the first concise descrip-tions of this type of tremor, which includes thalamic tremor. Some monosymptomatic and isolated tremors originally classified as possible ET type 2 by the TRIG group (Table

Table 12.1 Tremor definitions: the International Tremor Investigation Group's 1993 recommended definitions of tremor and the various components of tremor [2].

Tremor	A rhythmical oscillatory movement of a body part
Rest tremor	Tremor that is present when a limb is fully supported against gravity and the relevant muscles are not voluntarily activated
Action tremor	Any tremor occurring on voluntary contraction of muscle
Postural	Tremor apparent during the maintenance of a particular posture against gravity
Kinetic	Tremor evident during any type of movement
Intention	The pronounced exacerbation of kinetic tremor towards the end of a goal-directed movement
Isometric	Tremor occurring as the result of muscle contraction against a rigid, stationary object
Task-specific	Tremor that occurs to any significant extent during the performance of highly skilled activities, such as writing, playing a musical instrument or using a jeweller's screwdriver

Table 12.2 Classification of some common tremors (modified from [1]).

Frequency (Hz)	Disease or process or locus of lesion	Behavioural characteristics
2.5–3.5	Cerebellar/brainstem	Postural, kinetic
	Multiple sclerosis	
	Alcoholic degeneration	
	Post-traumatic	
	Dystonic	
4–5	Parkinson's disease	Rest
	Drug-induced (e.g. neuroleptics ?MPTP)	
	Cerebellar disease	Postural, kinetic
	Holmes tremor	Rest, postural, kinetic
5.5–7.5	Essential tremor Clonus	Postural, kinetic
	Parkinson's disease	
	Drug-induced (lithium, sodium valproate, tricyclics)	
8–12	Enhanced physiological tremor	Postural, kinetic
	Drug intoxications	
	Essential tremor	
	?Cerebrocortical	
13–18	Primary orthostatic	Postural

MPTP, 1-methyl-4-phenyl-1,2,3,6-tetrahydropyridine.

Table 12.3 Some common drugs producing tremor (modified from [2]).

Transmitter system affected	Drugs
Central cholinergic	Acetylcholine, muscarine and nicotine agonists, cholinesterase inhibitors, aminopropanols
Central monoaminergic	Neuroleptics, phenylethylamines, indoles
Peripheral adrenergic	Epinephrine (adrenaline), β-agonist, lithium, caffeine, amphetamine, corticosteroids
Other	Heavy metals, metal chelators, carbon tetrachloride

12.4 [2]) have been more clearly defined as subcategories including primary writing tremor, occupational tremor, primary orthostatic tremor and voice tremor.

Rest tremor

Parkinsonism including idiopathic PD is responsible for most rest tremors, which present with low frequency, alternating supination and pronation of the forearm, sometimes accompanied by adduction and abduction of the thumb, the so-called 'pill-rolling tremor'. Some postural ET tremors cause confusion as they continue at rest even when the limb is fully supported. PD rest tremor usually attenuates during target-directed voluntary movements but voluntary movements accentuate action/postural tremors. Many patients with PD have a tremulous jaw, foot or leg. Head and neck tremor is rare in PD, but common in ET. A postural or action tremor indistinguishable from 'pure' ET can occur in PD. Postural tremor has a higher frequency than rest tremor and is physiologically distinct [4–6].

Action tremor

Action tremor is produced by *voluntary* contraction of muscle and includes postural and movement or kinetic tremor. It is very common, with a range of underlying causes (see Table 12.2). Kinetic tremor can be simple non-target directed or target directed (intention tremor). The commonest action tremor is enhanced physiological tremor, and virtually everyone has experienced it when anxious or stressed. It is mainly postural with a high frequency and is usually reversible. It may occur with fatigue or metabolic changes including thyrotoxicosis and drug withdrawal states.

Essential tremor

ET is the most common action tremor, with a prevalence between 0.3 and 5% in people over 40 years of age. There may be a million patients in the US with symptomatic ET [7]. It is often labelled benign but it can produce serious physical and psychological handicap

Table 12.4 Tremor Investigation Group's definition of essential tremor (ET) [2].*

Inclusions	Exclusions
Definite ET	
Tremor	
Bilateral postural tremor, with or without kinetic tremor, which is visible and persistent, involving hands or forearms	Other abnormal neurological signs
	Presence of known causes of enhanced physiological tremor
Tremor of other body parts may be present in addition to upper limb tremor	Concurrent or recent exposure to tremorgenic drugs or the presence of drug withdrawal state
Bilateral postural tremor may be asymmetrical	
Tremor is reported by patient to be persistent, thought amplitude may fluctuate. Tremor may or may not produce disability	Direct or indirect trauma to the nervous system 3 months preceding reported onset of tremor
	Historical or clinical evidence of psychogenic origins in tremor
	Convincing evidence of sudden onset or evidence of stepwise deterioration
Duration	
Relatively long-standing (i.e. >5 years)	
Probable ET	
Tremor	
As for definite ET. Tremor may be confined to body parts other than hands. These may include head and postural tremor of the legs. However, abnormal postures of the head would suggest the presence of dystonic head tremor	As for definite ET
	Primary orthostatic tremor
	Isolated voice tremor
	Isolated position-specific or task-specific tremor including occupational tremors and primary writing tremor
	Isolated tongue or chin tremor
Duration	
Relatively long-standing (i.e. >3 years)	
Possible ET	
Type 1	
Subjects who satisfy the criteria of definite or probable ET but exhibit other recognizable neurological disorders, such as parkinsonism, dystonia, myoclonus, peripheral neuropathy or restless leg syndrome	
Subjects who satisfy the criteria of definite or probable ET but exhibit other neurological signs of uncertain significance not sufficient to make the diagnosis of a recognizable neurological disorder. Such signs may include mild extrapyramidal signs (e.g. hypomimia, decreased arm swing or mild bradykinesia)	
Type II	
Monosymptomatic and isolated tremors of uncertain relationship to ET. This includes position-specific and task-specific tremors, such as occupational tremors, primary writing tremor, primary orthostatic tremor, isolated voice tremor, isolated postural leg tremor and unilateral postural hand tremor	

*Presence of ET: a phenomenological criterion, not a function of disability, pathophysiology or heredity.

[8]. There is a positive family history in 17.4 to 100% (average 50%) of patients and in them the inheritance is dominant with very high penetrance, and the phenotype has been defined [9]. Two groups, Gulcher *et al.* [10] and Higgins *et al.* [11] have recently established linkage of ET to different chromosome locations. They called them the FET1 gene and 'ETM' gene, respectively [12].

In ET, there is usually bilateral postural tremor of the arms, sometimes with an associated action tremor. Distressing head tremor in the absence of abnormal posturing occurs in about 30% of patients with ET [13]. It is distinct from dystonic head tremor with hand tremor. Dystonic head tremor shows abnormal neck posturing, often with irregular jerks, active neck muscle contraction and reduction of tremor amplitude by *gestes antagonistiques* [13]. These features are not seen in essential head tremors. Head tremor related to ET responds poorly to oral medication but reasonably well to botulinum toxin (Bt). It may be difficult to clinically separate ET from other causes of postural tremor and from enhanced physiological tremor (see Table 12.4). Tremors indistinguishable from ET may occur in other neurological disorders, such as PD or dystonia [14]. On the other hand ET can present with intention [15,16] or rest [16,17] tremor. Some monosymptomatic or isolated, position-specific or occupational task-specific tremors are thought to be related to ET but the new Movement Disorder Society consensus statement groups them separately [3].

Dystonic tremor

This is defined as tremor in a body part affected by dystonia [3]. These are usually postural/kinetic tremors and are not seen at rest. Tremulous spasmodic torticollis is a classic example (dystonic head tremor). Some tremors occurring in dystonic patients are associated with dystonia although the body part in which the tremor occurs may not be dystonic. e.g. patients with cervical dystonia often show postural tremor of the arms [18,19]. Isolated head tremor can occur in patients with a family history of spasmodic torticollis. Recently, a study in 114 consecutive cervical dystonia patients with and without head tremor [20] found that patients with head tremor were more likely to have a positive family history of head/hand tremor suggestive of ET. The authors postulated a possible genetic linkage between ET and cervical dystonia head tremor. Bt is the most effective treatment for dystonia and associated tremor.

Other action tremors

Cerebellar or brainstem lesions produce a postural and kinetic tremor, which is most evident during goal-directed movements such as the finger to nose test. Whenever a tremor increases during the pursuit of a target or a goal there is likely to be a disturbance of the cerebellum and its afferent or efferent pathways [21,22]. Lesions of the dentate nucleus or superior cerebellar peduncle can produce pure tremors, but if there are multiple or less discrete lesions, the tremor is frequently contaminated by dysmetria. Rubral or midbrain tremor (now called Holmes tremor) may resemble the rest tremor of PD except that it persists in posture and throughout movement. Primary writing tremor is when tremor occurs specifically during writing. The current definition excludes tremor associated with writer's cramp, the so-called dystonic writing tremors. There are two forms of primary writing tremor. Type A occurs with actual writing (task specific) and type B is when the hand adopts a writing position without actually writing (position specific) [23]. Primary orthostatic tremor occurs mainly in legs on standing [24–26]. It improves with walking, sitting and lying. EMG typically showing 13–18 Hz high frequency pattern confirms the diagnosis [24–26]. This tremor frequency is higher than any other pathological tremor and it involves synchronized rhythmical activity of all lower limb muscles.

Pathophysiology of tremor

Tremor develops when the discharges of many motor units become synchronized rhythmically. There are complex interactions between the mechanical properties of the body appendage, the peripheral and long latency reflexes and the central oscillators [27]. The effects of perturbing the tremulous part mechanically often allow us to distinguish between tremors that arise mainly from synchronization around peripheral reflexes, and those from within the central nervous system. These behavioural techniques are not practical for routine clinical use [28].

Electromyography (EMG), accelerometry and computer technology have rapidly improved our understanding of tremor mechanisms over the last two decades, especially through the analysis of tremor frequency spectra [29, 30]. Oscillating systems and central oscillators are important in both physiological and pathological tremor [31, 32]. Neurones in the inferior olives and other brainstem nuclei have spontaneous oscillatory activity [32]. In PD, nigrostriatal dopamine deficiency probably disinhibits central oscillators in the basal ganglia and thalamus [15]. In ET, the relative contributions of central oscillators and peripheral spinal and reflex mechanisms remain uncertain. Dynamic studies using positron emission tomography have implicated bilateral cerebellar and brainstem structures [33].

In general, the frequencies of pathological tremors resist peripheral manipulation and are relatively fixed over short periods of time. For tremors which mainly depend on peripheral reflexes and peripheral feedback, mechanically loading or weighting the limb reduces the frequency. The peak frequency of physiological tremor and cerebellar kinetic tremor decreases with mechanical loading [34], suggesting that peripheral reflex mechanisms are important [35]. The frequency of ET is more resistant to peripheral manipulation, compatible with an important central component.

Measurement of tremor

Any treatment for tremor must both reduce the tremor and improve function. Objective assessment requires practical, validated and repeatable measures. Although quantitative laboratory methods such as EMG and accelerometry are improving, they do not necessarily reflect disability.

Early clinical trials focused too much on accelerometry and neglected the effects of tremor on patients [36]. They probably overestimated the benefits of medical therapy. It is now possible to measure many facets of tremor and its impact on the patient. Trials of Bt should use such measures and should test each specific tremor type separately. Bain and colleagues [37,38] recently developed the first fully validated clinical rating scales which reflect disability and are reliable between and within individual observers. A 0–10 analogue rating scale assesses the behavioural characteristics of the tremor and body part. It rates simple handwriting and figures such as Archimedes spirals from 0 to 10 [38]. Measuring the volume of water displaced from a standard beaker is as good as the most complex and expensive computer techniques and is a fraction of the cost [29,37,38].

Treatment trials should also measure any changes in the quality of life. Many patients would consider a 50% reduction in hand tremor to be a major improvement but a similar reduction of head tremor is less helpful, perhaps because head tremors are psychologically more damaging and cause more embarrassment and distress.

Treatment of tremors

Management of tremor depends on accurate diagnosis. Many patients with enhanced physiological tremor or very mild ET do not need treatment and are satisfied with reassurance that they do not have more serious underlying pathology, such as PD. Treat any underlying cause in patients with intrusive tremor. Unfortunately, this is rarely an option. Drug therapy is the mainstay of treatment for most patients: Table 12.5 outlines drugs that may control tremor of different types. Bt injections are an alternative

Table 12.5 Drug treatment of tremor.

Disease/disorder	Effective drugs
Enhanced physiological tremor	Beta-blockers, alcohol
ET	Beta-blockers, primidone, phenobarbitone, topiramate, mirtazapine
'Kinetic-predominant' ET	Clonazepam
Primary orthostatic tremor	Clonazepam, gabapentin, levodopa
Parkinson's disease	
Rest tremor	Levodopa, dopamine agonists, anticholinergics, amantadine
Postural tremor	?Beta-blockers, ?alcohol, clozapine
Multiple sclerosis	Isoniazid
Wilson's disease	D-penicillamine

ET, essential tremor.

tremorlytic therapy. Various surgical procedures are available to control tremor in cases resistant to medical treatment.

Parkinson's disease

Optimal management of the underlying PD is the best treatment for rest tremor, and relies chiefly on anticholinergic, dopaminergic drugs [39,40] and amantadine [41]. It is not clear why tremor is controlled by levodopa in some patients but not others [42].

Higher frequency postural and kinetic tremors occur commonly in PD and may be indistinguishable from ET. There is no systematic study of the pharmacology of these tremors, which may be more functionally disabling than the rest tremor. Long-acting *propranolol* (160 mg daily) can reduce rest tremor by 70% and postural tremor by 50% in patients with PD [42]. Recently dopamine agonist drugs have been introduced to control PD tremor [43]. The atypical neuroleptic drug *clozapine* also improves parkinsonian tremor [44]. Clozapine was found to be as effective as *benztropine* in controlling PD tremor in another study [45]. Due to haematological side-effects clozapine is not recommended for tremor in the UK.

Budipine has been effective in some cases of PD tremor. Possible side-effects such as cardiac arrhythmias limit its use [46].

Surgery

Disabling Parkinsonian tremor that does not respond to drugs may improve dramatically after stereotactic ventrolateral thalamotomy [47]. About 80% improve, but about 3% sustain permanent neurological deficit, including contralateral hemimotor and hemisensory disturbances. There may be functional improvement of 30–50%. The risk is greater and speech disturbance is more likely with dominant hemisphere or bilateral lesions. Lesions at other sites, such as the posterior ventral portion of the medial globus pallidus and the subthalamic nucleus, may improve both tremor and bradykinesia [48,49].

Deep brain stimulation with electrodes implanted in the ventral intermediate nucleus of the thalamus is becoming an increasingly acceptable form of management in resistant Parkinsonian tremor [50–52].

Essential tremor

Functionally acceptable 'benign' tremor may still cause severe psychological and social distress. Beta-adrenergic blocking drugs acting through peripheral β2-receptors are the first choice for ET [39]. The non-selective drug *propranolol* is the most effective, and is used both as a single dose given acutely in specific predictable stressful situations and in chronic therapy [39,53].

Seventy per cent of patients prefer once-daily long acting propranolol, which is as effective as divided doses [54]. Patients with ET tolerate it well but 30% of those with full β-blockade complain of some side-effects, including weakness of the legs and fatigue [55].

Primidone is also a first-line treatment for ET [56], and may act centrally. It is about as effective as propranolol, though unlike propranolol it will occasionally abolish tremor completely. About 25% of patients have acute toxic effects including nausea, vomiting and ataxia, even with a small dose. Start treatment with a very small dose such as 62.5 mg daily, increasing within a three times a day regimen until a there is a good response or unacceptable dose-related side-effects occur. The usual effective dose is 375–750 mg daily, producing an average 55% reduction of tremor. The effects of primidone and propranolol may be additive in some patients.

Ethanol powerfully attenuates ET in about 50% of patients [57], but obvious problems include pharmacological tolerance, addiction and abuse. Ethanol may work by augmenting γ-aminobutyric acid (GABA) and glycine-induced neuronal inhibition at multiple levels of the neuraxis [39]. In placebo controlled, randomized, double blind trials [58,59] *clozapine* reduced tremor resistant to other drugs, but haematological complications limit its usefulness. *Gabapentin* at a dose of 400 mg three times per day was found to be effective in some studies [60] but ineffective in others [61]. An open label study of the novel antiepileptic drug *topiramate* in ET found improvement in hand, head and voice tremor [62]. The methylxanthene derivative *theophyllin* also helped in some cases of ET [63]. Nimodipine is effective in some patients with ET [64].

Surgery

Stereotactic thalamotomy can control ET in patients with severe unilateral or asymmetric ET who have marked functional disability and have not responded to maximum doses of antitremor drugs [65]. Recent studies show a high success rate for this procedure [66,67]. Long-term follow up continued to show benefit with less than 10% showing persistent morbidity. Chronic deep brain (thalamic) stimulation (DBS) of the VIM nucleus suppresses ET [67]. An obvious advantage of this procedure over thalomotomy is that it can be performed bilaterally without much increase in mortality or morbidity and it is potentially reversible.

Cerebellar tremors

The chemistry of cerebellar function is complex and poorly understood and no major neurotransmitter deficiency has been shown in cerebellar syndromes producing tremor. GABA is the most abundant neurotransmitter, but trials with GABAergic drugs, including baclofen, ethanol and benzodiazepines, have not shown any significant effect.

Isoniazid may be effective in cerebellar or brainstem tremors, including multiple sclerosis [68]. Combinations of membrane-stabilizing drugs, such as lidocaine, tocainide and hyoscine, help some complex and action tremors [69]. Thalamotomy may be effective symptomatic treatment [70].

Thalomotomy may help the action tremor of multiple sclerosis. In a recent review of 14 articles between 1960 and 1992, 75% of 234 patients experienced improvement in their tremor, and there was long-term benefit in 50–73% patients [71].

Task-specific tremors

Task-specific tremor occurs only during the specific activity, commonly writing. Primary writing tremor is considered a form of focal dystonia [23]. Its relationship to ET and dystonia is uncertain [72]. Pharmacological treatment of primary writing tremor is disappointing. Recently, Bt injections were used to treat primary writing tremor [73]. Dystonic patients may have tremor indistinguishable from ET, as well as a true DT (a tremor in the dystonic part). Treatments for dystonia, including anticholinergic drugs and Bt injections, may help both types of tremor [72].

Primary orthostatic tremor is interesting and the EMG appearances are diagnostic. It responds well to *clonazepam* [72]. Other drugs reported to be effective in this condition include *phenobarbital* [74], *primidone* [75], *valproic acid, levodopa* [76] and *gabapentin* [77].

Dystonic tremor

Dystonic tremor (DT) is distinct from ET. Isolated head or trunk tremor may be the initial manifestation of focal dystonia. DT may respond to clonazepam and anticholinergics but the results are generally disappointing. Bt treatment for DT often results in significant improvement of tremor and contributes to a better quality of life.

Conclusions on current pharmacological management of tremor

Whilst drug management of tremor is sometimes effective, it is often disappointing and causes side-effects. Our poor understanding of tremor mechanisms suggests that new antitremor drugs will only be found by chance. Although several new medications are currently under investigation, only primidone and propranolol have proven efficacy for ET. Bt may be effective in some patients with essential head and voice tremor but probably not hand tremor because of its side-effects. Surgical techniques include stereotaxic lesioning and chronic stimulation and can be highly effective, but the potential for serious side-effects is often unacceptable. Consider thalamic deep brain stimulation if oral drugs and Bt fail to reduce tremor in ET. DTs respond poorly to oral drugs but well to Bt.

Review of tremor treatment with botulinum toxin

Bt helps some tremors. Simplistically, the rationale for using Bt is that the chemical denervation of muscle interferes with the final common pathway of the neuronal activity causing tremor and reduces the amplitude of the tremor whether it is generated by a central oscillator or by oscillating peripheral systems. Alternatively, changing the gain of feedback activity could disrupt or subdue underlying tremorgenic circuits. This could occur directly through reduced contraction of somatic muscle fibres or indirectly via an effect on alpha-gamma coactivation if muscle spindles are affected.

Dystonic and related tremor

Bt is now a well-established treatment for dystonia, and often attenuates any accompanying tremors, whether they are true DTs occurring in the dystonic muscles or associated ET away from the dystonic part [78,79]. In patients with cervical dystonia and dystonic head 'tremor', the often distressing, irregular jerking movement commonly appears when the head is moved against the action of the dystonic muscle. Toxin injections into the dystonic muscles usually improve the tremor by reducing its amplitude. About 75% of the patients with dystonic head tremor improve. The response starts within the 1st week and lasts on average between 2 and 4 months [80]. Muscle strength recovers over 2–3 months, and as the dystonia returns the tremulous movement usually recurs and requires further treatment. However, many questions remain regarding the optimal technique of administration. Neutralizing antibodies occur in about 5–10% patients and appear to be related to the dose and the interval between doses [80].

Tremor associated with task-specific movement disorders such as dystonic writer's cramp may also be managed successfully with repeated Bt injections into the dystonic muscles. Injections need to be EMG guided to ensure that the activated muscles are injected [81].

An early open study by Jankovic and Schwartz [78] used video, EMG and clinical rating scales in patients with tremors of various types. Tremor was dystonic in 14 patients, essential in 12, mixed dystonic and essential in 52 and there were one each with parkinsonian tremor, peripherally induced and midbrain tremor. The mean age of the patients was 55 years and the mean duration of symptoms was 13.9 years. At 160 treatment visits, a mean of 242 mu Botox® was injected into cervical muscles of 42 patients with head tremor. 'No–no' tremors of the head were treated with injections into both splenii capitus muscles, and 'yes–yes' tremors were treated with injections into one or both sternocleidomastoids. Ten patients with hand tremor received a mean of 95 mu Botox® into forearm muscles. In typical postural arm tremors, wrist extensors (predominantly extensor carpi radialis and ulnaris) and wrist flexors (predominantly flexor carpi radialis and ulnaris) were injected. If there was additional dystonia, the dose was distributed asymmetrically and the primary dystonic muscles received a larger dose than their antagonists. Surface EMG did not help in localizing the involved muscles or guiding injections.

The results of this early open study were encouraging, and were compatible with our own experience. Using clinical ratings, 67% improved more than one grade on a 0–4 improvement scale. The mean latency of onset of response was 6.8 days and the mean duration of maximum improvement was 10.5 weeks. Although there was no formal objective analysis of function or disability, some patients noted improvement in daily activities, such as dressing, eating and writing. Objectively the toxin reduced the amplitude of EMG bursts. Complications lasting a mean of 21 days were noted in 17 patients (40%) injected for head tremor. There was dysphagia in 12 patients (29%), transient neck weakness in four (10%) and local pain in two (5%). Six patients (60%) with hand tremor had transient focal weakness.

Controlled trial evidence

Most of the randomized controlled trials of BtA and botulinum toxin type B (BtB) in cervical dystonia report that DT is significantly and usefully reduced, using Botox®, Dysport® or NeuroBloc® (see chapter 8 for details).

Essential hand tremor

In a randomized clinical trial, 25 patients with essential hand tremor received placebo or 50 mu Botox® to the wrist extensors and flexors in the dominant limb [82]. If they failed to respond 100 mu was injected 4 weeks later. At 4 weeks after treatment with BtA there were significant improvements in the tremor severity ratings compared to placebo. Hand weakness was the main adverse effect and was commoner in the treatment group. Randomized trials suffer from relatively rigid treatment protocols and open studies suggest that personalized injections are more effective, as shown in one study using Dysport® for essential hand tremor in 15 drug-resistant cases [83].

One multicentre, double blind, randomized, placebo controlled study of BtA in uncomplicated essential hand tremor [84] enrolled 133 patients (90 male and 43 female) from 10 centres. Forty-five patients received 100 mu Botox®, 43 patients 50 mu, and 45 patients received placebo. The patients stopped all antitremor therapy 2 weeks before the injections and took no alcohol or caffeine for 36 and 12 h, respectively. The trialists rated the severity of rest, postural and action/kinetic tremors. Both 100 mu and 50 mu Botox® improved postural tremor significantly at 6, 12 and 16 weeks, and kinetic tremor at 6 weeks. There were no changes in the placebo group. The trial report concluded that 50 and 100 mu Botox® per limb each reduce hand tremor severity in ET. Weakness of grip was common, perhaps made more likely by the relatively rigid treatment protocols required by the trial.

Expert reviews conclude that some patients with essential hand tremor benefit from BtA [85]. Tremor improves in 60% patients with an equal number developing hand weakness. This side-effect limits its use as most patients would rather have tremor than weakness. However in clinical practice individualization of dose and sites of injection may minimize weakness and achieve a satisfactory compromise.

Essential head tremor

Essential head tremor is very disabling and is seen in 30% patients with ET. It must be distinguished from dystonic head tremors with head tilt. The head tremors of ET respond poorly to oral medication and open studies suggest it is better to treat with Bt, which can reduce the head oscillations in about 50% of patients [78]. Horizontal head tremors respond better than vertical head tremors.

Parkinson's disease tremor

There is even less experience of treating the tremor of PD with Bt. In a pilot open study in seven patients with parkinsonian tremor, there was mild to marked improvement with a mean change of 2.6 on a 0–4 global rating scale. Three patients showed more than 50% reduction in tremor severity on a clinical rating scale and in objective measurements [86].

A double blind pilot study randomized seven patients with rest tremor to receive normal saline or 100 mu Botox® into the extensors. One patient with bilateral tremor received placebo in one arm and active toxin in the other. There was significant improvement in the treated arm after 1 month, with median improvements of 24% in time to spill water and in water spilt in 1 min, 38.6% in maximum accelerometric displacement and 1.25 and 1.5, respectively, for spiral and rest tremor grades (all $P < 0.05$). There was no significant change in writing speed or pegboard performance. The benefits had largely disappeared at 3 months. Finger extensor strength was reduced by a median of 20% at 1 and 3 months ($P < 0.05$) but this was rarely clinically significant. Normal saline had no effect. The authors concluded that BtA might be useful in parkinsonian tremor [87], but associated hand weakness seems to be the limiting factor.

Other tremors

Bt has a beneficial effect on voice tremor [88]. The toxin is already established in the management of spasmodic dysphonia, which may mimic essential voice tremor. This topic is covered in detail in Chapter 7.

Practice points in using botulinum toxin treatment for tremor

> ### DOSES: A HEALTH WARNING
>
> Please read the warning on p. 35 about doses of Bt. There are three preparations available. *Dysport®* and *Botox®* are type A toxins (BtA), *NeuroBloc®/MYOBLOC™* is type B (BtB). Even though the doses for each are quoted in mouse units (mu), the three preparations have different dose schedules: one mu of *Dysport®* is **not** the same as one mu of *Botox®*, and neither is equivalent to one mu of *NeuroBloc®/MYOBLOC™*.

Select muscles for injection based on the pattern of the tremor and dominant muscle activity. Chapter 8 describes methods of selecting Bt doses and appropriate neck muscles that also apply for dystonic and essential head tremors. Employ the techniques described in Chapter 9 for forearm muscle selection in essential hand tremor, writer's tremor and extrapyramidal tremor. In general, inject both agonist and antagonist muscles, dividing Botox® 50–100 mu or Dysport® 200–400 mu between two and three sites in the forearm flexor compartment and Botox® 50–75 mu or Dysport® 100–300 mu between one and three sites in the extensors.

Table 12.6 summarizes typical muscle patterns according to tremor type. Select muscles with visible or palpable hypertrophy or tremor-locked activity. EMG is not always needed, but can be useful in the following circumstances:

1 In complex forms of cervical dystonia associated with tremor.
2 In writer's cramp/tremor where several forearm muscles may be involved.

Table 12.6 Muscles injected according to the type of tremor.

Tremor type	Muscles injected
Head tremor 'No–No'	SM bilateral
	SC bilateral
Head tremor 'Yes–Yes'	SM bilateral
	SS bilateral
	SC bilateral
Dystonic head tremor with rotation	SM contralateral to rotation
	TR contralateral
	SC ipsilateral or bilateral
Essential hand tremor	FCR and FCU
	ECR and ECU
Writer's tremor/cramp	Forearm muscles under EMG guidance

ECR, extensor carpi radialis; ECU, extensor carpi ulnaris; EMG, electromyography; ET, essential tremor; FCR, flexor carpi radialis; FCU, flexor carpi ulnaris; SC, splenius capitis; SM, sternomastoid; SS, semispinalis; TR, trapezius.

3 For reassessing the patient after unsuccessful injection using clinical criteria.
4 To guide the injection into deep muscles.
5 When obesity makes muscles difficult to palpate.

Side-effects of botulinum toxin treatment into neck and forearm muscles

Chapters 8 and 9 describe the adverse effects of injections of Bt into neck and forearm muscles in detail. They include temporary injection site pain and soreness. Rarely, flu-like symptoms and local hypersensitivity reactions may occur.

After neck injections there may be dryness of the mouth, dysphonia or a feeling of neck weakness. Breathing difficulty is rare and should prompt a visit to the doctor. Dysphagia is dose related and affects up to 15–30% of patients following neck injections. It is less likely with doses below Botox® 200 mu, Dysport® 500 mu or NeuroBloc® 10 000 mu, and with unilateral rather than bilateral sternomastoid injections. Even if it occurs, dysphagia is only rarely serious enough to require medical treatment and it gradually improves as the toxin wears off. Rare cases of prolonged dysphagia occur.

After forearm injections the predominant complication and limiting factor is localized weakness. Minimize it by using the lowest effective doses and a good muscle selection strategy.

The future of botulinum toxin in the management of tremor

We clearly need further evaluation of Bt in the management of tremors. Efficacy studies must demonstrate significant improvement in functional ability and handicap as well as objective diminution of tremor [38]. It seems important to be able to adapt injection sites and doses individually to reduce complications and to get the maximum benefit.

We need a better understanding of which are the best muscles to inject and whether EMG control is helpful. For instance, in cerebellar tremors EMG may distinguish individual 'inductor' muscles that seem to control tremor spread [89]. It is possible that injecting these muscles will be more effective. We need a clearer understanding of whether it is important to inject near to the motor points (this seems not to be important in other conditions), which tremor types benefit, whether benefit is maintained with repeated injections and, most importantly, whether the toxin can control tremor long-term without increasing functional disability.

Although Bt does seem to help in the management of some tremors there are few studies of the long-term response after repeated injections, or of the overall effect on the pathophysiology of tremor. We need to define criteria predicting a good response. In the authors' experience about 80% of patients with head tremor stay on regular Bt treatment, suggesting that the patients perceive overall benefit. There are no comparable data on patients with hand tremors.

References

1 Findley LJ, Cleeves L. Classification of tremor. In: Quinn N, Jenner P. eds. *Disorders of Movement: Clinical Pharmacological and Physiological Aspects.* San Diego: Academic Press Ltd., 1989: 506–19.

2 Findley LJ, Koller WC, LeWitt P *et al.* Tremor Research Group (TRIG) classification and definition of tremor. In: Lord Walton of Detchant, ed. *Indications for and Clinical Implications of Botulinum Toxin Therapy.* Round Table Series 29. London: Royal Society of. Medicine Services Ltd, 1993: 22–3.

3 Deuschl G, Bain PG, Brin M, and ad hoc scientific committee. Consensus statement of the movement disorder society on tremor. *Mov Disord* 1998; **13**: 2–23.

4 Findley LJ, Gresty MA, Halmagyi M. Tremor, the cogwheel phenomenon and clonus in Parkinson's disease. *J Neurol Neurosurg Psychiatry* 1981; **44**: 534–46.

5 Geraghty JJ, Jankovic J, Zetusky WJ. Association between essential tremor and Parkinson's disease. *Ann Neurol* 1985; **17**: 329–33.

6 Cleeves L, Findley LJ, Koller WC. Lack of association between essential tremor and Parkinson's disease. *Ann Neurol* 1988; **24**: 23–6.

7 Findley LJ, Koller WC. Essential tremor: a review. *Neurology* 1987; **37**: 1194–7.

8 Bain PG, Mally J, Gresty M, Findley LJ. Assessing the impact of essential tremor on upper limb function. *Eur J Neurol* 1993; **241**: 54–61.

9 Bain PG, Findley LJ, Thompson PD *et al.* A study of hereditary essential tremor. *Brain* 1994; **117**: 805–24.

10 Gulcher JR, Jonsson P, Kong A *et al.* Mapping of a familial essential tremor gene FET1 to chromosome 3q. 13. *Nature Genet* 1997; **17**: 84–7.

11 Higgins JJ, Pho LT, Nee LE. A gene ETM for essential tremor maps to chromosome 2p 22-p25. *Mov Disord* 1997; **12**: 859–64.

12 Findley LJ. Epidemiology and genetics of essential tremor. *Neurology* 2000; **54** (Suppl.): S8–S13.

13 Jankovic J, Leder S, Warner D *et al.* Cervical dystonia: clinical findings and associated movement disorders. *Neurology* 1991; **41**: 1088–91.

14 Koller WC, Busenbark K, Milner K. The Essential Tremor Group. The relationship of essential tremor to other movement disorders. *Ann Neurol* 1994; **35**: 717–23.

15 Marsden CD. *Origins of Normal and Pathological Tremor.* In: Findley LJ, Capildeo R, eds. *Movement Disorders: Tremor.* London: Macmillan Press, 1984: 37–84.

16 Deuschl G, Koester B. Diagnose und behandlung des tremors. In: Conrad B, Ceballos-Baumann AO, eds. *Bewegungsstorungen in der Neurologie.* Stuttgart: Thieme-Verlag, 1996: 22–53 (English abstract).

17 Elble RJ, Koller WC. *Tremor.* Baltimore MD: Johns Hopkins University Press, 1990.

18 Couch JR. Dystonia and tremor in spasmodic torticollis. *Adv Neurol* 1976; **14**: 245–58.

19 Jedynak CP, Bonnet AM, Agid Y. Tremor and idiopathic dystonia. *Adv Neurol* 1988; **50**: 473–92.

20 Pal K, Samii A, Schulzer M, Mak E, Tsui JKC. Head tremor in cervical dystonia. *Can J Neurol Sci* 2000; **27**: 137–42.

21 Hallett M. Classification and treatment of tremor. *JAMA* 1991; **266**: 1115–7.

22 Hore J, Wild B, Diener HC. Cerebellar dysmetria at elbow wrist and fingers. *J Neurophysiol* 1991; **65**: 563–71.

23 Bain PG, Findley LJ, Britton TC *et al.* Primary writing tremor. *Brain* 1995; **116**: 203–9.

24 Heilman KM. Orthostatic tremor. *Arch Neurol* 1984; **41**: 880–1.

25 Britton TC, Thompson PD. Primary orthostatic tremor. *Br Med J* 1995; **310**: 143–4.

26 Thompson PD, Rothwell JC, Day BL *et al.* The physiology of orthostatic tremor. *Arch Neurol* 1986; **43**: 584–7.

27 Stein RB, Lee RG. Tremor and clonus. In: Brooks, BV, ed. *Motor Control: Handbook of Physiology.* Baltimore: William & Williams, 1981: 2, Section 1.

28 Marsden CD. Origins of normal and pathological tremor. In: Findley LJ, Capildeo R, eds. *Movement Disorders: Tremor.* London: Macmillan Press, 1984: 37–85.

29 Elble RJ, Koller WC. The measurement and quantification of tremor. In: Elble RJ, Koller WC, eds. *Tremor.* Baltimore MD: Johns Hopkins University Press, 1990: 10–36.

30 Gresty M, Buckwell D. Spectral analysis of tremor: understanding the results. *J Neurol Neurosurg Psychiatry* 1990; **53**: 976–81.

31 Lamarre Y. Animal models of physiological, essential and parkinsonian-like tremors. In: Findley LJ, Capildeo R, eds. *Movements Disorders: Tremor.* London: Macmillan Press, 1984: 183–94.

32 Llinas RR. The intrinsic and electrophysiological properties of mammalian neurones: insight into central venous system functions. *Science* 1988; **242**: 1654–64.

33 Jenkins IH, Bain PG, Colebatch JG *et al.* A positron emission tomography study of essential tremor: evidence for over activity of cerebellar connections. *Ann Neurol* 1993; **34**: 82–90.

34 Elbe RJ. Physiologic and essential tremor. *Neurology* 1986; **36**: 225–31.

35 Sanes JN, LeWitt PA, Mauritz KH. Visual and mechanical control of postural and kinetic tremor in cerebellar system disorders. *J Neurol Neurosurg Psychiatry* 1988; **56**: 123–6.

36 Bain PG. The effectiveness of treatments for essential tremor. *Neurologist* 1997; **3**: 305–21.

37 Bain PG, Findley LJ, Atchison P *et al.* Assessing tremor severity. *J Neurol Neurosurg Psychiatry* 1993; **56**: 868–73.

38 Bain PG, Findley LJ. *Assessing Tremor Severity. A Clinical Handbook.* London: Smith–Gordon & Co., 1993.

39 Findley LJ. The pharmacology of tremor. In: Clifford Rose F, ed. *Advances in Neuropharmacology.* London: Smith–Gordon & Co, 1993: 191–204.

40 Jankovic J, Marsden CD. Therapeutic strategies in Parkinson's disease. In: Jankovic J, Tolosa E, eds. *Parkinson's Disease and Movement Disorders,* 2nd edn. Baltimore: Williams & Williams, 1993: 115–44.

41 Koller WC. Pharmacological treatment of parkinsonian tremor. *Arch Neurol* 1986; **43**: 126–7.

42 Koller WC, Herbster G. Adjuvant therapy of parkinsonian tremor. *Arch Neurol* 1987; **44**: 921–4.

43 Kunig G, Pogarell O, Moller JC, Delf M, Ocrtel WH. Pramipexole a non-ergot dopamine agonist is effective against rest tremor in intermediate to advanced Parkinson's disease. *Clin Neuropharmacol* 1999; **22**: 301–5.

44 Pakkenberg H, Pakkenberg B. Clozapine in the treatment of tremor. *Acta Neurol Scand* 1986; **73**: 295–7.

45 Friedman JH, Koller WC, Lannon MC, Busenbark K, Swanson-Hayland E, Smith D. Benztrophine versus clozapine for the treatment of tremor in Parkinson's disease. *Neurology* 1997; **48**: 1077–81.

46 Spieker S, Breit S, Klockgether T, Dichgans J. Tremorlytic activity of budipine in Parkinson's disease. *J Neural Transmission (Supplementum)* 1999; **56**: 165–72.

47 Burnett L, Jankovic J, Grossman RG. Thalamotomy in movement disorders: an update. *Neurology* 1992; **42** (Suppl. 3): 198.

48 Laitinen LV, Bergenheim AT, Harris MI. Leskell's posteroventral pallidotomy in treatment of Parkinson's disease. *J Neurosurg* 1992; **76**: 53–61.

49 Aziz TZ, Peggs D, Sambrook MA, Crossman AR. Lesion of the subthalamic nucleus for the alleviation of 1-methyl-4-phenyl-1236-tetrahydropyridine (MPTP)-induced parkinsonian in the primate. *Mov Disord* 1991; **6**: 288–92.

50 Benabid AL, Pollack P, Gervaron C. Long-term suppression of tremor by chronic stimulation of the ventral intermediate thalamic nucleus. *Lancet* 1991; **1**: 403–6.

51 Benabid AL, Pollak P, Gao D *et al.* Chronic electrical stimulation of the ventral intermedial nucleus of the thalamus as a treatment of movement disorders. *J Neurosurg* 1996; **84**: 203–14.

52 Hubble JP, Busenbark KL, Wilkinson S *et al.* Effects of thalamic deep brain stimulation based on tremor type and diagnosis. *Mov Disord* 1997; **12**: 337–41.

53 Findley LJ. Pharmacological management of essential tremor. In: Marsden, CD, Fahn, S, eds. *Movement Disorders 2.* Butterworth-Heinemann, Oxford, 1986: 438–58.

54 Koller WC. Long-acting propranolol in essential tremor. *Neurology* 1985; **35**: 108–10.

55 Stone R. Proximal myopathy during beta blockade. *Br Med J* 1989; **2**: 1583.

56 Findley LJ, Calzetti S, Cleeves L. Primidone in essential tremor of hands and head: double blind controlled study. *J Neurol Neurosurg Psychiatry* 1985; **48**: 911–5.

57 Koller WC, Biary N. Effect of alcohol on tremors. Comparison with propranolol. *Neurology* 1984; **34**: 221–2.

58 Ceravolo R, Salvetti S, Piccini P *et al.* Acute and chronic effects of clozapine in essential tremor. *Mov Disord* 1999; **14**: 468–72.

59 Thompson C, Lang A, Parlees JD, Marsden CD. A double blind trial of clonazepam in benign essential tremor. *Clin Neuropharmacol* 1984; **7**: 83–8.

60 Gironell A, Kulisevsky J, Barbanoj M *et al.* A randomized placebo controlled comparative trial of gabapentin and propranalol in essential tremor. *Arch Neurol* 1999; **56**: 475–80.

61 Pahwa R, Lyons K, Hubble JP *et al.* Double blind control trial of gabapentin in essential tremor. *Mov Disord* 1998; **13**: 465–7.

62 Galvez-Jimenez N, Hargreave M. Topiramate and essential tremor. *Ann Neurol* 2000; **47**: 837–8.

63 Mally J, Stone TW. Effect of theophyllin on essential tremor: possible role of GABA. *Pharmacol Biodem Behav* 1991; **39**: 345–9.

64 Biary N, Bahou Y, Sofi MA, Thomas W, Al-Deeb SM. Effect of Nimodipine on essential tremor. *Neurology* 1995; **45**: 1523–5.

65 Narabayashi H. Surgical approach to tremor. In: Marsden, CD, Fahn, S, eds. *Movement Disorders 1.* London: Butterworths, 1982: 292–9.

66 Niranjan A, Kondziolka D, Baser J, Heyman R, Lunsford LD. Functional outcomes after gamma knife thalamotomy for essential tremor and multiple sclerosis related tremor. *Neurology* 2000; **55**: 443–6.

67 Pahwa R, Lyons K, Koller WC. Surgical treatment of essential tremor. *Neurology* 2000; **54** (Suppl. 4): S39–S44.

68 Hallett M, Lindsey JW, Adelstein BD, Riley PO. Controlled trial of isoniazid therapy for severe postural cerebellar tremor in multiple sclerosis. *Neurology* 1985; **35**: 1374–7.

69 Elle JS, Findley LJ, Gresty MA. Pendular nystagmus (ocular myoclonus) and related somatic tremors: their pharmacological modification and treatment. In: Findley LJ, Capildeo R, eds. *Movement Disorders: Tremor.* London: Macmillan Press, 1984: 421–61.

70 Nagaseki Y, Shibazaki T, Hirai T. Long-term follow up results selective VIM-thalamotomy. *J Neurosurg* 1986; **65**: 296–302.

71 Haddow LJ, Mumsford C, Whittle IR. Stereotactic treatment of tremor due to multiple sclerosis. *Neurosurg Q* 1997; **7**: 23–4.

72 Cleeves L, Findley LJ, Marsden CD. Odd tremors. In: Marsden CD, Fahn S, eds. *Movement Disorders 3.* London: Butterworth–Heinemann, 1994: 434–58.

73 Bain PG, Findley LJ, Britton TC *et al.* Primary writing tremor. *Brain* 1995; **118**: 1461–72.

74 Papa SM, Gershanik OS. Orthostatic tremor: an essential tremor variant. *Mov Disord* 1988; **3**: 97–108.

75 Deuschl G, Lucking CH, Quintern J. Orthostatic tremor. Clinical signs, pathophysiology and therapy. *EEG EMG* 1987; **18**: 13–9.

76 Willis AJ, Bursa L, Wang HC, Brown P, Marsden CD. Levodopa may improve orthostatic tremor. Case report and trial of treatment. *J Neurol Neurosurg Psychiatry* 1999; **65**: 681–4.

77 Evidente VG, Alder CH, Caviness JN, Gwinn KA. Effective treatment of orthostatic tremor with gabapentin. *Mov Disord* 1998; **13**: 829–31.

78 Jankovic J, Schwartz K. Botulinum toxin treatment of tremors. *Neurology* 1991; **41**: 1185–8.

79 Jankovic J. Treatment of tremors with botulinum toxin. In: Jankovic J, Hallett M, eds. *Therapy with Botulinum Toxin.* New York: Marcel Dekker Inc, 1994: 494–50.

80 Dauer WT, Burke RE, Green P, Fahn S. Current concepts on clinical features, aetiology and management of idiopathic cervical dystonia. *Brain* 1998; **121**: 547–60.

81 Cohen LG, Hallett M, Geller BD, Hochberg F. Treatment of focal dystonias of the hand with botulinum toxin injections. *J Neurol Neurosurg Psychiatry* 1989; **52**: 355.

82 Jankovic J, Schwartz K, Clemence W, Aswad A, Mordaunt J. Randomized double blind placebo controlled study to evaluate BoNT/A in essential hand tremor. *Mov Disord* 1996; **11**: 250–6.

83 Mancini F, Pacchetti C, Bulgheroni M, Martignoni E, Nippi G. Individualized treatment with BoNT/A for hand tremor. *Mov Disord* 1998; **13** (Suppl. 2): 205.

84 Brin MF, Lyons KE, Doucette J *et al*. A randomized, double masked, controlled trial of botulinum toxin type A in essential hand tremor. *Neurology* 2001; **56**: 1523.

85 Koller WC, Hristora A, Brin M. Pharmocologic treatment of essential tremor. *Neurology* 2000; **54**(11) (Suppl. 4): 530–8.

86 Trosch R, Pullman SL. Botulinum toxin A injections for the treatment of hand tremors. *Ann Neurol* 1992; **32**: 250 (Abstract).

87 Bain PG, Gregory R, Hyman N. Treatment of parkinsonian tremor with botulinum toxin: results of a pilot study. Presented to Dystonia Forum, London, 1994.

88 Ludlow CL, Sedory SE, Fujita M, Naunton RF. Treatment of voice tremor with botulinum toxin injections (Abstract). *Neurology* 1989; **39** (Suppl. 1): 353.

89 Rondot P, Bathien N. Motor control in cerebellar tremor. In: Findley LJ, Capildeo R, eds. *Movement Disorders: Tremor*. London: Macmillan Press, 1984: 365–76.

Tics, myoclonus, stiff person syndrome, gait freezing and rigidity

MADHAVI THOMAS & JOSEPH JANKOVIC

Introduction

The indications for botulinum toxin (Bt) have broadened markedly since its original use for strabismus, blepharospasm and other facial spasms in the 1980s [1,2]. In this chapter we briefly review the use of botulinum toxin type A (BtA) in the treatment of relatively uncommon or unusual conditions, including tic disorders, myoclonus, stiff person syndrome, gait freezing and rigidity. A variety of reports suggest that Bt could be a valuable treatment option for some of these disorders, which are characterized by abnormal, involuntary, excessive or inappropriate muscle contractions. However, many of the publications involve single case reports or small series and there are few randomised controlled trials, making it difficult to draw firm conclusions. Unless stated otherwise, the term Bt in this chapter refers to botulinum toxin A (Botox® or Dysport®).

Tics and tourette syndrome

Tourette syndrome is a familial neurobehavioural disorder named after the French neurologist Georges Gilles de la Tourette who first described it in 1885. The diagnosis of Tourette syndrome is based on history of motor and vocal tics, behavioural abnormalities, obsessive-compulsive disorder, lack of impulse control and attention deficit hyperactivity disorder [3].

Clinical features and diagnosis

Tics are rapid, brief, jerk like movements (motor tics) or sounds produced by moving air through the nose, mouth or throat (phonic or vocal tics). Tics can be simple (focal, involving single muscles) or complex (sequential, coordinated movements involving many muscles). Characteristic features of tics include premonitory feelings or sensations, temporary suppressibility, exacerbation with stress and during relaxation after stress, remission with distraction and concentration, waxing and waning, transient remissions, and occurrence during sleep. Tics are rarely disabling, but some patients have troublesome tics that cause local discomfort, embarrassment or other problems such as functional blindness (due to excessive blinking and blepharospasm) or radiculopathy (from 'whiplash' jerking of the neck). Differential diagnosis of tics includes stereotypy, myoclonus, dystonia, chorea, mannerisms, rituals and habitual manipulations [4].

Pathogenesis

There is a growing body of scientific evidence to support the notion that Tourette syndrome is a genetic, developmental disorder of synaptic neurotransmission resulting in disinhibition of the cortico–striatal–thalamic–cortical circuitry. This is most likely to be due to abnormal innervation of striatum and limbic systems [5]. Magnetic resonance imaging (MRI) studies are usually normal except for subtle loss of normal asymmetry of the basal ganglia and decrease in the volume of the caudate nucleus. Functional imaging studies show activation of sensorimotor cortex in motor tics, and in vocal tics there has been increased activation of Broca's area, frontal operculum and the head of the caudate [6]. Functional MRI studies show decreased neuronal activity during periods of suppression in the ventral globus pallidus, putamen, and thalamus, and increased activity in the caudate, frontal cortex and other cortical areas normally involved in the inhibition of unwanted impulses (prefrontal, parietal, temporal and cingulate cortical areas) [7]. Positron emission tomography (PET) scans with 18 F-fluorodeoxyglucose showed evidence of increased metabolic activity in the lateral premotor and supplementary motor cortexes in the midbrain, and decreased metabolic activity in the caudate and thalamic areas (limbic basal ganglia-thalamocortical projection system) [8]. Postmortem examinations on patients with Tourette syndrome have not revealed any specific abnormalities.

Treatment

Medications

Dopamine receptor blocking drugs (neuroleptics), such as risperidone, haloperidol, pimozide and fluphenazine, are the most commonly used medications for treatment of tics. While usually effective in controlling the tics, they frequently provoke adverse effects such as sedation, weight gain, school phobia and a variety of movement disorders including acute dystonic reactions, akathisia and tardive dyskinesia. Pimozide has an added risk of QT prolongation. Other medications used to treat tics include tetrabenazine, clonidine and guanfacine [9–12]. It is unclear if atypical neuroleptics such as clozapine, olanzapine or quetiapine will be effective in treatment of tics, but ziprasidone was found to decrease the severity of tics by 35% in one study [13].

BOTULINUM TOXIN

Experience with a large number of patients in various studies has confirmed the beneficial effects of Bt in treatment of both motor and vocal tics and coprolalia (Table 13.1 [14–18]). Bt has been shown to be useful in the treatment of both clonic and dystonic

Table 13.1 Botulinum toxin (Bt) for tics.

Author	Diagnosis	Muscle groups treated	Dose range (mu)	Side-effects	Duration of benefit (weeks)
Jankovic [14] (Botox®)	Dystonic tics 10 patients	Eyebrow and eyelids	30–70	Ptosis	12–20
		Eyebrow, face	40–60		
		Eyebrow, face & masseters	45–80		
		Trapezius	100–200	Neck weakness	
		Rhomboid	75–100	Neck pain	
		Splenii	75–200	Neck stiffness	
Kwak et al. [15] (Botox®)	Tics 35 patients		Mean dose±SD 149.6±49.1		0.3–45.0 (mean 14.4±10.3)
		Cervical	57.4±18.4	Neck weakness	
		Upper face	79.3±52.5	Ptosis	
		Lower face	17.8±6.5	Dysphagia	
		Vocal cords	121.7±92.4		
		Other			
Salloway et al. [16] (Botox®)	Vocal tics 1 patient	Thyroarytenoid muscle	1.25–3.75	Breathy voice Difficulty swallowing liquids	9
Scott et al. [17] (Botox®)	Coprolalia with Tourette syndrome 1 patient	Left vocal cord	25–30	Moderate Hoarseness of voice	5
Trimble et al. [18] (Dysport®)	Coprolalia 1 patient	thyroaretynoid muscles	3.75–5	Breathy weak voice and slight aspiration for few days	12

tics [14]. The initial pilot study with Bt (Botox®) included 10 male patients 13–53 years of age with Tourette syndrome manifested by severe focal tics. Five patients had frequent blinking and severe blepharospasm rendering them functionally blind. Five other patients had intense painful repetitive dystonic tics involving their neck and shoulder muscles. The injection target was the anatomic location of the premonitory sensation. The dosages were similar to those used in dystonia in a comparable location. All patients in this study obtained some relief and improvement in the tics and also the premonitory sensation. Side-effects included ptosis, neck pain, neck weakness, and neck stiffness.

DOSES: A HEALTH WARNING

Please read the warning on p. 35 about doses of Bt. There are three preparations available. *Dysport®* and *Botox®* are type A toxins (BtA), *NeuroBloc®/MYOBLOC™* is type B (BtB). Even though the doses for each are quoted in mouse units (mu), the three preparations have different dose schedules: one mu of *Dysport®* is **not** the same as one mu of *Botox®*, and neither is equivalent to one mu of *NeuroBloc®/MYOBLOC™*.

In another open study from our centre, 35 patients (30 male; mean age of 23.3 ± 15.5 years; range 8–69 years) received Bt (Botox®) into muscles affected by the tics [15]. Sites of injections were: cervical (17), upper face (14), lower face (7), voice (4), other: upper back, shoulder (3), scalp (1), forearm (1), leg (1) and rectus abdominis (1). Response to Bt was based on a 0–4 clinical rating scale (0 = no improvement, 4 = marked improvement in severity and function). Questionnaires were administered to evaluate patients' impression of overall efficacy and degree of benefit for premonitory sensations. The mean latency to onset of benefit was 3.8 days (0–10), mean peak effect response in 115 treatment sessions was 2.8 (0–4), and the mean duration of benefit was 14.4 weeks (0–45). Twenty-one of 25 patients (84%) with premonitory sensations derived marked relief of these symptoms (mean benefit: 70.6%). The mean cumulative dose was 502.1 mu (range 15–3550), the mean number of visits was 3.3 (range 1–16) and the mean dose per visit was 119.9 mu (range 15–273). Complications included neck weakness (4), dysphagia (2), ptosis (2), nausea (1), hypophonia (1), fatigue (1), and generalized weakness (1) which were all mild and transient. This study and our subsequent experience led us to conclude that Bt is an effective and well-tolerated treatment of tics and that, besides improving the motor component of tics, it also provides relief of premonitory sensations.

In a placebo-controlled study of 15 patients with simple motor tics, Marras *et al.* [19] found a 42% reduction in the number of tics per minute in patients treated with Bt (type not specified) as compared to an 8% increase in the placebo group. In addition, there was a 0.57 reduction in 'urge scores' with Bt (compared to a 0.4 increase in the placebo group). This trial lacked the power to show statistically significant differences. Additional patients and longer follow-up are needed to clarify the efficacy of Bt in the treatment of tics, and the study continues.

Awaad [20] used BtA to treat 186 patients with tics and noted improvement in symptoms. Problems with this study include inadequate description of patient selection and the nature of the tics. Furthermore, the patients also received baclofen and it is not clear what additional effect this had. Injections were given into facial muscles such as levator labii superioris, depressor labii inferioris and depressor anguli oris, which could cause asymmetric facial weakness as a side-effect that is likely to be cosmetically unacceptable [21]. There were important methodological problems which the authors did not clarify and they reported unexpectedly few patients with side-effects (6).

There are two case reports of treatment of coprolalia with Bt. Scott *et al.* [17] used Bt (Botox®) injections into the left thyroaretynoid muscle in a 13-year-old-patient with severe, disabling coprolalia. Although the patient experienced transient hypophonia, there was marked and sustained reduction in the intensity and frequency of the coprolalia as well as marked improvement in urge and premonitory sensation. Trimble *et al.* [18] also used Bt injection for coprolalia, which resulted in a softer voice and more manageable coprolalia. Bt was also used by Salloway *et al.* [16] for refractory vocal tics with 40–50% improvement of symptoms. Transient side-effects noted in these studies include hoarseness, aspiration and reduced voice volume.

Myoclonus

Myoclonus is an abrupt, sudden, jerk-like movement encountered in a large number of systemic and central nervous system diseases. Not associated with loss of consciousness, myoclonus may be generalized, segmental, or focal involving limbs, face, and trunk.

Clinical features and diagnosis

Most myoclonic jerks are caused by abrupt muscle contractions (positive myoclonus), but brief jerk-like movements may be also caused by a sudden *cessation* of muscle contraction associated with a silent period on electromyography (EMG) (negative myoclonus). Myoclonus may be related to motor activity as in action or intention myoclonus, or it can occur at rest. Myoclonus is often stimulus sensitive, triggered by a wide variety of stimuli including light, muscle stretch, unexpected noise, and other sudden stimuli [22–24]. Palatal myoclonus is a form of segmental myoclonus produced by 1–3 Hz rhythmical contractions of either tensor veli palatini (essential or idiopathic myoclonus) or levator palatini (symptomatic myoclonus, secondary to a brainstem lesion).

Electrophysiological studies are useful in evaluating myoclonus from both a clinical and a physiological perspective. Electroencephalogram (EEG) studies often show complexes of atypical spike waves or polyspike waves commonly preceding myoclonic jerks with a latency of 7–32 ms, depending on the muscle involved. Cortical spikes are time locked to myoclonic jerks in cortical myoclonus [25,26]. Other investigations for myoclonus include pure tone and evoked response audiometry, often abnormal in brainstem myoclonus. Somatosensory evoked responses typically show giant potentials in patients with cortical myoclonus. MRI is also helpful, particularly in the assessment of brainstem and spinal segmental myoclonus. Differential diagnosis of myoclonus includes chorea, tics, and paroxysmal dyskinesias. Some of these abnormal movements can also accompany tremor or dystonia.

Pathogenesis

In patients with postanoxic myoclonus, the most common cause of generalized myoclonus, there are degenerative changes in the thalamus, subthalamic nucleus, basal ganglia, midbrain and pontine grey matter. Microscopic examination shows atrophic changes in the dentate nucleus and its projections. Purkinje cell loss and Bergman gliosis are particularly prominent in the outer aspects of the cerebellar hemispheres than in the folia [27]. Palatal myoclonus, the most common form of segmental myoclonus, is due to disconnection in the dentato–rubro–olivary pathway (the Guillain–Mollaret triangle). Brains of patients with secondary palatal myoclonus often show hypertrophic degeneration of the inferior olive.

Treatment

Medications

Conventional antiepileptics such as phenytoin, primidone or barbiturates have been reported to be effective in the treatment of generalized myoclonus, but the most effective drugs are 5-hydroxytryptophan and clonazepam. Sodium valproate is also effective in postanoxic myoclonus and progressive myoclonic epilepsy. Baclofen may be useful in patients with spinal myoclonus and in patients with Unverricht–Lundborg disease and myoclonus secondary to homocystinuria [28].

Piracetam is a nootropic drug which stimulates the synthesis and release of acetylcholine. Clinical trials show that it is effective in both cortical and subcortical myoclonus [29,30]. Medical treatments available for palatal myoclonus include anticholinergics, antidepressants, benzodiazepines, anticonvulsants, and 5-hydroxytryptophan have been used in the past, but none of these produce reliable control of the abnormal movements. More recently sumatriptan seemed effective for some patients [31].

BOTULINUM TOXIN

Bt has been reported to be useful in the treatment of myoclonus, but no controlled studies have been published (Table 13.2 [32–36]). Awaad *et al.* [37] described nine patients with childhood onset myoclonus from various aetiologies including trauma, mitochondrial disease, tumour, metabolic diseases and Lafora's disease. However, they fail to provide critical details and to document the long-term effects of treatment. Bt has been also reported to show improvement in a patient with propriospinal myoclonus following spinal cord infarction [36]. The patient had continuous painful and rhythmic contractions of her left quadriceps region. The patient also had complete resolution of pain, and significant reduction in myoclonus and marked decrease in the burst discharges on EMG. Lagueny *et al.* [35] reported a patient with stimulus sensitive spinal segmental myoclonus that improved with injection of Bt. Improvement began within 10 days and there was complete resolution of symptoms for 4 months. Symptoms re-

Table 13.2 Botulinum toxin (Bt) for myoclonus.

Author	Diagnosis	Muscle groups	Dosages (mu)	Side-effects	Duration of benefit (weeks)
Saeed & Brooks [32] Bt (product not specified)	Palatal myoclonus 3 patients	Insertion of tensor and levator veli palatini	2.5–5.0	Nasal regurgitation and dysphagia Speech problems	12–52
Varney et al. [33] BtA (Botox®)	Palatal myoclonus 1 patient	Insertion of tensor veli palatini	2.5	Mild nasal regurgitation	28
Bryce & Morrison [34] Bt (product not specified)	Palatal myoclonus	Tensor veli palatini	4–10	Aural fullness	8–16
Lagueny et al. [35] Bt (product not specified)	Stimulus sensitive spinal segmental myoclonus 1 patient	Left trapezius	100	None	16
Polo & Jabbari [36] Bt (Botox®)	Limb myoclonus of spinal origin 1 patient	Left quadriceps: rectus, vastus lateralis, and vastus medialis muscles	280	None	20

curred 6 months after the patient's initial treatment. Bryce et al. [34] reported two patients with palatal myoclonus who received Botox® at dosages of 7.5 mu and 10 mu, respectively. Complications included ear fullness on one side which required a tympanostomy tube and a hypernasal voice which persisted for 2 weeks. Other studies used Bt (Botox®)[32,33] 2.5 mu into the posterior aspect of palate at the insertion of tensor veli palatini and 2.5 mu laterally near the insertion of levator veli palatini on each side. Side-effects included transient nasal regurgitation and swallowing difficulties. Bt was thought to be safe and effective in palatal myoclonus. An average dose would be Botox® 2.5–5.0 mu on each side. There is only limited evidence to support treatment of other forms of myoclonus with Bt.

Stiff person syndrome

Moersch and Woltman described Stiff person syndrome in 1956. It is an autoimmune disorder characterized by a 'tin soldier' posture caused by continuous isometric contractions of the paraspinal and leg muscles [38]. Barker et al. [39] categorized patients into three types: (i) stiff trunk syndrome; (ii) stiff limb syndrome; and (iii) progressive encephalomyelitis with rigidity.

Clinical features and diagnosis

The symptoms usually begin between 30 and 70 years of age and women patients outnumber men patients. Stiffness spreads from axial to limb muscles and usually involves the leg. Noise, sudden movement or emotional stimuli precipitate superimposed episodic 'jerks' and painful muscle spasms. There is usually marked rigidity of back, abdominal and proximal extremity muscles. Kyphosis, lordosis, spastic gait, hyper-reflexia and cognitive dysfunction and brainstem signs have been noted. Other associated features include autonomic dysfunction, ocular involvement and cerebellar ataxia, myoclonus, and seizures [39–42].

EMG shows continuous motor activity in involved muscles, which is thought to be due to the failure of normal inhibitory mechanisms. It is abolished by intravenous or oral diazepam. Nerve conduction studies are normal [43]. Cerebrospinal fluid may show increased immunoglobulin (IgG) levels and oligoclonal bands and the diagnosis is generally confirmed by positive antiglutamic acid decarboxylase (antiGAD) and anti-amphiphysin antibodies (particularly in the paraneoplastic form) detected in the blood [43–46]. Antibodies to gephryn were described recently [47]. This is a protein selectively concentrated at the postsynaptic membrane of inhibitory synapses where it is associated with γ-aminobutyric acid A (GABA$_A$) and glycine receptors.

Pathogenesis

Stiff person syndrome is an autoimmune disorder [48]. Autopsies sometimes show evidence of brainstem disease, but there is no consistent evidence of cell destruction. The differential diagnosis includes spinal cord lesions, Isaac's syndrome, progressive supranuclear palsy, and chronic tetanus.

Treatment

Medications

Oral and intrathecal baclofen [49,50] has been used successfully in the treatment of stiff person syndrome, though it often provides only partial relief. Diazepam, clomipramine, clonidine, tizanidine, methocarbamol, vigabatrin and sodium valproate have also been used for spasms. Immunosuppressive therapies, such as corticosteroids, plasma exchange and intravenous immunoglobulin (IVIG) [51,52] have all been shown to be helpful in some patients. A recent double blind controlled trial of IVIG showed benefit in stiff person syndrome [53].

Table 13.3 Botulinum toxin (Bt) for stiff person syndrome.

Author	Diagnosis	Muscle groups	Dosages (mu)	Side-effects	Duration of benefit (weeks)
Davis & Jabbari [54] Bt (Botox®)	Stiff person syndrome 1 patient	L1–L5 paraspinal regions	200–560	None	16
Liguori et al. [55] (Dysport®) 50 U/0.1 mL)	Stiff person syndrome 2 patients	Adductor magnus	100	Flu-like syndrome	16–28
		Adductor longus	50		
		Rectus femoris	100		
		Vastus lateralis	50		
		Vastus medialis	50		
		Biceps femoris long head	100		
		Biceps femoris short head	50		
		Tibialis posterior	100		
		Soleus	50		
		Gastrocnemius	50		
		Trapezius	300		
		Deltoid	300		
		Biceps brachii	150		
		Coracobrachialis	50		
		Brachialis	100		
		Brachioradialis	100		

BOTULINUM TOXIN

Davis and Jabbari [54] first described the use of Bt as a treatment for stiff person syndrome in 1993 (Table 13.3 [54,55]). They injected Bt into five sites along the L1–L5 paraspinal regions with 16–20 units per site. The effect lasted about 4 months and the patient was reinjected at 6 months with relief of symptoms. Subsequently, Ligouri et al. [55] reported that repeat Bt (Dysport®) injections over a 2-year period provided a meaningful benefit to two patients with stiff person syndrome. The cumulative dose of Dysport® (50 mu/0.1 mL) for patient 1 was 4200 mu and for patient 2 was 5200 mu. They noted a progressive increase in the duration of benefit and the last injections provided relief for about 7 months. One of the patients had flu-like symptoms but this did not recur with a lower dose in subsequent treatments.

Bt was usually not sufficient to control the symptoms and nearly all patients were maintained on additional treatments including baclofen, diazepam and prednisone. However, they needed lower doses of these drugs after Bt injections. These anecdotal reports suggest that Bt may be useful for treatment of pain and spasms associated with stiff person syndrome.

Freezing

Freezing, a common symptom encountered in patients with Parkinson's disease, affects gait in the form of start hesitation and blocks during motion, in turns, when approaching an obstacle and in narrow spaces [56–58]. Freezing may occur in speech, writing and brushing teeth.

Clinical features and diagnosis

Patients describe freezing of gait as a sensation that both feet are suddenly glued to the floor making the next step impossible. It can occur during initiation of gait, turning, and walking through narrow passages. In patients with Parkinson's disease, freezing is sometimes associated with the end of dose phenomenon, underdose or excessive dopamine medication, or it can occur independently of levodopa and related therapy. Freezing episodes are transient and can last from seconds to several minutes. They are functionally disabling for the patient until the episode resolves. There are several other disorders in which freezing of gait may be prominent, including vascular parkinsonism, normal pressure hydrocephalus, progressive supranuclear palsy, multiple system atrophy and corticobasal ganglionic degeneration.

Pathogenesis

The pathophysiology of freezing is poorly understood. It is thought to result from a functional disruption in the pathways from frontal lobes to the basal ganglia or from the locomotor areas in the brainstem region. The observation that freezing can be easily overcome by visual cues suggests that the motor program for gait is intact but the patient has problems accessing it. Denny-Brown [59] postulated that mesial frontal lobe disease released grasp reflexes in the feet resulting in forceful toe flexion with feet being glued to the floor, and this hypothesis has served as a rationale for the use of Bt in freezing.

Treatment

Medications

Treatment options include cueing techniques [60] using cadence, a metronome, a suitable walking aid or even a laser pointer so patients can 'step over' the spot. Patients who have freezing during off periods may respond to dopaminergic agents. Although freezing is not considered as a primary indication for surgery, either pallidotomy or deep brain stimulation does sometimes help [61].

BOTULINUM TOXIN

Giladi *et al.* have conducted a pilot study using BtA (Allergan, USA) in 10 patients with

Table 13.4 Botulinum toxin (Bt) for freezing and rigidity.

Author	Diagnosis	Muscle groups	Dosages (mu)	Side-effects	Duration of benefit (weeks)
Giladi *et al.* [62] (Botox®)	Parkinsonism freezing of gait 10 patients	Soleus, tibialis posterior Extensor hallucis longus gastrocnemius	Max 300	Transient weakness	2–12
Polo & Jabbari [63] (Botox®)	Rigidity 2 patients	Biceps Brachioradialis	80–100 40–60	None	Not known
Grazko *et al.* [64] (Botox®)	Rigidity 8 patients	Biceps	80–100	None	12–16
		Brachioradaialis	20–60		
		Triceps	80–100		
		Supinator	5		
		Flexor carpi ulnaris	5–40		
		Flexor carpi radialis	5–40		
		Flexor digitorum fundus	5–20		
		Flexor digitorum sublimis	5–20		
		Extensor carpi radialis	5		
		Extensor carpi ulnaris	5		
		Extensor hallucis longus	40		

freezing of gait due of Parkinsonism. They injected gastrocnemius and soleus in all patients, and tibialis posterior and extensor hallucis longus in those with foot dystonia. Benefit was noted in seven patients with duration of benefit being two to 12 weeks [62] (Table 13.4).

We injected four patients with Bt (Botox®) for freezing of gait. One of the patients had foot dystonia with freezing; the other three patients had no foot dystonia. The muscles injected were plantaris, tibialis posterior and gastrocnemius at doses 100–300 mu (Botox®). While the three patients without foot dystonia reported no benefit, the patient with foot dystonia noted moderate improvement in freezing and was reinjected about 12 weeks later. The benefits noted in these few patients warrant more formal studies in patients with freezing, with and without foot dystonia.

Rigidity

Rigidity is a continuous and uniform increase in muscle tone, manifested by a constant resistance throughout the range of passive movement of a limb. It occurs in both distal and proximal muscles. Uniform resistance to movement in all directions is termed lead pipe rigidity. When tremor is superimposed on the background increase in tone, the ratchet-like quality of resistance to limb manipulation is called cogwheel rigidity.

Clinical features and diagnosis

Rigidity is one of the cardinal features of parkinsonism, but it be also occur in frontal lobe disorders where it is referred to as geggenhalten, and in disorders of the spinal cord (α-rigidity).

Pathogenesis

The mechanisms responsible for rigidity are not known. EMG recordings of rigid muscles reveal background motor unit discharge at low rates, increasing with rein-forcement and disappearing if complete relaxation is achieved. In patients with parkin-sonism, voluntary muscle activation recruits less electromyographic activity than normal subjects. Rigidity is selectively improved with surgical lesions of thalamus and pallidum. It is therefore most likely mediated by pathological changes in basal ganglia and the frontal lobes [65].

Treatment

Medications

In most patients dopaminergic drugs help rigidity [66]. Levodopa in combination with either carbidopa or bensarazide is one of the most commonly used medications. Dopamine agonists directly activate dopamine receptors and by-pass the presynaptic synthesis of dopamine. Bromocriptine, pergolide, pramipexole, cabergoline and apo-morphine are some of the useful dopamine agonists available.

BOTULINUM TOXIN

Although dopaminergic drugs provide the best relief, Bt may be a useful option for rigid-ity associated with Parkinson's disease and other parkinsonian disorders (see Table 13.4). Polo and Jabbari [63] used Bt for rigidity in two patients with progressive supranuclear palsy and noted marked improvement in rigidity within 1 week in both patients. They did not report the duration of benefit. In a second report they included patients with spasticity and rigidity [64]. There were a total of eight patients with pro-gressive supranuclear palsy, corticobasal ganglionic degeneration and Parkinson's dis-ease in this study. They reported improvement in seven out of eight patients in rigidity; four patients continued to receive additional treatments with Bt. The average duration of response was 3–4 months. We injected Bt into dystonic and painful areas in six pa-tients with corticobasal degeneration. Two experienced marked improvement of the dystonia and pain, and four had mild to moderate improvement [67]. There were no complications attributed to Bt. Bt may turn out to be a useful option for patients who re-spond poorly to standard dopaminergic therapy, but substantially more research is needed before we could recommend it generally.

Summary

Clinical experience in other fields, our understanding of the mechanism of action of Bt and the pathophysiology of the above disorders point to a reasonable chance of benefit with Bt. However, the literature is limited in most of these unusual indications and requires bolstering with randomized controlled trials.

References

1 Jankovic J. Botulinum toxin in movement disorders. *Curr Opin Neurol* 1994; **7**: 358–66.

2 Jankovic J, Brin MF. Botulinum toxin. Historical perspective and potential new indications. *Muscle Nerve Suppl* 1997; **6**: S129–S45.

3 Leckman J, Cohen D, Goetz C, Jankovic J. Tourette syndrome. Pieces of the puzzle. In: Cohen DJ, Jankovic J, Goetz CG, eds. *Tourette Syndrome, Advances in Neurology*, Vol. 85. Philadelphia: Lippincott, Williams & Wilkins, 2001: 369–90.

4 Jankovic J. Tourette's syndrome. *N Engl J Med* 2001; **345**: 1184–92.

5 Singer HS. Neurobiology of Tourette syndrome. *Neurol Clin* 1997; **15**: 357–79.

6 Stern E, Silbersweig D, Chee KY *et al.* A functional neuroanatomy of tics in Tourette's syndrome. *Arch. General Psychiatry* 2000; **57**: 741–8.

7 Peterson BS. Neuroimaging studies of Tourette syndrome. A decade of progress. In: Cohen DJ, Jankovic J, Goetz CG, eds. *Tourette Syndrome, Advances in Neurology*, Vol. 85. Philadelphia: Lippincott, Williams & Wilkins, 2001: 179–96.

8 Eidelberg D, Moeller JR, Antonini A *et al.* The metabolic anatomy of Tourette syndrome. *Neurology* 1997; **48**: 927–34.

9 Lang AE. Update on the treatment of tics. In: Cohen DJ, Jankovic J, Goetz CG, eds. *Tourette Syndrome, Advances in Neurology*, Vol. 85. Philadelphia: Lippincott, Williams & Wilkins, 2001: 355–62.

10 Scahill L, Chappell PB, King RA, Leckman JF. Pharmacologic treatment of tic disorders. *Child Adolesc Psychiatr Clin N Am* 2000; **9**: 99–117.

11 Robertson MM. Tourette syndrome, associated conditions and the complexities of treatment. *Brain* 2000; **123**: 425–62.

12 Kurlan R. Tourette syndrome. Treatment of tics. *Neurol Clin* 1997; **15**: 403–9.

13 Sallee FR, Kurlan R, Goetz CG *et al.* Ziprasidone treatment of children and adolescents with Tourette syndrome: a pilot study. *J Am Acad Child Adolesc Psychiatry* 2000; **39**: 292–9.

14 Jankovic J. Botulinum toxin in the treatment of dystonic tics. *Mov Disord* 1994; **9**: 347–9.

15 Kwak CH, Hanna PA, Jankovic J. Botulinum toxin in the treatment of tics. *Arch Neurol* 2000; **57**: 1190–3.

16 Salloway S, Stewart CF, Israeli L *et al.* Botulinum toxin for refractory vocal tics. *Mov Disord* 1996; **11**: 746–8.

17 Scott BL, Jankovic J, Donovan DT. Botulinum toxin injection into vocal cord in the treatment of malignant coprolalia associated with Tourette's syndrome. *Mov Disord* 1996; **11**: 431–3.

18 Trimble MR, Whurr R, Brookes G, Robertson MM. Vocal tics in Gilles de la Tourette syndrome treated with botulinum toxin injections. *Mov Disord* 1998; **13**: 617–9.

19 Marras C, Sime EA, Andrews DF, Lang AE. Botulinum toxin injections for simple motor tics: a randomized, placebo-controlled trial. *Neurology* 2001; **56**: 605–10.

20 Awaad Y. Tics in Tourette syndrome. New treatment options. *Journal of Child Neurology* 1999; **14**: 316–9.

21 Kwak C, Jankovic J. Tics in Tourette syndrome and botulinum toxin [letter]. *J Child Neurol* 2000; **15**: 631–4.

22 Hallett M, Chadwick D, Marsden CD. Cortical reflex myoclonus. *Neurology* 1979; **29**: 1107–25.

23 Brown P, Thompson PD, Rothwell JC, Day BL, Marsden CD. Axial myoclonus of propriospinal origin. *Brain* 1991; **114**: 197–214.

24 Brown P, Rothwell JC, Thompson PD, Marsden CD. Propriospinal myoclonus: evidence for spinal 'pattern' generators in humans. *Mov Disord* 1994; **9**: 571–6.

25 Shibasaki H. Electrophysiological studies of myoclonus. *Muscle Nerve* 2000; **23**: 321–35.

26 Ashby P, Chen R, Wennberg R, Lozano AM, Lang AE. Cortical reflex myoclonus studied with cortical electrodes. *Clin Neurophysiol* 1999; **110**: 1521–30.

27 Tijssen MA, Thom M, Ellison DW *et al*. Cortical myoclonus and cerebellar pathology. *Neurology* 2000; **54**: 1350–6.

28 Jankovic J, Pardo R. Segmental myoclonus. Clinical and pharmacologic study. *Arch Neurol* 1986; **43**: 1025–31.

29 Ikeda A, Shibasaki H, Tashiro K, Mizuno Y, Kimura J. Clinical trial of piracetam in patients with myoclonus: nationwide multiinstitution study in Japan. The Myoclonus/Piracetam Study Group. *Mov Disord* 1996; **11**: 691–700.

30 Obeso JA, Artieda J, Quinn N *et al*. Piracetam in the treatment of different types of myoclonus. *Clin Neuropharmacol* 1988; **11**: 529–36.

31 Jankovic J, Scott BL, Evans RW. Treatment of palatal myoclonus with sumatriptan [letter]. *Mov Disord* 1997; **12**: 818.

32 Saeed SR, Brookes GB. The use of clostridium botulinum toxin in palatal myoclonus. A preliminary report. *J Laryngol Otol* 1993; **107**: 208–10.

33 Varney SM, Demetroulakos JL, Fletcher MH, McQueen WJ, Hamilton MK. Palatal myoclonus: treatment with clostridium botulinum toxin injection. *Otolaryngol Head Neck Surg* 1996; **114**: 317–20.

34 Bryce GE, Morrison MD. Botulinum toxin treatment of essential palatal myoclonus tinnitus. *J Otolaryngol* 1998; **27**: 213–6.

35 Lagueny A, Tison F, Burbaud P, Le Masson G, Kien P. Stimulus-sensitive spinal segmental myoclonus improved with injections of botulinum toxin type A. *Mov Disord* 1999; **14**: 182–5.

36 Polo KB, Jabbari B. Effectiveness of botulinum toxin type A against painful limb myoclonus of spinal cord origin. *Mov Disord* 1994; **9**: 233–5.

37 Awaad Y, Tayem H, Elgamal A, Coyne MF. Treatment of childhood myoclonus with botulinum toxin type A. *J Child Neurol* 1999; **14**: 781–6.

38 Shaw PJ. Stiff man syndrome and its variants. *Lancet* 1999; **353**: 86–7.

39 Barker RA, Revesz T, Thom M, Marsden CD, Brown P. Review of 23 patients affected by the stiff man syndrome: clinical subdivision into stiff trunk (man) syndrome, stiff limb syndrome and progressive encephalomyelitis with rigidity. *J Neurol Neurosurg Psychiatry* 1998; **65**: 633–40.

40 Brown P, Marsden CD. The stiff man and stiff man plus syndromes. *J Neurol* 1999; **246**: 648–52.

41 Lorish TR, Thorsteinsson G, Howard FM Jr. Stiff man syndrome updated. *Mayo Clin Proc* 1989; **64**: 629–36.

42 McEvoy KM. Stiff man syndrome. *Semin Neurol* 1991; **11**: 197–205.

43 Meinck HM, Ricker K, Hulser PJ *et al*. Stiff man syndrome. Clinical and laboratory findings in eight patients. *J Neurol* 1994; **241**: 157–66.

44 Solimena M, Folli F, Denis-Donini S *et al*. Autoantibodies to glutamic acid decarboxylase in a patient with stiff man syndrome, epilepsy, and type I diabetes mellitus. *N Engl J Med* 1988; **318**: 1012–20.

45 Solimena M, De Camilli P. Autoimmunity to glutamic acid decarboxylase (GAD) in stiff man syndrome and insulin-dependent diabetes mellitus. *Trends Neurosci* 1991; **14**: 452–7.

46 Solimena M, Butler MH, De Camilli P. GAD, diabetes, and stiff man syndrome: some progress and more questions. *J Endocrinol Invest* 1994; **17**: 509–20.

47 Butler MH, Hayashi A, Ohkoshi N *et al*. Autoimmunity to gephyrin in stiff man syndrome. *Neuron* 2000; **26**: 307–12.

48 Blum P, Jankovic J. Stiff person syndrome: an autoimmune disease. *Mov Disord* 1991; **6**: 12–20.

49 Miller F, Korsvik H. Baclofen in the treatment of stiff man syndrome. *Ann Neurol* 1981; **9**: 511–2.

50 Silbert PL, Matsumoto JY, McManis PG *et al*. Intrathecal baclofen therapy in stiff man syndrome: a double-blind, placebo-controlled trial. *Neurology* 1995; **45**: 1893–7.

51 Harding AE, Thompson PD, Kocen RS *et al*. Plasma exchange and immunosuppression in the stiff man syndrome [letter]. *Lancet* 1989; **2**: 915.

52 Karlson EW, Sudarsky L, Ruderman E *et al*. Treatment of stiff man syndrome with intravenous immune globulin. *Arthritis Rheum* 1994; **37**: 915–8.

53 Dalakas MC, Fujii M, Li M *et al*. High-dose intravenous immune globulin for stiff person syndrome. *N Engl J Med* 2001; **345**: 1870–6.

54 Davis D, Jabbari B. Significant improvement of stiff person syndrome after paraspinal injection of botulinum toxin A. *Mov Disord* 1993; **8**: 371–3.

55 Liguori R, Cordivari C, Lugaresi E, Montagna P. Botulinum toxin A improves muscle spasms and rigidity in stiff person syndrome. *Mov Disord* 1997; **12**: 1060–3.

56 Fahn S. The freezing phenomenon in parkinsonism. *Adv Neurol* 1995; **67**: 53–63.

57 Giladi N, McDermott MP, Fahn S *et al*. The Parkinson Study Group. Freezing of gait in Parkinson's disease: prospective assessment of the DATATOP cohort. *Neurology* 2001; **56**: 1712–21.

58 Lamberti P, Armenise S, Castaldo V *et al*. Freezing gait in Parkinson's disease. *Eur Neurol* 1997; **38**: 297–301.

59 Denny-Brown D. The nature of apraxia. *J Nerv Ment Dis* 1958; **126**: 9–31.

60 Kompoliti K, Goetz CG, Leurgans S, Morrissey M, Siegel IM. 'On' freezing in Parkinson's disease: resistance to visual cue walking devices. *Mov Disord* 2000; **15**: 309–12.

61 Jankovic J, Lai EC, Ondo WG *et al*. Effects of pallidotomy on gait and balance. In: Ruzicka E, Jankovic J, Hallett M, eds. *Gait Disorders*. Philadelphia: Lippincott, Williams & Wilkins, 2001.

62 Giladi N, Gurevich T, Shabtai H, Paleacu D, Simon ES. The effect of botulinum toxin injections to the calf muscles on freezing of gait in Parkinsonism: a pilot study. *J Neurol* 2001; **248**: 572–6.

63 Polo KB, Jabbari B. Botulinum toxin A improves the rigidity of progressive supranuclear palsy. *Ann Neurol* 1994; **35**: 237–9.

64 Grazko MA, Polo KB, Jabbari B. Botulinum toxin A for spasticity, muscle spasms, and rigidity. *Neurology* 1995; **45**: 712–7.

65 Thompson PD. Rigidity and spasticity. In: Jankovic J, Tolosa E, eds. *Parkinson's Disease and Movement Disorders*. Baltimore MD: Williams & Wilkins, 1998: 755–62.

66 Olanow WC, Koller WC. An algorithm for the management of Parkinson's disease: treatment guidelines. *Neurology* 1998; **50** (Suppl. 3): S1–S57.

67 Vanek Z, Jankovic J. Dystonia in corticobasal degeneration. *Mov Disord* 2001; **16**: 252–7.

PART THREE

Autonomic disorders

Hypersecretory disorders

MARKUS NAUMANN

Focal hyperhidrosis and gustatory sweating

Introduction

Definition, symptoms, and differential diagnosis

Hyperhidrosis is excessive sweating and may be focal or generalized. Focal hyperhidrosis usually affects the face, axillae, palms or soles of the feet, and rarely other areas. It can be extremely disabling in both private and professional life. Focal hyperhidrosis affects up to 0.5% of the population and usually appears during the 2nd or 3rd decade of life. The simple qualitative definition of hyperhidrosis as excessive sweating is, of course, completely subjective. For research, hyperhidrosis is defined quantitatively, for example, as the production of more than 100 mg of sweat in one axilla over 5 min [1]. Focal hyperhidrosis is most often essential or idiopathic and caused by neurogenic overactivity of the sweat glands in the affected area. The palms and/or soles of the feet (palmoplantar hyperhidrosis) are affected in about 60% of patients, the axillae in 30–40% [2]. Facial sweating is less frequent and affects up to 10% of patients with idiopathic hyperhidrosis. It is different from *gustatory sweating* which occurs on the cheek in response to salivation or anticipation of food. Focal hyperhidrosis may arise following spinal cord injury and from some polyneuropathies. *Ross syndrome* is a rare form of focal hyperhidrosis of unknown aetiology characterized by progressive anhidrosis (loss of sweating) due to degeneration of sudomotor fibres. There may be disabling compensatory hyperhidrosis in areas in which sudomotor fibres remain intact (mostly trunk, sometimes extremities, neck, and face). *Generalized hyperhidrosis* with sweating occurring over the whole body has many causes (i.e. diabetes, chronic infectious diseases, malignancy). The consequences of hyperhidrosis include dehydration and maceration of the skin, which may result in secondary infections of the skin.

Pathophysiology

The cause of essential focal hyperhidrosis is unknown at present. The sweat glands and their innervation do not show any histological abnormalities. There may be dysfunction of the central sympathetic nervous system, possibly of hypothalamic nuclei, or prefrontal areas or their connections [3,4]. Sufferers display no other signs or symptoms of autonomic dysfunction. A positive family history for the condition in 30–50% of cases suggests a genetic component [5]. Gustatory sweating may result from misdirection of autonomic nerve fibres after surgery or in diseases of the parotid gland and may occur in diabetes and some other rare conditions. Generalized hyperhidrosis can be secondary to a variety of conditions including metabolic disease such as diabetes or hyperthyroidism or chronic infections such as tuberculosis, alcoholism and malignancy.

Severity rating scales/techniques

No validated severity rating scales are available for focal or generalized hyperhidrosis. In part, this is due to the known day-to-day variations of sweat secretion for any individual, often related to stress, exercise, or ambient temperature. Focal hyperhidrosis may be quantified qualitatively and quantitatively. The Minor's iodine starch test is a qualitative measure that visualizes and defines the extent of the hyperhidrotic area, irrespective of the amount of sweat produced. Gravimetry can quantify the volume of sweat secretion, typically by measuring the increase in weight of a filter paper absorbing sweat over a certain period of time (1–5 min).

Conventional treatment strategies

There are numerous and varied treatments for hyperhidrosis and none is completely satisfactory. If there is no obvious cause or if an underlying disease cannot be controlled sufficiently, current first-line treatment for focal hyperhidrosis is usually topical application of acids, aldehydes and metal salts. Anticholinergic drugs are quite effective but have unpleasant side-effects such as dry mouth and blurred vision. Tap water iontophoresis is a time-consuming procedure in which the hands are soaked in tap water and an electric current is passed for up to 30 min.

Many hyperhidrosis sufferers eventually resort to surgery. Excision and suction curettage of sweat glands are sometimes used in the axillae to remove the sweat coils in the skin. However, these methods may produce extensive scarring and cannot be applied to the palms. The neuronal innervation of the sweat glands in the palms can be blocked by destroying the second and third thoracic ganglia in a thoracic sympathectomy operation, resulting in correction of hyperhidrosis. Since the introduction of transthoracic endoscopic sympathectomy this operation has become the treatment of choice in severe cases of palmar hyperhidrosis as it provides a lasting relief in many cases. However, there may be serious complications including pneumothorax, compensatory sweating in other areas of the body or Horner's syndrome [6,7].

Botulinum toxin review

Hypo- or anhidrosis is a well known facet of botulism which was described in 1822 by

Table 14.1 Selection of larger studies (>10 patients) of BtA treatment of focal axillary or palmar hyperhidrosis.

Authors	Design	Region	n	Dose per side	Duration (months)
Botox®					
Glogau [20]	Open	Axillary	12	50 mu Botox®	4–7
Naver et al. [21]	Open	Axillary	55	32–100 mu Botox®	3–>14
Naumann et al. [13]	Open	Palmar + axillary	11	30–50 mu Botox®	>5
Naumann & Lowe [26]	Controlled*	Axillary	320	50 mu Botox®	>4
Naumann et al. [28]	Follow-up (open)	Axillary	207	50 mu Botox®	7 (mean)
Naver et al. [21]	Open	Palmar	94	120–220 mu Botox®	3–>14
Solomon & Hayman [23]	Open	Palmar	20	165 mu Botox®	4–9
Dysport®					
Schnider et al. [17]	Controlled*	Axillary	13	250 mu Dysport®	>3
Heckmann et al. [22]	Open†	Axillary	12	250 mu Dysport®	3–12
Heckmann et al. [27]	Controlled*‡	Axillary	145	100/200 mu Dysport®	>6
Schnider et al. [12]	Controlled*	Palmar	11	120 mu Dysport®	>3

*Controlled = double blind, placebo-controlled. †Side-controlled. ‡One axilla received BtA, the other axilla placebo.

Kerner [8] and was also noted as a side-effect of botulinum toxin A (BtA) used in treating hemifacial spasm. These observations formed the basis for the development of BtA as a therapy for hyperhidrosis. Subsequently BtA was shown to abolish physiological sweating in the axilla and the back of the hand in healthy volunteers [9,10]. After the first report of BtA use in a patient with palmar hyperhidrosis in 1997 [11] several small open and a few controlled studies were published [12–25]. All these studies dealt mainly with axillary and palmar sweating. More recently, two large placebo-controlled, double blind European multicentre studies on BtA in axillary hyperhidrosis reported their results [26,27]. Table 14.1 provides detailed information from this literature on the sites of injection, the doses used and the duration of action after injections of BtA for axillary and palmar hyperhidrosis [12, 13, 17, 20–23, 26–28].

Axillary sweating

BtA is a novel minimally invasive treatment option for axillary hyperhidrosis. Two recent large placebo-controlled, double blind studies, [26,27] and several open label studies, clearly documented the beneficial effect of botulinum toxin (Bt) treatment on reduction of sweat secretion [26,27] and improvement of quality of life [29] in patients suffering from axillary hyperhidrosis. One double blind, placebo-controlled study enrolled 320 patients and evaluated the safety, efficacy and impact on quality of life of intradermal administration of BtA (50 mu Botox® per axilla) or placebo for bilateral primary axillary hyperhidrosis [26]. Patients were followed for 16 weeks after treatment. At Week 4, 93.8% of patients treated with BtA were classified as responders

(>50% reduction in sweat production from baseline gravimetric measurement), compared with 35.9% of the placebo group ($P<0.001$). The mean percentage reduction in sweat production at Week 4 was 83.5% in the BtA group compared with only 20.8% in the placebo group ($P<0.001$). Mean patient satisfaction at Week 4, as assessed by the subject's global assessment of treatment satisfaction (+4 to −4), was significantly higher in the BtA group compared to the placebo group (+3.3 vs. +0.8; $P<0.001$). No major side-effects occurred.

In a 12-months follow-on study, 207 of these patients with axillary hyperhidrosis received up to three BtA injections [28]. Response rates and satisfaction with treatment remained consistently high with no diminution of effect with repeated treatments. Mean duration of benefit was about 7 months after a single treatment session. Twenty-eight per cent of patient did not require more than one injection, indicating a long-lasting benefit of more than 16 months in a substantial proportion of patients. No major side-effects occurred over the whole period of 16 months (initial and follow-up study). BtA treatment markedly improved the quality of life of patients afflicted with hyperhidrosis (Hyperhidrosis Impact Questionnaire [HIQ©] and the Medical Outcomes Trust SF-12 Health Survey™ [SF-12]) [29]. At baseline, participants reported a marked negative impact of their hyperhidrosis on various measures including: state of mind, emotional status, comfort in social situations, productivity at work, number of clothing changes needed per day, and their ability to engage in sex or participate in athletic activities. Post-treatment, significantly greater improvements were observed in all of these outcomes in the BtA group vs. the placebo group ($P<0.01$). Patients treated with BtA also exhibited significantly greater improvement in the physical component summary score of the SF-12 at 16 weeks than did placebo-treated patients ($P<0.019$).

Another placebo-controlled study in 145 patients tested 100/200 mu Dysport®/axilla [27]. One axilla was treated with BtA, the other side was injected with placebo. The two BtA doses proved equally effective in reducing axillary sweating but follow-up or quality-of-life data are not available. These studies supported the reports of several previous open studies [13,14,16,20–22,25] and one small controlled study on the treatment of axillary sweating with BtA [17]. In these former studies, injections were mostly given intracutaneously using a grid for orientation, or injecting at multiple sites evenly distributed over the identified hyperhidrotic area. The doses used ranged from 30 to 100 mu Botox® (250 mu Dysport®) per region). In most patients this was enough to abolish axillary sweating. The duration of BtA action was at least 4 months and reached 7–12 months in many cases. Side-effects included painful injections and small local haematomas. Injection of higher doses (200 mu Botox®) [24] did not convincingly prolong the effect on hyperhidrosis compared with lower doses, and is generally not recommended as it might cause more side-effects and increase the risk of antibody formation.

Palmar sweating

The positive effect of BtA on palmar hyperhidrosis has been demonstrated by several open studies [13,18,23,25] and by one single blind [30] and one small double blind placebo-controlled trial [12]. BtA was injected using a grid for orientation or by evenly distributing small amounts of the toxin over the palms. The required total doses were much higher than in the treatment of axillary hyperhidrosis because of the larger area. The earlier studies used between 120 and 220 mu Botox® per palm or 120 mu Dysport® per palm. The subsequent single blind dose ranging study found no objective difference in suppression of palmar sweating between 50 and 100 mu Botox® per palm [30]. Several studies demonstrated a significant decrease of the amount of sweating, in accordance with the patients' subjective reports. Sweating was reduced for between 4 and 12 months. Injections were often painful, and side-effects included small haematomas and slight transient weakness of small hand muscles due to diffusion of the toxin. Measured by dynamometer, thumb-index finger pinch strength was reduced by 23% (±27%) with 50 mu Botox® and 40% (±21%) with 100 mu Botox®, and weakness was detectable for 30–60 days. However, subjective weakness was mild and generally only lasted about 10 days [30]. Local nerve block of the median and ulnar nerves at the wrist prior to injection avoids the pain of injection.

Craniofacial hyperhidrosis

Craniofacial hyperhidrosis is a relatively rare form of essential focal hyperhidrosis that is also amenable to BtA treatment. One open label study showed a significant decrease of sweat production on the forehead after intradermal injections of BtA [31]. Botox® was injected at multiple sites evenly distributed over the forehead (mean total 86 mu). The effect lasted at least 5 months in nine of the 10 patients. Side-effects were rare and included painful injections and a transient weakness of forehead muscles with an inability to frown without ptosis. All patients subjectively judged the treatment as very effective. Similar results were obtained by another study injecting a total dose of up to 480 mu Dysport® along the forehead [32].

Ross syndrome

BtA has also been applied successfully to patients with excessive compensatory sweating in *Ross syndrome* [33].

Gustatory sweating (Frey's syndrome)

After the initial report in 1995 [34], BtA has also been used as a highly effective treatment for gustatory sweating. In a large open study of 45 patients, there was a significant reduction of local facial sweating after injection of Botox® (mean dose 21 mu, range 5–72 mu) and no recurrence of sweating was observed during the follow-up period of 6 months [35]. A marked long-lasting improvement was also observed in three other open

Table 14.2 Selected studies (>10 patients) on BtA treatment of gustatory sweating (Frey's syndrome).

Author	Year	Design	n	Dose (mean)	Duration
Naumann *et al.* [35]	1997	Open	45	21 mu Botox®	>6 months
Bjerkhoel & Trobbe [36]	1997	Open	15	37 mu Botox®	>13 months
Laskawi *et al.* [37]	1998	Open	19	31 mu Botox®	11–27 months
Laccourreye *et al.* [38]	1999	Open	33	86 mu Dysport®	12–36 months

studies [36–38] (Table 14.2 [35–38]). Benefit lasted from 11 to 36 months. Thus, BtA appears to have a particularly long-lasting effect on gustatory sweating. The reason for this prolonged benefit is unclear.

A single study has compared the effects and side-effects of needle injections with injections using a Dermojet device, in palmar and axillary hyperhidrosis [14]. With the same doses, the needle injection was more effective than the dermojet. Side-effects were more frequent with the dermojet, in particular irritation of digital nerve branches, so that the Dermojet is not recommended for palmar or axillary injections. It has yet to be shown whether it is safe in the treatment of plantar hyperhidrosis [39].

Treatment with botulinum toxin

First define the affected area using Minor's test. This is particularly important in the axillae, on the forehead, on the cheek and on the trunk.

MINOR'S TEST

Paint an iodine solution (2 g of iodine in 10 mL of castor oil and alcohol to 100 mL) over the area of skin under test. After it has dried, apply fine rice or potato powder. Sweat causes the mixture to turn dark blue (Figs 14.1–14.3). Photograph or draw the area affected for comparison after treatment, to show the therapeutic effect and to help identify possible causes for a relative treatment failure.

LOCAL ANAESTHESIA

In general, local anaesthesia is not needed when treating axillary or facial sweating. Some centres use local cooling with ice or apply local anaesthetic cream, but in our experience these are no more effective than placebo. In palmar hyperhidrosis, the injection may be very painful, and patients need median and ulnar nerve blocks at the wrist. In plantar hyperhidrosis, anaesthetize the tibial nerve in the tarsal tunnel. The injector must be familiar with the local anatomy and injection techniques to avoid nerve or blood vessel injuries.

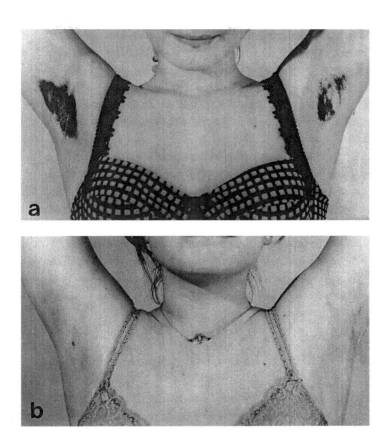

Fig. 14.1 Axillary hyperhidrosis (Minor's iodine starch test) before (a) and after (b) injection of BtA.

INJECTION TECHNIQUE AND DOSES APPLIED

DOSES: A HEALTH WARNING

Please read the warning on p. 35 about doses of Bt. There are three preparations available. *Dysport®* and *Botox®* are type A toxins (BtA), *NeuroBloc®/MYOBLOC™* is type B (BtB). Even though the doses for each are quoted in mouse units (mu), the three preparations have different dose schedules: one mu of *Dysport®* is **not** the same as one mu of *Botox®*, and neither is equivalent to one mu of *NeuroBloc®/MYOBLOC™*.

There are several possible ways to apply Bt. Based on the above studies and on personal experience, I recommend the following procedure. It is helpful to draw a grid on the skin to mark the injection fields. Use dilutions of 100 mu Botox® or 500 mu Dysport®/5 mL of sterile 0.9% saline.

In *axillary hyperhidrosis*, for each side inject a total of 50 mu Botox® or 100/200 mu

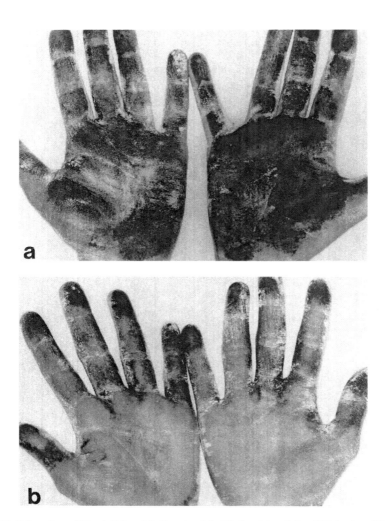

Fig. 14.2 Palmar hyperhidrosis (Minor's iodine starch test) before (a) and after (b) injection of BtA.

Dysport® intradermally, evenly distributed over the hyperhidrotic area and split between 10 and 15 injection sites (Fig. 14.4).

In *palmar or plantar hyperhidrosis*, the dose given varies from patient to patient and depends on the size of the hyperhidrotic area to be injected. Inject 2–3 mu Botox® or 8 mu Dysport® intradermally at sites 1.5–2.0 cm apart and evenly distributed over the affected area. In palmar hyperhidrosis, inject the fingers as well as the palms. In plantar hyperhidrosis, sweating frequently also occurs at the lateral and medial edges of the foot and these areas may need additional injections.

In *gustatory* and *forehead sweating (craniofacial hyperhidrosis)*, inject 2–3 mu Botox® or 8 mu Dysport® intradermally at sites 2.0–2.5 cm apart and evenly distributed over the affected area. Avoid ptosis (in forehead sweating) by not treating the caudal strip

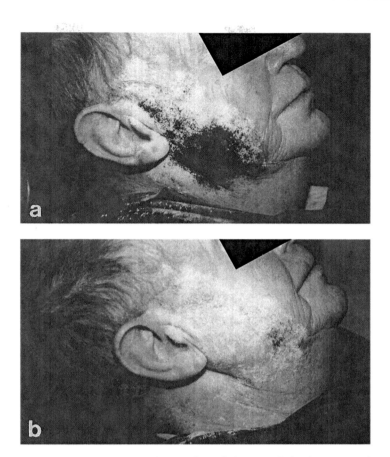

Fig. 14.3 Gustatory sweating (Minor's iodine starch test) before (a) and after (b) injection of BtA.

about 1.5 cm above the eyebrow. Prevent drooping of the mouth (in gustatory sweating) by sparing the region around the zygomatic muscle. Table 14.3 provides dose ranges for focal hyperhidrosis.

SIDE-EFFECTS

Specific side-effects of the injection of Bt for hyperhidrosis include pain on injection, local haematomas, and local muscle weakness due to diffusion of the toxin to adjacent muscles: small hand muscle weakening in palmar hyperhidrosis, drooping of the eyelid or mouth in craniofacial sweating, and inability to frown in forehead sweating. Local infections are extremely rare. Local side-effects are much more likely if there has been recent local trauma, presumably because of reduced barriers to diffusion.

REINJECTION

One single study prospectively evaluated the effect of repeated BtA injections in axillary hyperhidrosis [28]. Improvement of sweating and satisfaction with treatment remained

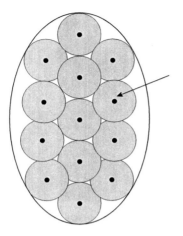

Fig. 14.4 Axillary hyperhidrosis: injection technique. Several injection sites are equally distributed over the affected area (which has to be stained using the Minor's test). After the injection at one site, the toxin spreads radially and results in an anhidrotic patch.

Table 14.3 Dose ranges for focal hyperhidrosis.

Region	Botox®	Dysport®
Axillary hyperhidrosis	50 mu per axilla	100–200 mu per axilla
Palmar hyperhidrosis	60–120 mu per palm (depending on size)	250–500 mu per palm (depending on size)
Other types of focal hyperhidrosis	2–3 mu/2 cm²	6–8 mu/2 cm²

consistently high with no diminution of effect with repeated (up to four) injection cycles. This confirms my personal experience where repeated injections over 5 years retain a relatively constant and reproducible effect. One of the main concerns about repeated BtA injections in any situation is triggering an immune response to BtA, thereby generating neutralizing antibodies. Thus on general grounds, avoid reinjection within 3 months.

SUMMARY

All studies performed so far indicate that BtA is a safe and effective treatment for focal hyperhidrosis of the axillae and palms, for gustatory sweating, and for some other rare conditions associated with focal hyperhidrosis. There is class I evidence for the efficacy of Bt in axillary hyperhidrosis, and class II evidence for palmar and gustatory sweating (according to American Academy of Neurology criteria [40]). At present, it appears that the benefit lasts at least 4–6 months, which is longer than in conditions in which it is used to weaken muscles. We still need to define the optimal and the lowest effective doses for axillary and palmar hyperhidrosis, to minimize dose related side-effects, to lower the costs of treatment, and to reduce the risk of antibody formation. Pregnant or breast-feeding women should not receive BtA. In summary, BtA has the potential to replace current invasive and surgical techniques and should at least be considered as a viable alternative.

Sialorrhea

Introduction

Definition, symptoms, and pathophysiology

Sialorrhea is a common and socially disabling symptom in degenerative diseases such as motor neuron diseases (e.g. bulbar amyotrophic lateral sclerosis (ALS)) and Parkinson's disease. About 70% of patients with Parkinson's disease and up to 20% of ALS patients suffer from excessive drooling. It is usually caused by swallowing dysfunction and can lead to choking, aspiration and chest infections. Primary sialorrhea due to an increased salivary secretion is rare.

Severity rating scales/techniques

Drooling can be evaluated subjectively using questionnaires comprising rating scales for severity (1 = dry; 2 = mild; 3 = moderate; 4 = severe; 5 = profuse) and frequency (1 = never drools; 2 = occasional drooling; 3 = frequent drooling; 4 = constant drooling) [41]. As a simple quantitative method to assess drooling, patients can document the amount of salivary secretion by counting the number of one brand of paper handkerchiefs used per day. For scientific purposes, salivary gland scintigraphy can quantify salivary secretion using the tracer technetium 99 m pertechnetate [42].

Conventional treatment

Anticholinergic drugs may reduce salivary secretion. Lack of efficacy or unacceptable adverse effects with higher doses often limit their use. Occasionally, surgical treatment or salivary gland radiation is carried out. The latter may cause local side-effects and increase the risk of malignancy.

Botulinum toxin review

In animals, immunohistochemical studies have shown a significant reduction of acetylcholinesterase in the salivary glands and a reduction of saliva production after local treatment with BtA [43,44]. There are only a few small uncontrolled published studies on Bt in the treatment of siallorhea in Parkinson's disease [45–48] and bulbar amyotrophic lateral sclerosis [42,45,46]. Up to two-thirds of the patients subjectively experienced a marked or moderate improvement of drooling following treatment of both parotid glands [46–48] or the parotid and submandibular glands combined [42,45]. The application techniques, doses applied and outcome measures varied considerably between the studies. Trials have used intraglandular injections of 10–40 mu Botox® per parotid gland [42,45,47,48], or subcutaneous injections of 20 mu Dysport® above the

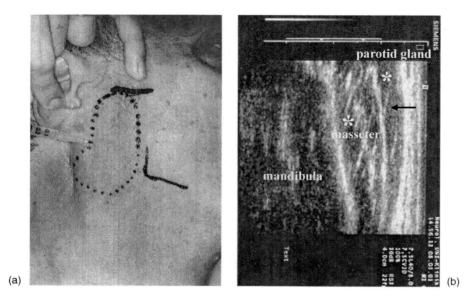

Fig. 14.5 Sialorrhea: (a) injection sites for the parotid gland. (b) Sonography of the parotid gland (arrow).

parotid gland [46]. Objective measures seem to be more sensitive in detecting reduction of sialorrhea than subjective estimation. Bt in salivary glands may suppress salivation for as long as 7 months. Side-effects include local muscle weakness, worsening of dysphagia and drying of the mouth.

Treatment with botulinum toxin

LOCAL ANATOMY

The parotid gland lies between the mastoid process and the ramus of the mandible. Cranially it reaches the zygomatic arch, caudally it ends at the level of body of the mandible, partly covering the dorsal part of the masseter muscle (Fig. 14.5a).

INJECTION TECHNIQUE AND DOSES APPLIED

There is limited experience with Bt injections into the salivary glands, and we do not yet know the best dose and way to inject. For the moment, we empirically inject Bt into 2–3 different sites on each side (Fig. 14.5a), preferably guided by ultrasound (Fig. 14.5b). A retrograde transductal approach in two ALS patients was followed by a marked deterioration of dysphagia and a local infection of the gland. Initially, use not more than 10–20 mu Botox® or 40–60 mu Dysport® per parotid gland, at a dilution of 100 mu Botox® or 500 mu Dysport®/2 mL of sterile 0.9% saline. Depending on the response, slowly increase the total dose by injecting the same or a lower amount of Bt after 8–10 weeks (risk of antibody formation if reinjections are given earlier). In the palliative treatment of sialorrhea in ALS, reinjections may be given after a shorter period of time. Sometimes, the submandibular glands also need injection using 5–10 mu Botox® or 20–30 mu Dysport® per submandibular gland. The highest safe individual dose is not known and may be very low in some patients, particularly in patients suffering from a motor neurone disorder, who may be unusually sensitive to BtA. We do not know the effect of repeated injections of Bt over time, or the risk of developing antibodies.

SIDE-EFFECTS

Reported side-effects of Bt injections into the salivary glands encompass local injection pain, local infection of the salivary gland, dry mouth, deterioration of dysphagia due to diffusion of the toxin into the pharyngeal muscles, and weakness of mouth closing and opening. Other potential adverse effects may include haematomas, salivary duct calculi, local injuries of the carotid artery or branches of the facial nerve. Empirically, I attempt to minimize the risk by cautiously increasing the dose and number of treated glands in successive treatment cycles.

SUMMARY

The results of pilot studies are encouraging. However, the optimal dose, best mode of application, side-effects, and duration of action of Bt in sialorrhea remain uncertain. We need further formal clinical trials to evaluate risks and benefits of BtA for palliative treatment in Parkinson's disease and bulbar ALS.

Pathological tearing (crocodile tear syndrome) and rhinorrhea

Introduction

Definition, symptoms, and differential diagnosis

Pathological tearing (crocodile tears syndrome) is a relatively rare syndrome which is characterized by inappropriate and sometimes excessive lacrimation provoked by eating. It should be distinguished from other local eye disorders associated with increased tearing.

Pathophysiology

Secretomotor fibres of the facial nerve innervate the lacrimal gland through the greater superficial petrosal nerve. Following any proximal facial nerve lesion, autonomic nerve fibres which originally supplied the salivary gland may missprout to the lacrimal gland and cause crocodile tears (gustolacrimal reflex). Most cases occur after incomplete recovery from peripheral facial nerve palsy [49] and acoustic neuroma surgery [50].

Severity rating scales/techniques

The Schirmer test can measure increased tearing. Insert one end of a 5-mm-wide and 25-mm-long strip of a thin filter paper into the lower conjunctival sac, while the other end hangs over the edge of the lower lid. The tears wet the strip of the filter paper, producing a moisture front [51].

Botulinum toxin review

There is no effective conventional treatment of hyperlacrimation. Since the lacrimal glands are innervated by cholinergic fibres, *hyperlacrimation* in crocodile tears syndrome may be effectively treated by intraglandular injections of Bt. So far, there are only a few reports on Bt use [51–54]. In one open study [52], injection of 20 mu Dysport® into the lacrimal gland or subcutaneous injection of a total of 75 mu Dysport® into the orbital part of the orbicularis oculi muscle for treatment of synkinesis produced a marked to moderate improvement of hyperlacrimation. In other reports [51,54], intraglandular injection of 2.5 or 5 mu Botox® normalized hyperlacrimation for more than 6 months. The dilutions used were 500 mu Dysport/2.5 mL 0.9% saline and 100 mu Botox®/5 mL 0.9% saline.

A single double-blind placebo-controlled study evaluated the effect of Bt on *rhinorrhea* in 60 patients with intrinsic rhinitis [55]. The dose of 4 mu Botox® given in each nasal cavity significantly improved rhinorrhea as judged subjectively and reduced the number of paper tissues needed per day. No side-effects occurred. The benefits lasted 4 weeks.

Treatment with botulinum toxin A

INJECTION TECHNIQUE AND DOSES APPLIED

Anaesthetize the conjunctival mucosa using eye drops before injecting the lacrimal gland. Ectropionize the upper lid and use a binocular lens for magnification. Inject 2.5–5.0 mu Botox® or 10 mu Dysport® into the palpebral part of the lacrimal gland between the secretory orifices (Fig. 14.6). Use dilutions of 100 mu Botox® or 500 mu Dysport®/2.0 mL 0.9% saline. If the effect is insufficient, a second injection with the same or a lower dose may be worthwhile. In view of the minute amounts of toxin needed, reinjections may be given within a few weeks without increasing the risk for antibody formation.

SIDE-EFFECTS

Injections of Bt into the lacrimal gland may cause dry eye symptoms, local infection, ptosis, or diplopia due to a diffusion of the toxin to the lateral rectus muscle.

SUMMARY

Based on the few reports published, Bt injections into the lacrimal gland for hyper-

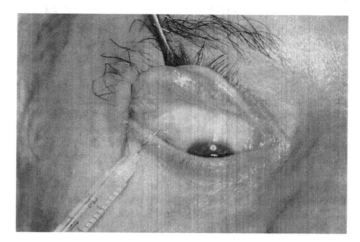

Fig. 14.6 Hyperlacrimation: injection into the right lacrimal gland.

lacrimation may be an elegant method to treat this sometimes disabling condition. However, we need larger studies to evaluate the risks and long-term benefits of this new treatment.

References

1 Hund M, Kinkelin I, Naumann M, Hamm H. Definition of axillary hyperhidrosis by gravimetric assessment. *Arch Dermatol* 2002; **138**: 539–41.

2 Naver H, Aquilonius S-M. The treatment of focal hyperhidrosis with botulinum toxin. *Eur J Neurol* 1997; **4** (Suppl. 2): S75–9.

3 Sato K, Hang H, Saga K, Sato KT. Biology of sweat glands and their disorders. I. Normal sweat gland function. *J Am Acad Dermatol* 1989; **20**: 537–63.

4 Sato K, Hang H, Saga K, Sato KT. Biology of sweat glands and their disorders. II. Disorders of sweat gland function. *J Am Acad Dermatol* 1989; **20**: 713–26.

5 Mosek A, Korczyn A. Hyperhidrosis in palms and soles. In: Korczyn A, ed. *Handbook of Autonomic Nervous System Dysfunction.* New York: Marcel Dekker, 1995: 167–77.

6 Claes G, Drott C. Hyperhidrosis. *Lancet* 1994; **1**: 247–8.

7 Drott C, Gothberg G, Claes G. Endoscopic transthoracic sympathectomy, an efficient and safe method for the treatment of hyperhidrosis. *J Am Acad Dermatol* 1995; **33**: 78–81.

8 Kerner J. *Das Fettgift oder die Fettsäure und ihre Wirkungen auf den thierischen Organismus, ein Beytrag zur Untersuchung des in verdorbenen Würsten giftig wirkenden Stoffes.* Stuttgart, Tübingen: Cotta, 1822.

9 Bushara KO, Park DM. Botulinum toxin and sweating. *J Neurol Neurosurg Psychiatry* 1994; **57**: 1437–8.

10 Chesire WP. Suncutaneous botulinum toxin type A inhibits regional sweating: an individual observation. *Clin Auton Res* 1996; **6**: 123–4.

11 Naumann M, Flachenecker P, Bröcker E-B, Toyka KV, Reiners K. Botulinum toxin for palmar hyperhidrosis. *Lancet* 1997; **349**: 252.

12 Schnider P, Binder M, Auff E *et al.* Double-blind trial of botulinum toxin for the treatment of focal hyperhidrosis of the palms. *Br J Neurol* 1997; **136**: 548–52.

13 Naumann M, Hofmann U, Bergmann I *et al.* Focal hyperhidrosis: effective treatment with intracutaneous botulinum toxin. *Arch Dermatol* 1998; **134**: 301–4.

14 Naumann M, Bergmann I, Hofmann U, Hamm H, Reiners K. Botulinum toxin for focal hyperhidrosis. technical considerations and improvements of application. *Br J Dermatol* 1998; **139**: 1123–4.

15 Odderson IR. Axillary hyperhidrosis: treatment with botulinum toxin A. *Arch Phys Med Rehabil* 1998; **79**: 350–2.

16 Naumann M, Hamm H, Kinkelin I, Reiners K. Botulinum toxin type A in the treatment of focal, axillary and palmar hyperhidrosis and other hyperhidrotic conditions. *Eur J Neurol* 1999; **6**: S111–15.

17 Schnider P, Binder M, Kittler H *et al.* A randomized, double blind, placebo-controlled trial of botulinum toxin for severe axillary hyperhidrosis. *Br J Dematol* 1999; **140**: 677–80.

18 Shelley WB, Talanin NY, Shelley ED. Botulinum toxin therapy for palmar hyperhidrosis. *J Am Acad Dermatol* 1998; **38**: 227–9.

19 Naumann M, Jost W, Toyka KV. Botulinum toxin in the treatment of neurological disorders of the autonomic nervous system. *Arch Neurol* 1999; **56**: 914–16.

20 Glogau RG. Botulinum A neurotoxin for axillary hyperhidrosis. *Dermotol Surg* 1998; **24**: 817–19.

21 Naver H, Swartling C, Aquilonius S. Treatment of focal hyperhidrosis with botulinum toxin type A. Brief overview of methodology and 2 years' experience. *Europ J Neurol* 1999; **6**: S117–20.

22 Heckmann M, Breit S, Ceballos-Baumann A *et al.* Side-controlled intradermal injection of botulinum toxin A in recalcitrant axillary hyperhidrosis. *J Am Acad Dermatol* 1999; **41**: 987–90.

23 Solomon B, Hayman R. Botulinum toxin type A therapy for palmar and digital hyperhidrosis. *J Am Acad Dermatol* 2000; **42**: 1026–9.

24 Karamfilov T, Konra H, Karte K, Wollina U. Relapse rate of botulinum toxin A therapy for axillary hyperhidrosis by dose increase. *Arch Dermatol* 2000; **136**: 487–90.

25 Naver H, Swartling C, Aquilonius S-M. Palmar and axillary hyperhidrosis treated with botulinum toxin: 1-year clinical follow-up. *Eur J Neurol* 2000; **7**: 55–62.

26 Naumann M, Lowe N. Botulinum toxin type A in the treatment of bilateral primary axillary hyperhidrosis: a randomized, double blind, placebo-controlled trial. *Br Medical J* 2001; **323**: 596–9.

27 Heckmann M, Ceballos-Baumann A, Plewig G. Botulinum toxin A for axillary hyperhidrosis (excessive sweating). *N Engl J Med* 2001; **344**: 488–93.

28 Naumann M, Lowe NJ, Hamm H. A multicenter, open label continuation study evaluating the safety and efficacy of botulinum toxin type A in the treatment of bilateral axillary hyperhidrosis. *JEADV* 2001; **15** (Suppl. 2): 130.

29 Naumann M, Hamm H, Lowe N. Effect of botulinum toxin type A on quality of life measures in patients with excessive axillary sweating. A randomized controlled trial. *Br J Dermatol* 2002, in press.

30 Saadia D, Voustianiouk A, Wang A, Kaufmann H. Botulinum toxin type A in primary palmar hyperhidrosis. Randomized, single blind, two-dose study. *Neurol* 2001; **57**: 2095–9.

31 Kinkelin I, Hund M, Naumann M, Hamm H. Effective treatment of frontal hyperhidrosis with botulinum toxin A. *Br J Dermatol* 2000; **143**: 824–7.

32 Böger A, Herath H, Rompel R, Ferbert A. Botulinum toxin for treatment of craniofacial hyperhidrosis. *J Neurol* 2000; **415**: 857–61.

33 Bergmann I, Dauphin M, Naumann M *et al.* Selective degeneration of sudomotor fibers in Ross syndrome and successful treatment of compensatory hyperhidrosis with botulinum toxin. *Muscle Nerve* 1998: **21**: 1790–3.

34 Drobik C, Laskawi R. Frey's syndrome: treatment with botulinum toxin. *Acta Otolaryngol* 1995; **115**: 459–61.

35 Naumann M, Zellner M, Toyka KV, Reiners K. Treatment of gustatory sweating with botulinum toxin. *Ann Neurol* 1997; **42**: 973–5.

36 Bjerkhoel A, Trobbe O. Frey's syndrome: treatment with botulinum toxin. *J Laryngol Otol* 1997; **111**: 839–44.

37 Laskawi R, Drobik C, Schönebeck C. Up-to-date report of botulinum toxin type A treatment in patients with gustatory sweating (Frey's syndrome). *Laryngoscope* 1998; **108**: 381–4.

38 Laccourreye O, Akl E, Gutierrez-Fonseca R *et al*. Recurrent gustatory sweating (Frey's syndrome) after intracutaneous injection of botulinum toxin type A. *Arch Otolaryngol Head Neck Surg* 1999; **125**: 282–6.

39 Vadoud-Seyedi J, Simonart T, Heenen M. Treatment of plantar hyperhidrosis with Dermojet injections of botulinum toxin. *Dermatology* 2000; **201**: 179.

40 American Academy of Neurology. Practice advisory on selection of patients with multiple sclerosis for treatment with Betaseron. Report of the Quality Standards Subcommittee of the American Academy of Neurology. *Neurology* 1994; **44**: 1537–40.

41 Crysdale WS, White A. Submandibular duct relocation for drooling. A 10-year experience with 194 patients. *Otolaryngol Head Neck Surg* 1989; **101**: 87–92.

42 Giess R, Naumann M, Werner E *et al*. Injections of botulinum toxin into the salivary gland improves sialorrhea in amyotrophic lateral sclerosis. *J Neurol Neurosurg Psychiatry* 2000; **69**: 121–3.

43 Shaari CM, Wu BL, Biller HF, Chuang SK, Sanders I. Botulinum toxin decreases salivation from canine submandibular glands. *Otolaryngol Head Neck Surg* 1998; **118**: 452–7.

44 Ellies M, Laskawi R, Götz W, Arglebe C, Tormählen G. Immunohistochemical and morphometric investigations of the influence of botulinum toxin on the submandibular gland of the rat. *Eur Arch Otorhinolaryngol* 1999; **256**: 148–52.

45 Porta M, Gamba M, Bertacchi G, Vaj P. Treatment of sialorrhea with ultrasound-guided botulinum toxin type injection in patients with neurological disorders. *J Neurol Neurosurg Psychiatry* 2001; **70**: 538–40.

46 Bhatia KP, Münchau A, Brown P. Botulinum toxin is a useful treatment in excessive drooling of saliva [letter]. *J Neurol Neurosurg Psychiatry* 1999; **67**: 697.

47 Pal PK, Calne DB, Calne S, Tsui JK. Botulinum toxin A as treatment for drooling saliva in PD. *Neurology* 2000; **54**: 244–7.

48 Jost W. Treatment of drooling in Parkinson's disease with botulinum toxin [letter]. *Mov Disord* 1999; **14**: 1057–9.

49 Yagi N, Nakatani H. Crocodile tears and thread test of lacrimation. *Ann Otol Rhinol Laryngol Suppl* 1986; **122**: 13–16.

50 Irving RM, Viani L, Hardy DG, Baguley DM, Moffat DA. Nervus intermedius function after vestibular schwannoma removal: clinical features and pathophysiological mechanisms. *Laryngoscope* 1995; **105**: 809–13.

51 Riemann R, Pfenningsdorf S, Riemann E, Naumann M. Successful treatment of crocodile tears by injection of botulinum toxin into the lacrimal gland. *Ophthalmology* 1999; **106**: 2322–4.

52 Boroojerdi B, Ferbert A, Schwarz M, Noth J. Botulinum toxin treatment of synkinesia and hyperlacrimation after facial palsy. *J Neurol Neurosurg Psychiatry* 1998; **65**: 111–14.

53 Hofmann RJ. Treatment of Frey's syndrome (gustatory sweating) and crocodile tears (gustatory epiphora) with purified botulinum toxin. *Ophthal Plast Reconstr Surg* 2000; **16**: 289–91.

54 Meyer M. Krokodilstränen und ihre Behandlung. In: Laskawi R, Roggenkämper P, eds. *Botulinumtoxin-Therapie im Kopf-Hals-Bereich*. Munich: Urban and Vogel, 1999: 245–55.

55 Kim K, Kim S, Yoon J, Han J. The effect of botulinum toxin type A injection for intrinsic rhinitis. *J Laryngol Otol* 1998; **112**: 248–51.

Pelvic floor and gastrointestinal uses

WOLFGANG JOST

Introduction

Many signs and symptoms of gastrointestinal and urogenital disease such as achalasia or neurogenic bladder disorders involve increased activity of striated or smooth muscles due to peripheral or central nervous system dysfunction. Botulinum toxin A (BtA) has closed several therapeutic gaps and contributed to the understanding of these diseases, and to new diagnostic and therapeutic procedures (Table 15.1). There are no reports yet of the use of botulinum toxin B (BtB) for this indication.

Botulinum toxin in urological disorders

Botulinum toxin for detrusor-sphincter dyssynergia

Definition, aetiology and pathogenesis

The lesion in detrusor-sphincter dyssynergia (DSD) lies in the spinal cord between the pontine and the sacral micturition centres and is often due to traumatic spinal cord injury or multiple sclerosis. The loss of descending input leads to insufficient relaxation and uncoordinated contraction of the vesical sphincter during detrusor contraction, leading to incomplete bladder emptying and residual urine. High intravesical pressure during voiding attempts may lead to ureteral reflux and renal damage.

Botulinum toxin review

All the published studies on BtA in DSD, from 1988 [1,2] onwards, are open studies (Table 15.2 [1–6]). Despite encouraging results, we cannot yet draw final conclusions as they include only small series of patients and use different combinations of outcome measures such as patients' subjective reports, residual urine volume or urodynamic test parameters. Taken singly, none of these provide sufficient evidence of treatment efficacy. The studies use a wide range of BtA doses [2,3] and the outcome seems to be independent of the dose. Trials including more than 10 patients report success rates of 58–88% of patients treated, as defined by a reduction of residual urine by more than 50% [3,4]. We still need controlled and longer term studies in well-defined patient popu-

Table 15.1 Indications for botulinum toxin in pelvic floor and gastrointestinal disorders.

Urogenital
Detrusor muscle
Vesical sphincter
Vagina (vaginismus)

Gastrointestinal
Oesophagus (achalasia, diffuse oesophageal spasm, diverticula, etc.)
Sphincter of Oddi
Stomach
Colon (e.g. Hirschsprung's disease, etc.)
Anal sphincters (anal fissure, anismus, outlet constipation)

Table 15.2 Publications on botulinum toxin in detrusor-sphincter dyssynergia.

Authors	n	Dose	Results
Dykstra *et al.* [1] Dykstra & Sidi [2]	11	140 mu (+240 mu) Botox®	Duration of action 2 months *(Urodynamic investigation, urinal residual volume measurement)*
Schurch *et al.* [3]	24	100 mu Botox®, 250 mu Dysport®	Improvement in 21–24 patients. Duration of action 3–9 months *(Urodynamic investigation, postvoiding urinal residual volume measurement)*
Petit *et al.* [4]	17	150 mu Dysport®	Improvement in 10 of 17 patients. Duration of action 2–3 months *(Urodynamic investigation, postvoiding urinal residual volume measurement)*
Jost *et al.* [5]	26	5–20 mu Botox®	Good result in 15, moderate improvement in 7 patients. Duration of action 4.2 months *(Patient report)*
Phelan *et al.* [6]	21	80–100 mu Botox®	Improvement in 14 of 21 patients. Postvoid residual decreased by 71% *(Urodynamic investigation, postvoiding urinal residual volume measurement)*

lations, using validated and reproducible outcome measures and preferably testing repeated injections over more than one injection cycle.

As a general principle, the lowest effective dose should be used, to minimize side-effects such as urinary incontinence and the costs of treatment. Some investigators recommend reinjection at monthly intervals [3], but this should be avoided as it may increase the risk of antibody formation.

Treatment with botulinum toxin

PATIENT SELECTION

Patients referred for BtA treatment require detailed neurological, urological and especially urodynamic examinations. Ensure that simple accepted measures such as toileting and drugs have been tried before considering BtA treatment.

The effect of BtA is completely reversible and adverse effects are generally minimal. A therapeutic trial may therefore be justified in patients with a high residual volume, at high risk for reflux-induced renal damage or if they fail to respond to conventional therapy. Injections are probably preferable to destructive surgical procedures, particularly in potentially reversible spinal cord lesions such as an acute exacerbation of multiple sclerosis or acute transverse myelitis. Patients must understand the range of treatment options before being asked to agree to BtA injections.

DOSE AND INJECTION TECHNIQUE

The goal of BtA injection is to decrease residual volume and minimize urinary urgency, frequency and incontinence. BtA weakens both the striated external sphincter and the smooth muscle internal sphincter because they lie close together. BtA can be injected either under visual guidance using an urethroscope, under electromyographic (EMG) control, or using imaging techniques like ultrasound, computerized tomography (CT) or magnetic resonance imaging (MRI). Urologists usually prefer to use the urethroscope, while neurologists prefer EMG guidance. Clinicians should use the technique with which they are most familiar.

For EMG guided injections the patient lies in the lithotomy or the left lateral decubitus position. Local anaesthesia is neither necessary nor helpful. In females, place the injection lateral to the urethral orifice (Fig. 15.1). In males, palpate the prostate and insert the needle into the perineum advancing it towards the fingertip until EMG activity is acquired (Fig. 15.2). Inject the external vesical sphincter muscle bilaterally, placing a single toxin depot on each side. Because EMG cannot identify the internal sphincter muscle it is not possible to target its injection precisely. Fortunately this does not prevent the toxin from working as there is enough passive diffusion to weaken the smooth internal sphincter satisfactorily.

If using the urethroscope place the patient in the lithotomy position, and identify the bladder neck first. The sphincter is easier to see if the operator asks the patient to contract it voluntarily, or asks him to cough, to induce a reflex contraction. Inject the sphincter under visual guidance in the left and right lateral position at the points of maximum visible muscle contractions.

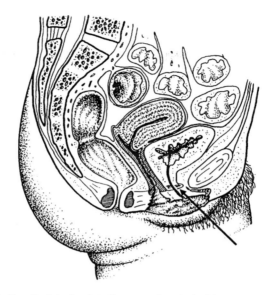

Fig. 15.1 Female injection site. Injection into the external vertical sphincter (arrow).

Botulinum toxin doses

DOSES: A HEALTH WARNING

Please read the warning on p. 35 about doses of botulinum toxin (Bt). There are three preparations available. *Dysport®* and *Botox®* are type A toxins (BtA), *NeuroBloc®/MYOBLOC™* is type B (BtB). Even though the doses for each are quoted in mouse units (mu), the three preparations have different dose schedules: one mu of *Dysport®* is **not** the same as one mu of *Botox®*, and neither is equivalent to one mu of *NeuroBloc®/MYOBLOC™*.

Doses used in trials vary greatly and range from 10 to 140 mu Botox® or from 40 to 750 mu Dysport® [3,5]. We start with a dose of 10 mu (2 × 5 mu) Botox® at a dilution 50 mu/mL 0.9% saline or 40 mu (2 × 20 mu) Dysport® at a dilution of 200 mu/mL 0.9% saline. If there is no clinical improvement after the initial treatment we reinject the same dose after a minimum of 2 months. If there was a minor but inadequate clinical response we increase the dose by about 50% of the previous dose. The maximum dose should not exceed 100 mu Botox® (4 × 25 mu) or 400 mu Dysport® (4 × 100 mu).

Onset of effect and duration of action

The effects of Bt usually appear within 24 h. Maximum sphincter paresis occurs typically after about 1 week, and the benefit lasts for between 2 and 6 months. There is a wide

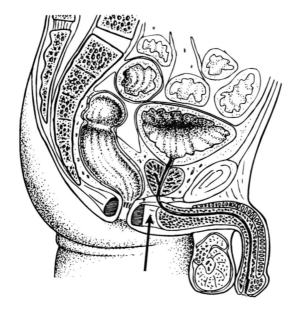

Fig. 15.2 Male injection site. Injection into the external vertical sphincter (arrow).

variation in the degree and duration of benefit, perhaps related to the dose used, the severity of the underlying condition and to any induced adverse effects such as an urinary incontinence.

Adverse effects

Adverse local or systemic effects are unlikely from the above doses (10–20 mu Botox® or 40–80 mu Dysport®). The needle pass may, however, cause local haematomas, urethral bleeding [4] and local infections. Sphincter haematomas may impair urinary flow. Dykstra et al. [1,2] reported transient limb weakness in one patient and in one further patient there was transient exacerbation of autonomic dysreflexia.

Patients should understand that transient urinary incontinence may occur in about one-third of treatments. It is more common in older patients and in women, especially if they are multiparous. Incontinence is usually much shorter-lived than the beneficial effect of the toxin.

Contraindications

Coagulation disorders are the main contraindications.

Botulinum toxin for hyperreflexic bladder

Botulinum toxin injections into the detrusor muscle may become useful for the treatment of hyperreflexic bladder. This treatment is a possible new therapeutic option in patients with severe detrusor hyperreflexia refractory to anticholinergic medication. Preliminary studies with up to 30 injections given cystoscopically into the detrusor muscle show encouraging results. In particular, BtA appears to significantly increase bladder volume.

In one typical study, average bladder volume increased from 261 mL to 490 mL and there were no side-effects. Seventeen of 21 patients improved [7]. Many injections are needed because there is a large bladder surface and the toxin must be distributed over many points, sparing the trigone. The doses used in trials vary from 2.5 to 10 mu of Botox® or from 10 to 40 mu of Dysport® injected per single site. The duration of action may be 4–6 months, in some cases 9 months [7]. Available studies suggest that patients need 200–300 mu Botox® or 700–1200 mu Dysport® per session, which is costly.

Potential untoward effects include haemorrhages, haematomas and bladder perforation.

Further studies are needed before this treatment can be widely recommended.

Botulinum toxin in urethrism/urethrospasm

Urethrism is defined as involuntary contraction of the voluntary sphincter on micturition, or — in some cases — at rest as well. This causes incomplete bladder evacuation and bears a risk of urinary retention. Staccato voiding is a clinical cardinal symptom and some patients also complain of pain. EMG of the sphincter confirms the diagnosis. Although there are no formal series on the treatment of urethrism with Bt, injection of the toxin may at least be an alternative to urethrotomy. The doses are usually somewhat higher than in DSD. We start with 5 mu Botox® (0.1 mL) or 20 mu Dysport® per injection side, injected into the external vesical sphincter muscle on both sides under electromyographic or cystoscopic guidance (total 10 mu Botox® or 40 mu Dysport®). On reinjection, we adjust the dose according to the therapeutic effect. Much higher doses are sometimes needed. The maximum dose should not exceed 100 mu Botox® (4× 25 mu) or 400 mu Dysport® (4×100 mu). The injections are given in the same way as those for DSD [8].

Again, urinary incontinence can occur, so it is important to keep the dose as low as possible. Haematomas in the sphincter may impair urinary outflow.

Botulinum toxin in spasticity of the external vesical sphincter

Damage to the upper motor neuron, e.g. multiple sclerosis or spinal cord injury, may cause spasticity of the striated muscles of the pelvic floor. Any intra-abdominal increase of pressure or dilatation of the urethra results in inappropriate contractions of the striated sphincter, which can be weakened by injections of Bt. Again, one should start out at a low dose to minimize the risk of incontinence.

Initial doses range from 5 to 10 mu Botox® or from 20 to 40 mu Dysport® per site, and may be higher in individual cases. Injections are performed under electromyographic or cystoscopic control on both sites of the sphincter. Possible urinary incontinence is the only relevant undesired side-effect of the injection. Spasticity of the anal sphincter is common in most of these patients, necessitating treatment of both regions this way.

Botulinum toxin in neobladder (artificial bladder)

Increased residual urine is a possible complication in neobladders. Medication is frequently ineffective. The installation of an artificial bladder eliminates reflex contraction and coordination between detrusor contraction and sphincter relaxation, and the sphincter fails to relax. Bt may help by weakening the sphincter muscle. Bt is injected urethroscopically into the internal vesical sphincter under visual guidance. We inject 5 mu Botox® or 20 mu Dysport® on each side [9]. For subsequent injections, the dose is adjusted depending on the result of the first trial. The dose required may be higher in some cases. Possible urinary incontinence constitutes a problem. It takes patience and perseverance from both the patient and the physician to find the optimal dose. So far there is no controlled study of this indication.

Botulinum toxin in the therapy of vaginismus

Vaginismus, sometimes called dystonic vaginismus, means narrowing of the vaginal introitus by involuntary contraction of the pelvic musculature and the outer third of the vaginal musculature in response to a real or imagined attempt to introduce an object into the vagina. In severe cases, even insertion of a finger or a tampon is difficult or impossible because of discomfort and elicits a typical defence response. Some patients, especially when afflicted by 'psychogenic' vaginismus, present with adduction and inward rotation of the thighs and hyperlordosis. Take care to distinguish true vaginismus from coitophobia without vaginal spasm, which is often incorrectly termed vaginismus.

All patients should have a thorough gynaecological evaluation before treatment. Exclude psychological causes if there is any doubt about the diagnosis of dystonic vaginismus and patients should try adequate conventional treatment.

Besides surgical interventions and vaginal dilatations, options include various muscle relaxing drugs, psychotherapy and relaxation exercises. If these fail, injections of Bt into the muscles of the vagina and pelvic floor [10] are a promising symptomatic option for vaginismus and have few adverse effects. Even though the direct benefit related to induced muscle weakness lasts only 3–4 months, the experience of being asymptomatic may sometimes heal mental or even physical scars and permit much longer benefit.

A gynaecologist experienced in sexual medicine should take the decision to treat. Treatment is usually carried out by either the gynaecologist or a neurologist familiar with sexual disorders and with the anatomy of the pelvic floor.

A low dose is recommended for initial treatment, e.g. 4×5 mu Botox® or 4×20 mu Dysport® (4×0.1 mL) injected into each quadrant of the paravaginal musculature [11]. The treatment thus requires several injections which women with vaginismus may find unpleasant and stressful. The dose may be increased on subsequent injections. Transitory incontinence may occur due to muscular weakness. Larger open or controlled studies are not available.

Botulinum toxin for gastroenterological disorders

Botulinum toxin in achalasia

Achalasia is a well-known indication for Bt in gastroenterology [12–14]. It occurs most often between the 2nd and 4th decade of life and is characterized by inadequate relaxation of the lower oesophageal sphincter. The aetiology is unclear, though there is usually degeneration or absence of ganglion cells in the myenteric plexus. Neuropathic changes also occur in the dorsal vagal nucleus. Clinical symptoms include dysphagia, retrosternal pain, nocturnal regurgitation, non-cardiac chest pain, and secondary weight loss. Conventional treatment is with Heller's myotomy or pneumatic dilatation, with its attendant risk of perforation.

More than 30 study groups have replicated Pasricha's [13] excellent results in the treatment of achalasia with BtA although no controlled trials are available (Table 15.3 [13,15–20]).

The treatment is only practical for gastroenterologists as injections must be given endoscopically into the quadrants of the lower oesophageal sphincter using a sclerotherapeutic syringe. The usual starting dose is 20 mu Botox® (0.8 mL) or 60–80 mu Dysport® (0.6–0.8 mL) per injection site [15] (total dose: 80 mu Botox®, or 240–320 mu Dysport®). Some patients need even higher doses. The initial success rate ranges from 60 to 90%, the good improvement for some months ranges from 32 to 78% (Table 15.3). Some patients respond for as long as 15 months after a single treatment.

In view of the limited duration of benefit and the costs of treatment, Bt in achalasia may be mainly indicated for moribund patients, for patients who are at high risk for more invasive procedures, after complications following other treatments, or at the patient's request. Children with achalasia and patients suffering from achalasia due to Chagas' disease may be treated as well [21]. Possible side-effects are chest pain immediately after Bt injection and reflux.

Table 15.3 Selection of studies on botulinum toxin in achalasia.

Authors	n	Dose mu (Botox®)	Initial success (%)	Long-term success (%)
Cullière et al. [13]	55	80	85	60
Annese et al. [15]	36	100	90	78
Annese et al. [16]	38	100	82	68
Fishman et al. [17]	60	80	70	36
Pasricha et al. [18]	31	80	90	68
Vaezi et al. [19]	22	100	64	32
Wehrmann et al. [20]	22	100	64	32

Bt in upper gastrointestinal disorders

Other rare indications for Bt include oesophageal disorders such as insufficient relaxation of the upper oesophagus, cricopharyngeal dystonia, diffuse oesophageal spasm [22–25], infantile oesophageal diverticulitis [12], hypertrophic pyloric stenosis [12], postoperative pylorospasm [12], sphincter of Oddi dysfunction [12], and undiagnosed non-cardiac chest pain [12].

Diffuse oesophageal spasm

Typical symptoms are chest pain and dysphagia. They are often refractory to symptomatic treatment using antispasmodic drugs (nitrates, calcium channel blockers). Oesophagomyotomy or balloon dilatation of the oesophagus may be performed in severe cases. Bt injections may be an alternative to these more invasive options. Only open studies with small patient groups are available, so the evidence for benefit remains weak. Use the same total dose as in achalasia (i.e. 80 mu Botox® and 250 mu Dysport®, respectively), with circular injections at multiple levels of the oesophagus [23,24]. One study reported a good response to treatment in 11 of 15 patients [24]. Other authors used higher doses [12].

Injections of Bt may be beneficial in the rare disorder of inadequate relaxation of the upper oesophagus or cricopharyngeal dystonia [26]. In inadequate relaxation of the upper oesophagus the dose is similar to achalasia, in patients with cricopharyngeal dystonia therapy should start with smaller doses. Early studies on infantile hypertrophic pyloric stenosis have not been convincing [12]. BtA has been tried for postoperative pylorospasm, for oesophageal diverticulitis, and for non-cardiac chest pain, but experience remains limited [12].

Dysfunction of the sphincter of Oddi

There are several anecdotal reports on treatment of dysfunction of the sphincter of Oddi using Bt [12,27]. This condition produces a biliary- or pancreatic-type pain. Endoscopic manometry can confirm or refute the diagnosis. Endoscopic sphincterotomy is the current treatment of choice. However, in small open studies, endoscopic Bt injection into the papilla of Vater appeared to be safe and provided short-term relief in about 80% of the patients. Patients responding to Bt may subsequently be cured by sphincterotomy. Benefit from Bt lasted about 3–8 months. The doses of up to 100 mu Botox® reported in some studies seem relatively high, and 20 mu Botox® or 80 mu Dysport® may be sufficient [12]. In the absence of larger studies it is not possible to be definitive about efficacy, safety or duration of benefit.

Treatment of obesity using gastric injections of botulinum toxin

Treatment of obesity with botulinum toxin [28] remains an embryonic indication. In rats, injection of the toxin at several sites in the gastric antrum can block propulsive gastric contractions, delay emptying, and thereby prolong the sensation of fullness. This approach is somewhat analogous to gastric banding. However, at present Bt injection into the gastric antrum is experimental. It is not clear how effective it is in reducing obesity, and there are many possible adverse consequences. For instance, we do not know how well a paralysed gastric wall protects itself against gastric acid. This is a potentially important indication which deserves a fuller preclinical assessment and, if appropriate, properly powered and controlled clinical trials.

Botulinum toxin in proctology

Anal fissure

Bt is more than a symptomatic treatment for anal fissure, since the toxin decisively interferes with the pathogenic mechanisms causing chronic fissure, and thereby heals the majority of patients. Extensive studies have led to Bt becoming standard treatment in many hospitals.

Pathogenesis and clinical picture

After haemorrhoids, anal fissure is the most frequent ailment in proctology. It is defined as a longitudinal ulcer of the dry sensitive anoderm between the dentate line and anocutaneous line. In about 90% of cases the fissure occurs at the posterior median line (Fig. 15.3). The aetiology remains unclear and it is probably multifactorial. There is thought to be a vicious circle of inflammation, pain, sphincter spasm, and tissue ischaemia leading to 'chronic' anal fissure (Fig. 15.4).

The disease is marked by severe and often prolonged anal pain on defecation. Burning sensations, oozing and bleeding may occur and the pain commonly provokes constipation.

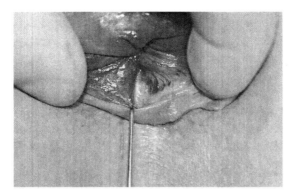

Fig. 15.3 Anal fissure in the posterior midline.

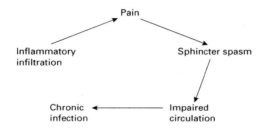

Fig. 15.4 The cycle of events leading to chronic anal fissure.

The diagnosis is made from the typical history and findings on inspection. The fissure can be seen by gently parting the buttocks/natal cleft, and frequently presents with an inflammatory border at the inferior margin, the so-called sentinel tag. Proctoscopy and rectoscopy are needed for differential diagnosis.

Conventional treatment

Therapeutic interventions all start at one point of the vicious circle. Conservative treatment, for instance with unguents, suppositories, anal plugs and sitzbaths, is mainly directed at inflammation and pain (including the spasm). Various drug therapies are include topical application of nitroglycerine unguents, which help to reduce sphincter tone. Lateral sphincterotomy is still performed to reduce the sphincter tone in chronic uncomplicated fissures. However, lateral sphincterotomy carries a substantial risk of early and prolonged incontinence.

In chronic complicated fissures, the fissure, any ulcer and secondary lesions are often excised, and this results in secondary or consecutive reduction in sphincter tonus.

Possible later incontinence apart, problems with these surgical treatments include the need for hospitalization, and the likelihood of pain and complications of wound healing.

Botulinum toxin in anal fissure

In 1990, BtA was injected for the first time to treat anal fissure [29,30]. Meanwhile, more than 10 open studies on the treatment of anal fissure with Bt have been completed world-wide, all of them with comparable success [29–42]. The results in a controlled trial [33] were similar to the results in the open trials. Detailed information on these studies is given in Table 15.4 [30–35,37,38,40–42].

In early attempts to use BtA for anal fissure we injected Bt into the internal anal sphincter, which was thought to play the major role in sphincter hypertonus. We found that diffusion of the toxin lead to paralysis of both sphincters. We decided to switch and to limit the injection to the external anal sphincter since it is easier to inject accurately, and diffusion does produce adequate weakness of the internal sphincter. As it happens, subsequent studies showed that both the internal and the external sphincter muscles are involved in sphincter hypertonus [43]. Many injectors still inject into the internal sphincter [e.g. 31], although it cannot be targeted precisely. These injections risk delivering the toxin into the intersphincteral cleft, which leads to an unwanted diffusion to adjacent regions, e.g. the puborectal muscle.

COMPARISON WITH NITROGLYCERIN PREPARATIONS

Shortly after publication of early therapeutic successes with Bt, good results were also described using topical application of gylceryl trinitrate (GTN) cream. Unfortunately, glyceryl trinitrate often produces headaches, and patients need to apply the cream several times a day for several weeks. Most patients tend to carry on treatment just until they are pain-free, subsequently forgetting about their ointment, thus delaying healing or even leading to chronic changes. By contrast, BtA injections last for several weeks, active patient cooperation is not required and there are no systemic effects. A comparative study showed that treatment with BtA alone was more effective and convenient than nitroglycerine alone [37]. A recent publication showed that topical nitrates can potentiate BtA injections [44], but this combination is probably not necessary.

PATIENT SELECTION

Patients referred for BtA therapy need detailed proctologic examination, which must exclude fistulas, abscesses or underlying disease. An injection should only be given after allowing time for spontaneous remission (a few weeks) or topical applications (e.g. GTN) have failed. Since BtA works by abolishing sphincter hypertonus, patients should only be selected for treatment with BtA if they have increased sphincter tonus. When sphincter tone is already low there is a risk of faecal incontinence if the sphincters are further weakened. Manometry may be misleading since pain artificially inflates the readings: clinical assessment of sphincter tone usually suffices.

Table 15.4 Publications on botulinum toxin in anal fissure.*

Authors	n	Sphincter	Dose	Improvement (%)	Side-effects
Jost & Schimrigk [30]	12	EAS	5 mu Botox®	Healing in 83%	None
Gui et al. [31]	10	IAS	15 mu Botox®	Healing in 70%	1 × mild transient faecal incontinence
Maria [32]	57	IAS	15 mu & 20 mu Botox®, possible retreatment with higher doses	Healing in 43.5% (15 mu). 67.6% (20 mu)	No side-effects
Maria et al. [33]	15	IAS	20 mu Botox®	Healing in 53.3% after 1 month: healing in 73.3% after 2 months	1 × transient incontinence for gas (in the control group)
Jost [34]	100	EAS	5–10 mu Botox®	Healing 82% after 3 months; 79% after 6 months	7 × transitory faecal incontinence
Jost & Schrank [35]	50	EAS	20 vs. 40 mu Dysport®	Healing in 76% resp? 80%	3 × transient incontinence for flatus
Minguez et al. [40]	69	IAS	10 mu, 15 mu and 21 mu Botox®, with possible reinjection (52%, 30%, 37%)	Without reinjection: 26% (10 mu). 48% (15 mu), 58% (21 mu) With reinjection: 83% (10 mu). 78% (15 mu). 90% (21 mu)	1 × subcutaneous infection 1 × small perianal haaematoma
Gonzales Carro et al. [41]	40	AS	15 mu Botox®	42.5% after 3 months. 50% after 6 months	2 × transitory incontinence for gas
Brisinda et al. [37]	25	IAS	20 mu Botox®	Improvement in 96%	No side-effects
Fernandez Lopez et al. [38]	76	AS	80 mu Botox®	Healing 67%	2 × transitory gas incontinence 1 × haemorrhoidal thrombosis
Maria et al. [42]	50	IAS	40 mu Botox®	Healing 60% resp. 88%	No side-effects

*All open studies, except for Maria et al. [33].
AS, anal sphincter; EAS, external anal sphincter; IAS, internal anal sphincter.

Coagulation disorders, anticoagulation treatment and complicated fissures with formation of fistulas constitute relative contraindications.

Patients should understand the advantages and possible disadvantages of BtA treatment.

The decision to offer BtA therapy should be made by a proctologist. Usually, either the proctologist or a neurologist familiar with the technique will give the injections.

RISK–BENEFIT CONSIDERATIONS

The side-effects of BtA injections for anal fissure are minimal and temporary. The primary benefit in anal fissure is healing, and the secondary benefit is avoidance of surgery with possible incontinence. The sphincter system is preserved. Therefore, Bt therapy should be considered before any operation. All potential candidates for surgery should not only be aware of the risks involved but should also know about the alternative of treatment with BtA.

PRACTICAL APPLICATION OF BOTULINUM TOXIN INJECTION

Patient preparation: dose and injection sites The dose depends somewhat on the degree of muscle hypertonus, and should be increased if the tone is very high. Local anaesthesia is not required. The injection technique is simple and can be learned easily.

A typical procedure is to dissolve 100 mu Botox® in 4 mL of isotonic saline solution, or 500 mu Dysport® in 2.5 mL. The toxin is injected via an insulin syringe and a fine needle (27 g), pierced about 1 cm into the external anal sphincter on each side laterally and distal to the fissure just lateral to the anocutaneous line. Deeper injections bear the risk of incontinence due to diffusion of the toxin into the puborectalis muscle. A typical dose is 2.5–5.0 mu Botox® (0.1–0.2 mL) or 10–20 mu Dysport® (0.05 mL–0.1 mL) per injection site (5–10 mu Botox®, 20–40 mu Dysport® in total). In some centres the internal anal sphincter is also injected. Some authors recommend higher doses. In our experience these are unnecessary, and merely increase adverse effects and the cost. Neither is it necessary to give a third injection site below the fissure. That some authors obtained better results with higher doses [32,33] might be related to different patient referral patterns and selection. In our studies [30,34], the injection was only made after surgery had been suggested by the proctologist.

No specific measures are needed after the injection. Patients simply pursue normal anal hygiene, such as showering with lukewarm water after defaecation.

Onset and duration of action The effect usually appears within a few days, with reduced pain frequently within the first 2 days. Maximum muscle paralysis occurs after 4–7 days, lasts about 4 weeks, and gradually recovers. Benefit may last several months, depending on a variety of factors, especially the injected dose. The period of maximal action may be associated with marked paralysis and atrophy of the injected sphincters.

On inspection the anus looks like a funnel, since the puborectalis muscle continues to contract normally.

Side-effects Major side-effects are unlikely with the doses recommended above. The main possible undesired effect is incontinence of faeces. The patient must be fully informed about this possibility. The likelihood of anal incontinence is increased with low baseline tonus, and is higher in females, after several deliveries and in old age. Using the above doses the overall incontinence rate in our group was less than 5%. Incontinence is transitory (lasting for up to 2 weeks) and limited to incontinence of flatus and faecal soiling. To date, we have never seen local haematomas or incontinence of solid stools. The world-wide published experience in 300 patients does not describe infections. Some early cases developed perianal thrombosis [45], which has not occurred in our last 200 consecutive cases.

RESULTS OF BOTULINUM TOXIN A

There is marked alleviation of pain in 75% of patients within the first few days. With the above doses most patients have significantly reduced sphincter tonus and with only a few developing significant reduction of puborectal tone [34,35]. Just under 80% of patients are cured after initial therapy [34]. Some authors report even higher cure rates.

We screen our patients carefully to rule out spontaneous remission and to make sure that conservative management had been exhausted. The higher cure rate described by other authors could also be due to their patient selection procedures. No relevant clinical differences have been observed between the two preparations of BtA.

If initial therapy fails to produce the desired outcome, reinjection is worthwhile after the effect of the initial toxin has worn off. Reinject if the fissure recurs [35].

RELAPSE

Repeat injections of BtA produced pain relief within a week in 95% of patients presenting with relapse after BtA injection. Seventy per cent of fissures resolved and were still healed 3 months later. No undesired effects were reported. Among the patients not responding to their first injection [36], 73.3% were pain-free within the 1st week after a second injection. Mild transitory incontinence occurred in 6.7% of patients. After 3 months, healing was evident in 70%.

Our results suggest that repeated BtA is effective in treating both relapse and inadequate initial response [36].

When patients undergo fissurectomy without sphincterectomy, it may be worth pretreating with BtA to decrease muscle tone and improve healing (see below).

Further use of botulinum toxin in proctology

Other anal canal disorders such as anismus [46], spasticity of the anal sphincter and insufficient relaxation of the sphincter muscles with straining and defecation (paradoxical puborectalis syndrome) are also amenable to BtA treatment [47]. The use of BtA to treat constipation is restricted to outlet constipation [47]. Constipation in Parkinson's disease is predominantly characterized by slow transit and will not respond to BtA.

Preoperative use of botulinum toxin

Postoperatively, increased sphincter tone due to pain is found in many candidates for proctologic surgery such as patch grafts in fistulas, conventional haemorrhoidectomies and sphincter reconstruction. A refractory raised sphincter tone frequently leads to impaired wound healing, thereby prolonging hospitalization, increasing costs, and sometimes requiring reoperation. Transient paralysis of the muscles responsible for increased sphincter tone might be helpful, and can be achieved using BtA injection [48].

We advise circumferential injections preoperatively at four sites of the external anal sphincter muscle. Due to diffusion, the internal muscle is paralysed as well. Minor paralysis of the puborectalis muscle occurs with deeper injection. The dose is determined according to the degree of paralysis desired. If mild to moderate paralysis is intended, injections of 4×2.5 mu of Botox® or, alternatively, 4×10 mu of Dysport® will suffice. Higher doses are rarely needed and they may lead to a higher rate of anal incontinence lasting several weeks.

CONTRAINDICATIONS

Abscesses in the area of injection are a definite contraindication. Coagulation disorders and intake of anticoagulants constitute a relative contraindication. The patients must be informed about possible temporary incontinence.

ADVERSE EFFECTS

From our personal experience patients indicate less pain postoperatively, impaired healing is less common, and the rate of relapse is significantly reduced after preparatory BtA treatment. There are no published larger studies. So far we have not seen any adverse effects. Incontinence in the form of flatulence and thin stools has been quite rare, and lasted for a few days to a maximum of 2 weeks.

Outlet constipation

From a pathophysiological point of view chronic constipation is due to slow transit or outlet obstruction. Outlet obstruction is often functional. Unfortunately, the term 'anismus' is frequently used indiscriminately to describe spastic pelvic floor syndrome, pelvic floor incoordination, paradoxical puborectalis contraction or neuromuscular outlet obstruction [49]. Neuromuscular outlet obstruction is defined as a paradoxical involuntary contraction of the external anal sphincter and/or the puborectalis muscle during defecation, when there should be relaxation of these muscles. Patients are more likely to receive optimal treatment if outlet constipation is classified pathophysiologically as this clarifies the underlying mechanism. There are three different types of outlet constipation:

1   The most frequent form of paradoxical contraction of the voluntary anal sphincter is sphincter dyscoordination. This is a benign disorder without underlying structural changes and responds to behavioural therapy, particularly when combined with biofeedback.

2   Spasticity of the striated anal sphincter due to an upper motor neurone lesion is also quite common. Treatment options include antispasticity medication, local BtA injection and surgery (see below).

3   Dystonia of the anal sphincter muscle is characterized clinically by irregular involuntary contractions both at rest and during defecation, and is rare in our experience. The term 'anismus' should be reserved for this situation, which is a true extrapyramidal motor disorder and is treated primarily with local BtA injection (see below).

In sphincter dyscoordination outlet constipation is due to a behaviour failure, in dystonia the symptom is due to involuntary contractions.

Spasticity

Spasticity of the voluntary sphincter muscles occurs in upper motor neuron lesions, and leads to reflex contraction when the sphincter muscle is dilated (triggered contraction) — analogous to limb muscle spasticity. The commonest cause is spinal cord disease, e.g. traumatic spinal cord injury, inflammation (e.g. multiple sclerosis) or space-occupying lesions (cervical disk prolapse, tumours). Spasticity of the pelvic floor can also occur with bihemispheric cerebral lesions (tumours, strokes). During each stimulus, such as dilatation of the muscle during defecation, dilatation during clinical examination (manometry, electromyography, digital examination) or Valsalva's manoeuvres the muscle contracts much more vigorously than normally. The term 'spastic pelvic floor syndrome' is reserved for this condition. Neurological examination is compulsory and may identify the aetiology.

The treatment of choice in spasticity is injection of BtA into the voluntary sphincters. Circular injections are advised in four sites of the external anal sphincter muscle (total of 10–20 mu Botox® or 40–80 mu Dysport®). Especially in spasticity of recent onset, injections should be the primary treatment since surgical measures (e.g. myotomy) are irreversible. For reinjection increase the dose if benefit was inadequate. The risk of anal incontinence depends on the dose.

Dystonia (anismus)

Anismus is a form of focal dystonia analogous to blepharospasm and is a true extrapyramidal motor disorder. Dystonia of the external sphincter and/or the puborectalis muscle is extremely rare. There are sudden, involuntary contractions of the striated external anal sphincter and/or the puborectal muscle. It is independent of defecation, and it is thus not a merely paradoxical contraction. Sphincter contractions characteristically increase with defecation and with straining, thereby causing constipation. The patients frequently also suffer from staccato micturition, which implies that dystonia may affect additional pelvic floor muscles.

Highly focal dystonia of the pelvic floor muscles or dystonia of the pelvic floor may occur in generalized dystonia or in Parkinson's disease.

Injections of BtA are the treatment of choice for focal dystonia of the anal sphincter (anismus). Inject 10–20 mu Botox® or 40–80 mu Dysport® in a circle at four sites of the external anal sphincter muscle. Transitory faecal incontinence may result, but systemic effects are quite unlikely. Because of their systemic action, anticholinergics and atypical neuroleptics are indicated only if there is more widespread dystonia involving other parts of the body, such as the trunk, face or the extremities.

If only the puborectal muscle is affected (diagnosed clinically, and with EMG), it is appropriate to confine BtA injections to puborectalis. Puborectalis is best punctured in the posterior commissure, and we recommend injection of 5–10 mu of Botox® or 40–80 mu of Dysport® on each side the posterior commissure. Faecal incontinence may occur and the initial dose should thus be as small as possible.

Outlet constipation in Parkinson's disease

Approximately 80% of patients with Parkinson's disease suffer from constipation [50] which is mostly compatible with slow-transit constipation. Outlet constipation is present in a few individual cases and should be managed as outlined above. Again, the dose of BtA selected should not be too high, in order to prevent incontinence.

Although paralysing the sphincter can produce a modest effect in slow-transit constipation, the primary objective should be restoration of normal transit times. The diagnosis may be supported by manometry, sphincter EMG and measurement of the colonic transit time.

Hirschsprung's disease

In Hirschsprung's disease, there is an 'aganglionic' segment in the bowel, predominantly in the rectum or sigmoid. This leads to dilatation of the intestine proximal to the narrow, aperistaltic segment. Resection of this segment is the current treatment of choice. Injection of BtA into the aganglionic segment offers an alternative. BtA may be worthwhile particularly in less severe cases, or when surgery is impossible. There are no conclusive studies available. Doses employed so far are 5–10 mu Botox® or 20–40 mu Dysport® per injection site. We apply circular injections over the entire area of the narrow segment (the distance being 2 cm). The longer the segment, the more injection sites are needed, with higher doses accordingly. Haemorrhage is a rare complication.

Summary

BtA has become a well-established and accepted indication and routine treatment for anal fissure, backed by several open and controlled studies. Because it is straightforward to use, with few contraindications and unwanted side-effects, it might become a first-line treatment. All the other BtA indications discussed above remain experimental.

In detrusor sphincter dyssynergia, detrusor hyperactivity and achalasia, the toxin is an alternative to try when standard treatments have failed. We still do not have controlled studies with well-founded outcome measures and adequate follow up. Current studies will probably permit clearer recommendations. It is too early to judge the benefits in detrusor hyperactivity, sphincter of Oddi dysfunction or outlet constipation.

Other gastroenterological and urological uses of BtA are limited to problem cases and rare instances. For many of the indications such as vaginismus, only case reports or open studies are available, and some of these have been published only as abstracts. We need better information before drawing definitive conclusions. Some possible indications such as gastric injection of BtA in obesity will probably never make their way into clinical routine practice, either because of their potential adverse effects or a weak rationale. Treatment with BtA prior to rectal surgery is more promising for a range of conditions.

References

1 Dykstra DD, Sida AA, Scott AB, Pagel JM, Goldish GD. Effects of botulinum A toxin on detrusor-sphincter dyssynergia in spinal cord injury patients. *J Urol* 1988; **139**: 912–22.

2 Dykstra DD, Sidi AA. Treatment of detrusor-sphincter dyssynergia with botulinum A toxin: a double-blind study. *Arch Phys Med Rehabil* 1990; **71**: 24–6.

3 Schurch B, Hauri D, Rodic B *et al.* Botulinum-A toxin as a treatment of detrusor-sphincter dyssynergia: a prospective study in 24 spinal cord injury patients. *J Urol* 1996; **155**: 1023–9.

4 Petit H, Wiart L, Gaujard E *et al.* Botulinum A toxin treatment for detrusor-sphincter dyssynergia in spinal cord disease. *Spinal Cord* 1998; **36**: 91–4.

5 Jost WH. Treatment of detrusor sphincter dyssynergia with botulinum toxin. *J Neurol* 1999; **246**: I/89.

6 Phelan MW, Franks M, Somogyi GT *et al.* Botulinum toxin urethral sphincter injection to restore bladder emptying in men and women with voiding dysfunction. *J Urol* 2001; **165**: 1107–10.

7 Schurch B, Stöhrer M, Kramer G *et al.* Botulinum A toxin for treating detrusor hyperreflexia in spinal cord injured patients: a new alternative to anticholinergic drugs? Preliminary results. *J Urol* 2000; **164**: 692–7.

8 Jost WH, Merkle W, Müller-Lobeck H. Urethrismus accounting for voiding disorder. *Urology* 1998; **52**: 352.

9 Jost WH, Ziegler M, Bewermeier H, Schimrigk K. Botulinum toxin in the treatment of insufficient neobladder emptying. *Mov Disord* 1995; **10**: 404.

10 Brin MF. Treatment of vaginismus with botulinum toxin injections. *Lancet* 1997; **349**: 252–3.

11 Jost WH, Selbach O. Vaginismus—Therapie mit Botulinumtoxin A. *Sexualmedizin* 1998; **4**: 37–49.

12 Wehrmann T, Jost WH, eds. *Treatment with Botulinum-Toxin in Gastroenterology.* Bremen/London/Boston: Uni-Med, 2002.

13 Cuillière C, Ducrotté P, Zerbib F *et al.* Achalasia: outcome of patients treated with intrasphincteric injection of botulinum toxin. *Gut* 1997; **41**: 87–92.

14 Pasricha PJ, Ravich WJ, Kalloo AN. Botulinum toxin for achalasia. *Lancet* 1993; **341**: 244–5.

15 Annese V, Bassotti G, Coccia G *et al.* Comparison of two different formulations of botulinum toxin A for the treatment of oesophageal achalasia. *The GISMAD Achalasia Study Group Aliment Pharmacol Therap* 1999; **13**: 1347–50.

16 Annese V, Bassotti G, Coccia G *et al.* A multicentre randomized study of intrasphincteric botulinum toxin in patients with oesophageal achalasia. *GISMAD Achalasia Study Group Gut* 2000; **46**: 597–600.

17 Fishman VM, Parkman HP, Schiano TD *et al.* Symptomatic improvement in achalasia after botulinum toxin injection of the lower oesophageal sphincter. *Am J Gastroenterol* 1996; **91**: 1724–30.

18 Pasricha PJ, Rai R, Ravich WJ, Hendrix TR, Kalloo AN. Botulinum toxin for achalasia. Long-term outcome and predictors of response. *Gastroenterology* 1996; **110**: 1410–5.

19 Vaezi MF, Richter JE, Wilcox CM *et al.* Botulinum toxin versus pneumatic dilatation in the treatment of achalasia: a randomized trial. *Gut* 1999; **44**: 149–50.

20 Wehrmann T, Kokabpick H, Seifert H, Lembcke B, Caspary WF. Long-term results of endoscopic injection of botulinum toxin in elderly achalasic patients with tortuous megaesophagus or epiphrenic diverticulum. *Endoscopy* 1999; **31**: 352–8.

21 Brant CQ, Nakao F, Ardengh JC, Nasi A, Ferrari AP Jr. Echoendoscopic evaluation of botulinum toxin intrasphincteric injections in Chagas' disease achalasia. *Dis Esophagus* 1999; **12**: 37–40.

22 Alberty J, Oelerich M, Ludwig K, Hartmann S, Stoll W. Efficacy of botulinum toxin A for treatment of upper oesophageal sphincter dysfunction. *Laryngoscope* 2000; **110**: 1151–6.

23 Katz PO, Richter JE. Diffuse oesophageal spasm. Diagnostic and therapeutic strategies. *Am J Med* 1991; **67**: 401–8.

24 Miller LS, Parkman HP, Schiano TD *et al.* Treatment of symptomatic non-achalasia oesophageal motor disorders with botulinum toxin injection at the lower oesophageal sphincter. *Dig Dis Sci* 1996; **41**: 2025–31.

25 Schneider I, Thumfahrt WF, Pototschnig C, Eckel HE. Treatment of dysfunction of the cricopharyngeal muscle with botulinum A toxin: introduction of a new, non-invasive method. *Ann Otol Rhinol Laryngol* 1994; **103**: 31–5.

26 Brant CQ, Siqueira ES, Ferrari AP Jr. Botulinum toxin for orophargeal dysphagia: a case report of flexible endoscope-guided injection. *Dis Esophagus* 1999; **12**: 68–73.

27 Wehrmann T, Schmitt TH, Arndt A *et al.* Endoscopic injection of botulinum toxin in patients with recurrent acute pancreatitis due to pancreatic sphincter of Oddi dysfunction. *Aliment Pharmacol Ther* 2000; **14**: 1469–77.

28 Gui D, De Gaetano A, Spada PL *et al.* Botulinum toxin injected in the gastric wall reduces body weight and food intake in rats. *Aliment Pharmacol Ther* 2000; **14**: 829–34.

29 Jost WH, Schimrigk K. Use of botulinum toxin in anal fissure. *Dis Colon Rectum* 1993; **36**: 974.

30 Jost WH, Schimrigk K. Therapy of anal fissure using botulinum toxin. *Dis Colon Rectum* 1994; **37**: 1321–4.

31 Gui D, Caessetta E, Anastasio G *et al.* Botulinum toxin for chronic anal fissure. *Lancet* 1994; **344**: 1127–8.

32 Maria G, Brisinda G, Bentivoglio AR *et al.* Botulinum toxin injections in the internal anal sphincter for the treatment of chronic anal fissures: long-term results after two different dosage regimens. *Ann Surg* 1998; **228**: 664–9.

33 Maria G, Cassetta E, Gui D *et al.* A comparison of botulinum toxin and saline for the treatment of chronic anal fissure. *N Engl J Med* 1998; **338**: 217–20.

34 Jost WH. One hundred cases of anal fissure treated with botulin toxin: early- and long-term results. *Dis Colon Rectum* 1997; **40**: 1029–32.

35 Jost WH, Schrank B. Chronic anal fissures treated with botulinum toxin injections: a dose-finding study with Dysport®. *Colorectal Dis* 1999; **1**: 26–8.

36 Jost WH, Schrank B. Repeat botulin toxin injections in anal fissure. In patients with relapse and after insufficient effect of the first treatment. *Dig Dis Sci* 1999; **44**: 1588–9.

37 Brisinda G, Maria G, Bentivoglio AR *et al.* A comparison of injections of botulinum toxin and topical nitroglycerin ointment for the treatment of chronic anal fissure. *N Engl J Med* 1999; **341**: 65–9.

38 Fernandez Lopez F, Conde Freire R, Rios Rios A *et al.* Botulinum toxin for the treatment of anal fissure. *Dig Surg* 1999; **16**: 515–8.

39 Mason PF, Watkins MJG, Hall HS, Hall AW. The management of chronic fissure *in-ano* with botulinum toxin. *J R Coll Surg Edinb* 1996; **41**: 235–8.

40 Mínguez M, Melo F, Espí A *et al.* Therapeutic effects of different doses of botulinum toxin in chronic fissure. *Dis Colon Rectum* 1999; **42**: 1016–21.

41 Gonzalez Carro P, Perez Roldan F, Legaz Huidobro ML *et al.* The treatment of anal fissure with botulinum toxin. *Gastroenterol Hepatol* 1999; **22**: 163–6.

42 Maria G, Brisinda G, Bentivoglio AR *et al.* Influence of botulinum toxin site of injections on healing rate in patients with chronic anal fissure. *Am J Surg* 2000; **179**: 46–50.

43 Jost WH, Schimrigk K, Mlitz H. The riddle of the sphincters in anal fissure (letter). *Dis Colon Rectum* 1995; **38**: 555.

44 Lysy J, Israelit-Yatzkan Y, Sestiery-Ittah M *et al.* Topical nitrates potentiate the effect of botulinum toxin in the treatment of patients with refractory anal fissure. *Gut* 2001; **48**: 221–4.

45 Jost WH, Schanne S, Mlitz H, Schimrigk K. Perianal thrombosis following injection therapy into the external anal sphincter using botulin toxin (letter). *Dis Colon Rectum* 1995; **38**: 781.

46 Joo JS, Agachan F, Wolff B, Nogueras JJ, Wexner SD. Initial North American experience with botulinum toxin type A for treatment of anismus. *Dis Colon Rectum* 1996; **39**: 1107–11.

47 Maria G, Brisinda G, Bentivoglio AR, Cassetta E, Albanese A. Botulinum toxin in the treatment of outlet obstruction constipation caused by puborectalis syndrome. *Dis Colon Rectum* 2000; **43**: 376–80.

48 Jost WH, Müller-Lobeck H. Preoperative use of botulinum toxin in coloproctology: hypothesis and first results. *Colorectal Dis* 2000; **2**: 55.

49 Jost WH, Schrank B, Herold A, Leiß O. Functional outlet obstruction. Anismus, spastic pelvic floor syndrome, and dyscoordination of the voluntary sphincter muscles. *Scand J Gastroenterol* 1999; **34**: 449–53.

50 Jost WH. Gastrointestinal motility problems in patients with Parkinson's disease. Effects of antiparkinsonian treatment and guidelines for management. *Drugs Aging* 1997; **10**: 249–58.

PART FOUR

Other indications

CHAPTER 16

Ophthalmic indications

JOHN LEE

Introduction

Strabismus is an ancient condition, mentioned in the Ebers Papyrus and the works of Hippocrates. The first authenticated operation for the treatment of strabismus was performed by Dieffenbach in Berlin in 1839, and much of our current repertoire of surgical procedures was already invented by the end of the 19th century. In 1973, Alan Scott, an ophthalmologist in San Francisco with an interest in strabismus, published a paper [1] in which he evaluated four different agents for their ability to induce strabismus when injected into the extraocular muscles of primates, arguing that an agent that could induce strabismus safely and effectively could be used to treat human strabismus without the need for conventional incisional surgery. He tried di-isopropyl-flurophosphate (an anticholinesterase), alpha-bungarotoxin, absolute alcohol and botulinum toxin A (BtA), concluding that only the botulinum toxin gave results that lasted a satisfactory period without any significant deleterious side-effects. Little notice was taken of this communication, but a great deal of interest greeted his report of 1979 [2], in which he reported detailed clinical results of 67 injections in 19 patients, establishing treatment techniques, dosages and indications for an entirely novel non-surgical method for the modification of ocular alignment.

Strabismus or *squint* is a relatively common condition, with a reported incidence of 2–4% in most populations. Nearly all cases are *concomitant*, i.e. not associated with muscular paralysis or mechanical restriction of ocular rotation, and the onset is typically in childhood. Adult concomitant strabismus is usually due to failure of development of the binocular vision reflexes, causing lifelong instability of ocular posture, and frequently the development of a divergent squint to replace the common convergent squint of childhood. Adult concomitant squint may also be secondary (sensory) due to temporary or permanent uniocular loss of vision.

About 95% of squint is concomitant, but it may also be caused by neurogenic causes such as cranial nerve palsy, supranuclear or internuclear lesions. Such squint is normally termed *paralytic*. A small subgroup of strabismus is caused by specific *muscular* disorders, such as the chronic progressive external ophthalmoplegias, thought to be due in the main to mitochondrial defects, or myasthenia gravis.

Finally, as the basis of ocular rotation involves not only the contraction of agonist muscles but also the simultaneous relaxation of antagonist muscles, any process that reduces the ability of an extraocular muscle to relax will cause *restrictive* strabismus. Common causes for this condition include dysthyroid eye disease, and the sequelae of trauma or surgery within the orbit, in particular multiple operations for squint and surgery for the treatment of retinal detachment.

Depending on the severity of the squint and the state of the fusion reflexes which maintain binocular vision, typical symptoms of strabismus are diplopia, ocular asthenia ('eye-strain') and social difficulties related to misalignment of the visual axes. Conventional therapies include spectacles, particularly to correct hypermetropia in children, prisms to control diplopia in relatively small angles of squint, and surgery, where combinations of muscle weakening procedures (recession, tenotomy) and strengthening procedures (resection, advancement, plication) may be supplemented by transposition of muscles to change their line of action. In adult patients, an extra degree of accuracy may be gained by the use of adjustable suture squint surgery, with postoperative manipulation of the ocular position under local anaesthetic in the alert patient. *Disadvantages of surgery* are minor in most cases, being largely due to minor surface discomfort in the immediate postoperative period. However, multiple surgical procedures carry the disadvantage of accumulating scar tissue, leading to chronic redness of the eye and restriction of ocular rotations. In addition, patients with no real potential for restoration of binocular vision will not be likely to stay well-aligned over an extended period of time, so the issue of multiple surgery may be very relevant to many cases of adult strabismus.

Botulinum toxin for ophthalmic indications

Botulinum toxin for strabismus

Our toxin treatment clinic at Moorfields Eye Hospital began in 1982 and, up to November 2000, we had treated a total of 4760 patients for a variety of disorders of ocular motility. The vast majority of our cases are adults with strabismus, so the discussion will largely concern them, but the treatment of childhood strabismus, the treatment of nystagmus and the induction of therapeutic ptosis will be covered. Figures 16.1–16.4 summarize the diagnostic breakdown of our cases treated for strabismus. The basic principle of treatment of strabismus is shown in Fig. 16.5.

A patient has an ocular deviation (see Fig. 16.5). The 'over-acting' muscle is injected with botulinum toxin (Bt) under electromyographic (EMG) control. Once the paralysis has become established (typically 2 days later) the tone in the antagonist muscle will cause an alteration in ocular alignment, often a reversal in the direction of the deviation. The over correction, if it occurs, will last a few weeks at most. The eyes will then be essentially straight for a period which, although it varies between patients, is usually several months. In patients with good binocular vision potential there may be permanent restoration of ocular alignment, but such cases of functional cure are relatively rare in our clinic. This is discussed further below. In most cases, the deviation recurs after

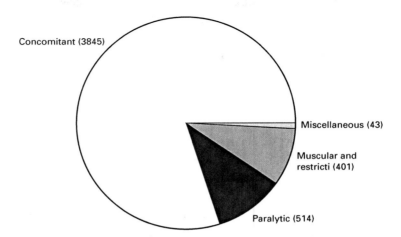

Fig. 16.1 Toxin clinic 1982–2000: cumulative data.

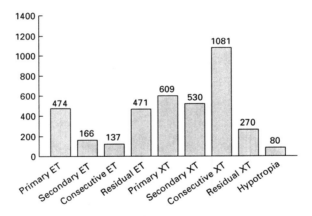

Fig. 16.2 Toxin clinic 1982–2000: concomitant strabismus. ET, esotropia; XT, exotropia.

several months and the patient can then decide whether they wish to continue with this line of treatment or elect for an alternative.

In theory, any extraocular muscle may be injected with BtA, but in practice we only treat, in descending order of frequency, the lateral, medial and inferior recti. Injection of the superior rectus nearly always induces an accompanying severe ptosis. Injection of the superior oblique tends to induce paralysis of the medial rectus and injection of the inferior oblique, while technically easy, has little lasting effect in the treatment of unilateral fourth nerve palsy.

The *indications* for therapy may be divided into *diagnosis, maintenance, palliation, cure* and *as an adjunct to surgery.*

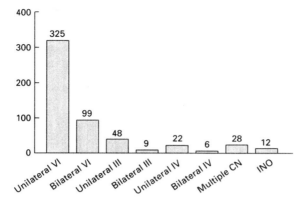

Fig. 16.3 Toxin clinic 1982–2000: paralytic strabismus. Multiple CN, multiple cranial nerve palsy; INO, internuclear ophthalmoplegia with exotropia.

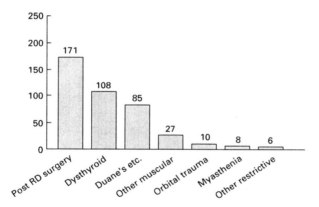

Fig. 16.4 Toxin clinic 1982–2000: muscular and restrictive strabismus. RD surgery, retinal detachment surgery.

Diagnosis

PREDICTION OF POSTOPERATIVE DIPLOPIA

Standard preoperative assessment of concomitant strabismus in older children and adults without binocular vision involves a test for postoperative diplopia. This is done because the patient may have learned to suppress the image seen by the retina of the non-dominant eye, but when alignment is changed by surgery, suppression may be lost, with consequent diplopia. As diplopia is not only a nuisance, but may affect the right to a driving licence, it is prudent to assess this risk. The test is done by neutralizing the angle of squint with prisms and then asking the patient to view a light or target. If the patient reports diplopia, the test is positive. Unfortunately, false positive results are very common and a large proportion of those reporting diplopia with prisms will have either triv-

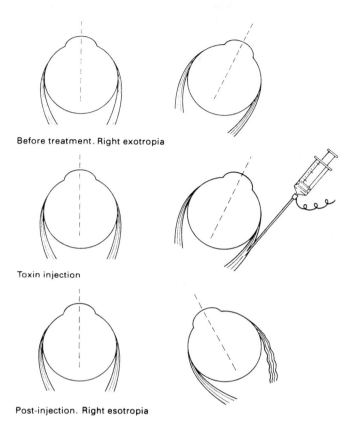

Before treatment. Right exotropia

Toxin injection

Post-injection. Right esotropia

Fig. 16.5 Rational of strabismus treatment. Diagram of the effect of BtA injected into one horizontal rectus muscle.

ial, easily ignored diplopia or no diplopia at all. The aim is to identify those few cases at risk of troublesome diplopia, and counsel them appropriately, while those not at risk can proceed with surgery. Temporary realignment with an injection of Bt allows both surgeon and patient to assess the risk of bothersome diplopia, and make a realistic decision on further treatment. Figures 16.6–16.8 show the results of a study conducted in our unit in 1995 [3], where we compared patient awareness of diplopia when tested with prisms, following Bt realignment, and in a proportion of the group, following surgery.

It is evident that if all those reporting diplopia on prism testing had been refused surgery on these grounds, many perfectly safe operations would not have been performed. Practically speaking, it is not essential to obtain perfect alignment for assessment of diplopia. It is frequently sufficient to produce enough paralysis of the target muscle to limit its function. If the patient is then asked to look in the direction of action of the injected muscle, the visual axes can usually be aligned, and resulting absence of diplopia is sufficient evidence to allow surgery to proceed.

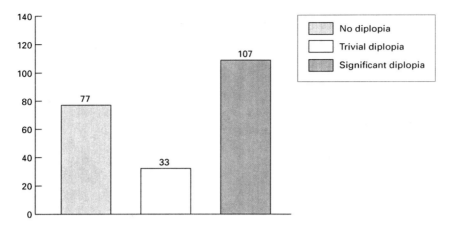

Fig. 16.6 Prediction of postoperative diplopia with prisms.

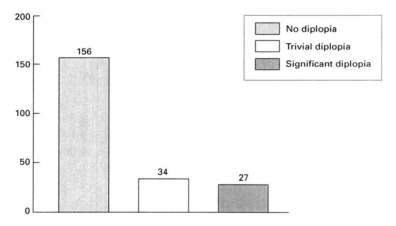

Fig. 16.7 Prediction of postoperative diplopia by toxin alignment.

INVESTIGATION OF FUSION POTENTIAL

Secondary strabismus typically follows temporary unilateral visual deprivation. If a patient sustains a penetrating ocular injury, say with a traumatic cataract, it may be several months at the latest before the eye may suitable for visual rehabilitation with an intraocular implant. By this time, the eyes may have slipped out of alignment, typically into exotropia, and optical correction with a contact lens induces diplopia. Patients may lose their binocular reflexes over a period of ocular misalignment. Alignment with an injection of BtA and contact lens wear will show which patients may be truly functionally rehabilitated and those who may not.

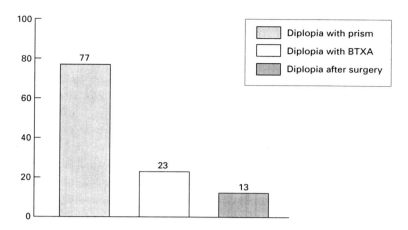

Fig. 16.8 Outcome after surgery in 117 cases vs. preoperative sensory tests.

RELIEF OF COMPENSATORY HEAD POSTURE

In Duane's syndrome [4], a congenital type of incomitant squint where one eye has a defect of abduction, patients often adopt a compensatory face turn to the side with the abduction deficit, to maintain binocular vision. Such patients often present as adults asking if anything can be done about their head posture. Again, BtA will transiently improve ocular alignment, permitting the patient to make a rational choice of therapy.

SYMPTOMATIC LATENT NYSTAGMUS

A rare diagnostic application is in patients with strabismus and manifest latent nystagmus, which is reducing visual acuity. The best surgical results in this situation are obtained by operating on the dominant, better-sighted eye, but patients are often justifiably apprehensive about this approach, fearing damage to their better eye. A diagnostic injection of BtA, to medial rectus of the fixing eye, will usually demonstrate the effectiveness of surgery [5].

It should be clear from the foregoing discussion that the main aim of diagnostic use of BtA is to allow the *patient* rather than the doctor to make a rational choice of therapy. This saves a great deal of time and effort for all concerned.

Maintenance

Maintenance therapy for strabismus accounts for the majority of the injections performed in our unit. Patients who are past the age of visual maturity (around 8 years old) and who have no vestige of binocular vision are likely to squint. More importantly, they have no rational prospect of ever having permanently straight eyes, as the squint will always recur, although it may reverse in its direction, becoming a consecutive deviation. Many of our patients have had multiple temporarily successful operations. There is an increasing literature on the social and psychological problems of manifest strabismus, so it is no surprise that patients seek therapy.

BtA does not permanently straighten eyes, but it can be administered very easily in the outpatient clinic setting, as many times as required, without the induction of scar tissue or other significant complication. Patients treated long-term, over many years [6], may show an increase in the duration of the effect, and an increasing interval between injections.

BtA is also particularly suitable for the management of *secondary (sensory)* strabismus in blind eyes [7]. Such eyes are often blind because of end-stage disease, such as glaucoma or retinal detachment, and may have undergone multiple previous procedures for the primary disease process. Many of these eyes are also *hypotonic* (intraocular pressure below 10 mmHg). In this circumstance, conventional squint surgery is contraindicated as it will further lower the intraocular pressure, which may make the eye phthisical and unsightly.

Palliation

BtA may be used palliatively when surgery is contraindicated, perhaps by serious cardiac or respiratory disease, or inoperable intracranial tumours or metastases causing cranial nerve palsies. The first patient we treated with BtA was a woman with carcinoma of the breast with a petrous temporal metastasis causing a partial sixth nerve palsy affecting her dominant eye, which she could not easily occlude. BtA treatment allowed her a valuable area of single binocular vision without an abnormal head posture for the remainder of her life.

Cure

Genuine cure of strabismus with BtA treatment is rather rare in our experience. However, there are patients with good binocular vision potential where there has been a temporary disruption, either of the motor system, e.g. acquired sixth nerve palsy, or the sensory system, e.g. penetrating ocular injury with traumatic cataract, or both, e.g. retinal detachment with successful surgical reapposition of the retina. In these circumstances, restoration of ocular alignment and balancing of muscular forces may permit the patient to re-establish binocularity without any further therapy, and avoid either surgery or chronic wearing of prisms.

In a recent review of our computer database, we found 110 cases which met our criteria of functional cure (no evidence of spontaneous improvement for a minimum of 6 months preinjection; lasting realignment with binocular single vision postinjection for a minimum of 12 months). This was 2.4% of our total number of treated cases, although we may have slightly underestimated the percentage, as some cases, having been cured, were then lost to follow up. In an audit of all cases treated in 1 year with retrospective case note review we found 3.6% functional cures.

We found the highest relative cure rate in patients with consecutive esotropia (9.3%), these being patients with intermittent exotropia who underwent surgery which led to an over correction. As most cases of intermittent exotropia have good sensory binocular function, but problems with maintaining their motor alignment, repositioning of the eye by medial rectus BtA injection is frequently of value and may avoid subsequent surgery. We have reported our experience with consecutive esotropia elsewhere [8]. Other conditions with a good percentage cure rate were unilateral partial sixth nerve palsy (8.3%) and strabismus following surgery for retinal detachment (6.3%).

Adjunct to surgery

Complete unrecovered sixth nerve palsy presents a difficult problem for the strabismus surgeon. In order to obtain realignment of the eyes with a useful field of binocular single vision, it is necessary to relieve the restriction of the contracted unopposed medial rectus, and also to provide some abducting force to replace the action of the paralysed lateral rectus. In theory, this may be achieved by recessing the medial rectus and at the same time transposing the vertical rectus muscles laterally, so they provide abducting force to the eye. However, the blood supply to the anterior segment of the eye is derived from the long posterior ciliary arteries and from the terminal branches of the arteries of the rectus muscles, the anterior ciliary arteries. Those of the vertical recti make the greatest contribution, with the medial rectus next, but almost no contribution from the lateral rectus. Therefore, any operation where the superior, inferior and medial recti are removed from the globe is liable to cause problems with anterior segment blood supply. In a child, the long posterior ciliary perfusion is adequate to maintain the supply, but in an older patient (over 25 years old) such surgery may precipitate the highly undesirable complication of *anterior segment ischaemia* with ocular hypotony, pupillary paralysis, corneal oedema and cataract. Although this is treatable, it is still best avoided, and much ingenuity has gone into devising techniques for its avoidance, such as partial transpositions or techniques of muscle transposition which leave the ciliary vessels still in connection with the globe.

An alternative approach which we described in 1988 [9] is to use BtA to paralyse the medial rectus without affecting its contribution to anterior segment perfusion, and transpose the vertical recti. This markedly reduces the risk of anterior segment ischaemia and also allows later surgery on the medial rectus, when anastamoses have developed and there is no further risk of inducing perfusion problems. We administer the BtA preoperatively, 4–14 days before surgery, but others obtain good results with peroperative and postoperative administration.

Other aspects of botulinum toxin therapy in paralytic strabismus

In sixth nerve palsy BtA may achieve a functional cure, cases with contraindications to surgery may benefit from BtA as a palliative agent, and cases of complete unrecovered sixth nerve palsy may be managed by combined BtA and transposition surgery. The suggestion has been made that BtA may have a *prophylactic* role in the management of paralytic strabismus and sixth nerve palsy in particular. The rationale for therapy is the suggestion that in acute acquired sixth nerve palsy immediate injection of the ipsilateral medial rectus may prevent contracture of the muscle, so that when the sixth nerve and lateral rectus recover there is a lower incidence of manifest strabismus. Although this was suggested in two uncontrolled observational series [10,11], we showed no prophylactic effect in a prospective randomised study of 47 largely microvascular sixth nerve palsies [12] and Holmes *et al.* have also shown no prophylactic effect in traumatic sixth nerve palsy [13]. Patients may benefit symptomatically from improved alignment and relief of compensatory head posture, but there is no evidence of a prophylactic effect.

BtA has a limited place in the management of third nerve palsy. Clearly, in the context of complete third nerve palsy with paralysis of four out of six extraocular muscles, ptosis and internal ophthalmoplegia, BtA has nothing to offer. There is, however, a subgroup of partial third nerve palsy with fairly good ocular rotations but a large angle exotropia which may do rather well with BtA treatment, with even some cases of functional cure [14].

In fourth nerve palsy, whether unilateral or bilateral, congenital or acquired, BtA has little to offer over conventional surgery, possibly because even when the antagonist is adequately paralysed, the paretic superior oblique muscle cannot 'take up the slack' and improve ocular alignment in the long term. Paralysing the contralateral inferior rectus [15] may help, but this is very bothersome for patients during the early postinjection period and we have largely abandoned the use of BtA in such cases, preferring surgery.

Multiple cranial nerve palsies, which are commonly posttraumatic, nearly always have some component of sixth nerve palsy, and may derive some benefit from BtA, but usually also require surgery when stable.

Botulinum toxin for strabismus in children

BtA seems to be valuable in three main groups of childhood strabismus. It is the treatment of choice in children with acquired strabismus and a high likelihood of potential binocular vision [16]. Such cases include consecutive esotropia after surgery for exotropia, sixth nerve palsy, acute normisensorial esotropia and strabismus following uniocular sensory deprivation. A second group of older children, aged 9 years or more, and visually mature, may be treated for concomitant strabismus with exactly the same indications and technique as adults. Typical diagnoses are consecutive exotropia and residual esotropia. A further group of children with complex strabismus may be realigned for diagnostic indications, usually to decide whether further surgery might be of value.

Other investigators [17–20] have used BtA to manage primary childhood strabismus, in particular essential infantile esotropia. It seems probable that in experienced hands, BtA be at least as effective as surgery in primary congenital esotropia, residual congenital esotropia, and primary exotropia.

However, all treatment in younger children requires admission to hospital and some type of sedation or anaesthesia. Conventional general anaesthesia is contraindicated, as it abolishes spontaneous eye movements and makes EMG monitoring of electrode position impossible. We use intravenous ketamine 1 mg/kg to induce dissociated anaesthesia, in addition to the usual topical ocular anaesthesia with drops. Although this medication has a reputation for inducing nightmares, we have never encountered this problem. Others have used nitrous oxide inhalation or intravenous propofol.

Botulinum toxin treatment for nystagmus and oscillopsia

Patients with congenital nystagmus typically have poor vision for a variety of sensory and motor reasons. Although some attempts have been made to treat such cases with BtA, little improvement has been shown. However, patients with acquired nystagmus note severe oscillopsia, the subjective sensation of constant movement of the perceived visual environment, which is extremely unpleasant. The commonest diagnosis is advanced multiple sclerosis, in which case there is usually also poor visual acuity due to consecutive optic atrophy and maybe also supranuclear ocular motility problems. Other causes include vascular or traumatic brainstem disease which may cause oculopalatal myoclonus with constant nystagmus, usually vertical or oblique, but otherwise normal eyes and therefore good potential vision. Helveston and Pogrebniak [21] suggested that such cases might be treated by retrobulbar injection of BtA to paralyse all the extraocular muscles and relieve the oscillopsia. Retrobulbar or individual muscle injection may improve the objective severity of their nystagmus in most cases [22,23]. Regrettably, although treatment is easy and can be repeated at will, not many patients derive real benefit. Patients with multiple sclerosis usually find that their other ocular problems limit the benefits of treatment. In those with good potential vision, the treatment has some serious limitations. It can only be done to one eye at a time, as bilateral retrobulbar injection would simply place the eyes in a position of exotropia with diplopia. The other eye must therefore be occluded. There is quite a high incidence of ptosis.

Most importantly, the vestibulo-ocular reflexes are abolished. In ambulatory patients this means that even small head movements are not compensated by reflex eye movements, so a whole new set of symptoms are induced. In short, BtA can be tried for any case of oscillopsia, if only to allow the patient to experience the effect. On balance [24] the main value is in patients who are immobile, with good potential vision, and who wish to read or watch television. In this subgroup the therapy may be repeated as often as required, which is typically every 2 months.

Success rate and indications for cessation of treatment

Success rate of Bt treatment for strabismus is difficult to define. At its simplest, it may be judged by the fact that the target muscle is injected and a muscular paralysis then ensues. Using this criterion, the 'success rate' is probably around 99%, with the only reasons for failure being technical, i.e. failure to find the target muscle, or mechanical restriction by scar tissue, which is not affected by the muscle paralysing action of Bt.

However, when treating individuals with strabismus the aim is improved ocular alignment, lasting a satisfactory period of time, which either relieves diplopia or improves the appearance for social interaction. Bt may be used in the hope of achieving a cure and avoiding surgery and, as has already been noted, this is not a common outcome in our patient population. Alternatively, it may be used to clarify the likely outcome of surgery, in particular the risk of postoperative diplopia. Here the success rate in terms of accurate prediction far exceeds that of neutralization of the squint with prism testing, which grossly over predicts diplopia.

In the group who are seeking maintenance therapy to keep their eyes straight for social reasons, those who obtain an adequate response from toxin treatment will tend to continue with the treatment, assuming that it provides an adequate period of alignment and that injections do not have to be given too frequently. This particularly applies to those with unilateral visual loss and a poorly sighted eye with a secondary squint. 'Failure' with Bt therapy means that except in the very rare cases of sight-threatening ocular perforation, the patient is in the same situation as they were prior to injection and can either be discharged or try another therapy.

Typically, treatment is discontinued when it does not work, when the patient wishes to try another therapy, during pregnancy, when the patient moves his or her home and is too far away for convenient attendance, or when the increasing interval between injections in the long-term maintenance group becomes so long that the patient may be suspended from attendance with instructions to reattend as required.

Botulinum toxin for therapeutic induction of ptosis

It has long been known that various forms of corneal disease, in particular neurotrophic keratitis and indolent epithelial defects, may be extremely resistant to treatment unless a central tarsorraphy is performed. In this procedure, the upper and lower lids are sutured together. It is unclear whether the improvement that occurs is due to simply reducing the size of the palpebral aperture, or whether the effect is due to stopping the lids moving across the cornea and inhibiting reepithelialization. Nevertheless, striking improvement is almost invariable.

Unfortunately, patients are understandably resistant to the idea of having an eye sewn closed, and it is extremely hard to judge when it is safe to open the tarsorraphy once the cornea has improved.

From the earliest reports of the use of BtA for strabismus indications, one of the commonest minor complications has been ptosis. In 1988 [25] we reported the use of BtA for the deliberate therapeutic induction of ptosis for patients with corneal epithelial problems. It continues to be a mainstay of the management of such cases.

The majority of such cases have poor vision due to their primary corneal disease, but patients who have good visual acuity should be warned of the risk of induction of persisting hypotropia due to an effect on the superior rectus. We have reported three cases of this complication [26].

Treatment

DOSES: A HEALTH WARNING

Please read the warning on p. 35 about doses of Bt. There are three preparations available. *Dysport®* and *Botox®* are type A toxins (BtA), *NeuroBloc®/MYOBLOC™* is type B (BtB). Even though the doses for each are quoted in mouse units (mu), the three preparations have different dose schedules: one mu of *Dysport®* is **not** the same as one mu of *Botox®*, and neither is equivalent to one mu of *NeuroBloc®/MYOBLOC™*.

Technique

Adult strabismus

We run two treatment clinics per week at Moorfields Eye Hospital. All new patients receive an information leaflet to read at their own convenience (see Appendix, p. 402). After appropriate measurement and orthoptic assessment, the patient discusses the treatment with the ophthalmologist and signs a standard hospital consent form.

Topical anaesthesia is induced with amethocaine 1% (4 drops at 5-min intervals). The forehead skin is lightly abraded with Omniprep™ to remove dead skin and improve electrical contact. Ground and reference electrodes (standard 10 mm 'EEG' silver/silver chloride disk electrodes, secured using 25 mm Micropore adhesive tape with electrolyte gel (Dracard™) are attached to the patient's forehead, with the pregelled ground electrode in the midline of the forehead and the reference electrode above the eye to be injected. The electrodes are checked for impedance (less than 5000 ohms) with a hand-held meter. A single drop of epinephrine (adrenaline) 0.1% is instilled in the eye to be injected. The purpose of this is to blanch the conjunctiva, which may become hyperaemic during the amethocaine instillation. It also allows visualization of the target muscle through the conjunctiva and may reduce the incidence of subconjunctival haemorrhage.

The patient sits in an inclinable chair and is reclined at about 45°. The brow electrodes are connected to the monitor. We use a Medelec MS6 polygraph with both audible and oscilloscope signals, but portable monitors are available and work well.

The injection electrode is a monopolar electrode manufactured by taking a

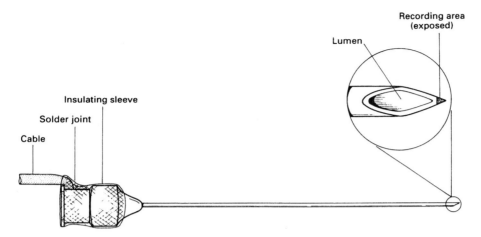

Fig. 16.9 A monopolar EMG/injection electrode.

27-gauge 38 mm needle with a metal Luer-lock, soldering an insulated lead to the Luer-lock hub, and coating the entire electrode except the extreme tip with an insulating resin. The electrode is shown in Fig. 16.9.

For horizontal rectus muscle injection, the patient is asked to look into a position opposite to the action of the muscle to be injected, i.e. for a left lateral rectus muscle, the patient will be asked to look to the right. The tip of the electrode is introduced into the muscle at roughly the equator of the globe. Once the electrode is engaged, the patient is asked to rotate their gaze to the opposite side, i.e. into the direction of action of the target muscle. The electrode is then advanced along the line of the muscle (envisaging a computed tomogram [CT] or magnetic resonance imaging [MRI] scan is very helpful for this) until the maximum EMG signal is detected. This is usually found when the tip of the electrode is in the area of maximum density of motor end-plates, about 30 mm from the insertion. Typical EMG amplitudes are from 300 to 600 microvolts.

For inferior rectus injection, the electrode is introduced transcutaneously through the lower eyelid while the patient maintains upward gaze. The electrode is then advanced through the orbital septum and inferior orbital tissues, aiming upwards and nasally, to engage the inferior rectus. As the inferior oblique is often encountered, it is essential to locate a muscle whose EMG increases only on depression, which must be the inferior rectus. Typical amplitudes are 200–500 microvolts.

Approximately 0.1 mL (2.5 U) of solution is then injected into the target muscle. The reason for having 0.2 mL in the syringe is to allow for leakage round the Luer-lock and dead space within the needle. The electrode is kept in place for 40 s. This gives time for the injected solution to diffuse into the muscle, and minimizes reflux back up the needle track. The needle and brow electrodes are then removed. The patient is either told to wear their own glasses or an eyepad is placed on the injected eye. This protects the anaesthetized eye from a possible corneal foreign body during the period when the anaesthetic is wearing off. The pad is discarded after 2 h. We see all new patients 1–2 weeks after injection, to check the effect, detect complications and assess the need for a repeat injection.

Strabismus in children under ketamine

This should be performed in the operating theatre suite and an anaesthetist expert in the use of ketamine is essential, as the child needs to be unaware but still have spontaneous ocular movements, and so must be in a very shallow plane of anaesthesia. The nominal dose of ketamine is 1 mg/kg, by intravenous injection, but this requires constant balancing to maintain the correct level. The electrodes are attached in the standard fashion and topical anaesthetic and epinephrine instilled. The tip of the needle should be introduced, and the operator should then wait for a spontaneous eye movement in the correct direction and take advantage of this to make the injection. Considerable experience is required. The child recovers extremely quickly and may be discharged a few hours later.

Nystagmus

EMG monitoring is not required. The volume to be injected is 1 mL (25 U = strabismus dose × 10). The patient is instructed to look up and medially and the lower lid wiped with a sterile alcohol swab. A standard retrobulbar needle is used. This is inserted through the lateral lower lid and advanced into the extraocular muscle cone, keeping the point low to reduce the risk of ptosis. The plunger should be withdrawn slightly to check a vessel has not been perforated and the injection performed. The needle is withdrawn and firm pressure maintained for a few minutes over the site of needle entry. Local anaesthesia and pads are unnecessary.

Induction of ptosis

EMG monitoring is not required. The volume to be injected is 0.3 mL (strabismus dose × 3). The upper lid is cleaned with a sterile alcohol injection swab. The operator palpates the lid to find the apex of the upper bony orbital rim, and introduces the needle (25 mm long, 25-gauge) through the skin. The needle is angled upwards and introduced to its full depth, to touch the roof of the orbit. There are no vessels or nerves in this area, so the injection is given without delay and the needle withdrawn, and digital pressure applied over the injection site for a few seconds. As the effect does not develop for 2 days, supportive therapy needs to be continued.

Doses

We originally started the clinic using BtA from Professor Edward Schantz, Alan Scott's supplier. We then changed around 1987 to BtA supplied by Professor Jack Melling at CAMR (Centre for Applied Microbiological Research), Porton Down. This latter formulation later acquired the trade name of Dysport® and we have used it since for all strabismus indications. Our standard dose for strabismus is 2.5 mu Dysport® for a rectus muscle, although we occasionally give 5 mu. (The dilution is made by first drawing up 10.5 mL of sterile 0.9% sodium chloride solution which is placed in a sterile rubber-topped vial. One mL of this is then injected into the Dysport® vial which contains 500 mu. Then 0.5 mL of the resulting solution is reinjected into the rubber-topped vial, giving a concentration of 250 mu/10 mL or 2.5 mu/0.1 mL.) Colleagues in the US and elsewhere use Botox® in doses between 2 and 5 mu for similar indications (Table 16.1 [27]). This appears paradoxical, as it is generally held that the Botox® mu is roughly equivalent to 3 Dysport® mu, and we have no explanation for this anomaly.

We do not store solutions overnight and all dilutions are made up on the day of use. For retrobulbar injection for nystagmus we use the same concentration and inject 1 mL, i.e. 10 times the strabismus dose. For induction of ptosis, we use the same concentration and inject 0.3 mL or 7.5 mu Dysport®.

Complications and side-effects

The main side-effect of rectus muscle injection is awareness of muscular paralysis, which may be accompanied by past-pointing, disorientation and diplopia, even in patients who suppress. The effects are more intrusive when the dominant eye is treated.

Ptosis is usually partial and always transient. It seems more common when medial recti are injected and when inexperienced medical staff do injections. However, its incidence is around 5% overall for adults, although for children treated under ketamine the incidence is about 25%. This difference is probably due to better muscle localization in the awake, cooperative patient and the fact that adults are treated reclined at 45°, whereas the children are lying flat.

Hypertropia is due to toxin affecting the ipsilateral inferior rectus, and is also commoner in difficult injections or when inexperienced operators inject. It is rarely a major problem, and a prism will help binocular patients.

Ciliary ganglion blockade is infrequent, and causes pupillary dilatation and blurring of near vision due to accommodative paralysis. It always resolves, usually over a few weeks.

Perforation of the globe is uncommon, and has never occurred in our clinic. The author is

Table 16.1 Suggested initial botulinum toxin A (BtA) doses for Botox® and Dysport®* (adapted from [27]).

		Botox® (mu)	Dysport® (mu)
Horizontal strabismus†	Under 25 PD	2.5	2.5
	Over 25 PD	2.5–5.0	2.5–5.0
MR injection for LR palsy	Early (1–3 months)	1.0–2.0	2.5
	Later, or together with transposition surgery or with MR contracture	2.5	2.5
Vertical muscles	IR for concomitant deviation	2.5	2.5
	IR for thyroid disease	5.0	2.5
	IO	2.5	2.5
	SR (rare)	2.5	2.5
Infantile esotropia or exotropia	Bilateral injections	2.5	2.5
Weak muscles	Myasthenia, aberrant regeneration	1.0–2.0	2.5
Retrobulbar	Nystagmus	25	25
Levator	For therapeutic ptosis	5	7.5

IO, inferior oblique; IR, inferior rectus; LR, lateral rectus; MR, medial rectus; PD, prism dioptres; SR, superior rectus.
*No doses are given for Neurobloc as there are no published data.
†May be adjusted proportionately to degree of squint. Small women are occasionally very sensitive and need smaller doses.

aware of four cases of this complication in the UK over the last 18 years, and in no case was there a persisting loss of visual acuity, although two patients had temporary diminution of vision due to vitreous haemorrhage, and one required a vitrectomy to clear the vitreous blood. Perforation may be more likely to happen in highly myopic eyes and when inexperienced personnel give injections.

Retrobulbar haemorrhage is also very rare, but we have had one case, with no effect on visual acuity, which resolved over 2 weeks.

Systemic complications do not occur when strabismus doses are used.

Data recording in the toxin clinic

Despite the fact that Alan Scott introduced BtA therapy specifically for treatment of strabismus, neither Dysport® nor Botox® has been given a product licence for treatment of strabismus or allied conditions in the UK, and probably never will be given one. The treatment is therefore given on a 'named patient' basis and all injections are entered on a computer database (DBase4), with recording of name, age, sex, diagnosis, strabismus data, EMG data, complications and disposal.

Future prospects

In the 21 years since Alan Scott's first clinical report Bt has gained a secure place in the management of strabismus, particularly adult strabismus. The principle of non-surgical modification of muscular action has a particular appeal in the oculomotor system, with its eight rectus muscles and four oblique muscles and the possibility of altering their relative power to alter or restore ocular alignment. However, Bt is not the ideal agent for all applications of this approach. For diagnostic use, to establish the likely outcome of planned surgical therapy, the effect of BtA lasts rather too long and wears off too slowly. Alpha-bungarotoxin, which Scott investigated in his original animal study, only paralyses extraocular muscles for a few days. BtA paralyses muscles and alters ocular alignment for weeks to months.

An ideal diagnostic agent would have a duration of a few weeks with speedy resolution of effect, to allow prompt progress to definitive surgical treatment.

A further disadvantage of BtA is the necessity to return again and again for maintenance injections. Although this therapy is well understood and tolerated by our patients, it places a significant burden on our hospital outpatient resources. The ideal situation would be to establish the practicality of injection therapy with BtA, and then inject the target muscle with a 'magic bullet' which accurately and predictably reduced the muscle fibre count, and thereby the power of a muscle, in order to provide long-term ocular alignment without either surgery or further injections. The recent report of Christiansen and colleagues [28] on the use of monoclonal antibodies to extraocular muscles linked to ricin to produce precise localized muscular damage may show a possible pointer to future therapeutic possibilities.

References

1 Scott AB, Rosenbaum AL, Collins CC. Pharmacologic weakening of extraocular muscles. *Invest Ophthalmol Vis Sci* 1973; **12**: 924–7.
2 Scott AB. Botulinum toxin injection into extraocular muscles as an alternative to strabismus surgery. *Ophthalmology* 1979; **87**: 1044–9.
3 White JES, Dawson E, Lee JP, Bunce C. The effect of visual acuity on the predictive value of the postop diplopia test and on botulinum A treatment. In: Lennerstrand G, ed. *Advances in Strabismology*. Buren, The Netherlands: Aoelus Press, 1999: 81–4.
4 White JES, Lee JP. The role of botulinum A injections in the management of patients with Duane's retraction syndrome. In: Tillson G, ed. *Trans VIIth International Orthopt Congress*. Germany: fahner Verlag, 1991: 341–5.
5 Liu C, Gresty M, Lee JP. Management of symptomatic latent nystagmus. *Eye* 1993; **7**: 550–3.

6   Horgan SE, Lee JP, Bunce C. The long-term use of botulinum toxin for adult strabismus. *J Ped Ophthalmol Strab* 1998; **35**: 9–16.

7   Woodruff S, Dawson E, Lee JP. The role of botulinum neurotoxin type A (BTXA) in secondary strabismus. In: Spiritus M, ed. *Trans 25th Meeting European. Strabismological Association*. Buren, The Netherlands: Aeolus Press, 2000: 84–9.

8   Dawson ELM, Marshman WE, Lee JP. Role of botulinum toxin A in surgically over corrected exotropia. *JAAPOS* 1999; **3**: 269–71.

9   Fitzsimons R, Lee JP, Elston JS. Treatment of sixth nerve palsy in adults with combined botulinum toxin chemodenervation and surgery. *Ophthalmology* 1988; **95**: 1535–42.

10 Metz HS, Mazow M. Botulinum toxin treatment of acute sixth and third nerve palsy. *Graefe's Arch Clin Ophthalmol* 1988; **226**: 141–4.

11 Murray AD. Early botulinum toxin treatment of acute sixth nerve palsy. *Eye* 1991; **5**: 445–7.

12 Lee JP, Harris S, Cohen J *et al*. Results of a prospective randomized trial of botulinum toxin therapy in acute sixth nerve palsy. *J Ped Ophthalmol Strab* 1994; **31**: 283–6.

13 Holmes JM, Beck RW, Kip KE *et al*. Botulinum toxin treatment versus conservative management in acute traumatic sixth nerve palsy or paresis. *JAAPOS* 2000; **4**: 145–9.

14 Saad N, Lee JP. The role of botulinum toxin in third nerve palsy. *Aust NZ J Ophthalmol* 1992; **20**: 121–7.

15 Garnham L, Lawson JM, O'Neill D, Lee JP. Botulinum toxin in fourth nerve palsies. *Aust & NZ J Ophthalmol* 1997; **25**: 31–5.

16 Rayner S, Hollick EJ, Lee JP. Botulinum toxin in childhood strabismus. *Strabismus* 1999; **7**: 103–11.

17 McNeer KW, Spencer RF, Tucker MG. Observations on bilateral simultaneous botulinum toxin injection in infantile esotropia. *J Ped Ophthalmol Strabismus* 1994; **31**: 214–9.

18 Gomez de Liano R, Rodriguez JM, Gomez de Liano P, DeAndres ML. Botulinum toxin in esotropic patients up to 3 years of age. In: Lennerstrand G, ed. *Update on Strabismus and Pediatric Ophthalmology*. Boca Raton: CRC Press, 1996: 429–32.

19 Campos EC. Indicazioni e aspettative nel trattiamento con tossina botulinica. *Bolletino Di Oculistica* 1996; **75** (Suppl. 4): 73–9.

20 McNeer KW, Tucker MG, Spencer RF. Management of essential infantile esotropia with botulinum toxin A. Review and recommendations. *J Ped Ohthalmol Strab* 2000; **37**: 63–7.

21 Helveston EM, Pogrebniak AE. Treatment of acquired nystagmus with botulinum A toxin. *Am J Ophthalmol* 1988; **106**: 584–6.

22 Ruben ST, Lee JP, O'Neill D, Dunlop I, Elston JS. The use of botulinum toxin for treatment of acquired nystagmus and oscillopsia. *Ophthalmology* 1994; **101**: 783–7.

23 Leigh RJ, Tomsak RL, Grant MP, *et al*. Effectiveness of botulinum toxin administered to abolish acquired nystagmus. *Ann Neurol* 1992; **32**: 633–42.

24 Tomsak RL, Remler BF, Averbuch-Heller L, Chandran M, Leigh RJ. Unsatisfactory treatment of acquired nystagmus with retrobulbar injection of botulinum toxin. *Am J Ophthalmol* 1995; **119**: 489–96.

25 Kirkness C, Adams GW, Dilley PN, Lee JP. Botulinum toxin A-induced protective ptosis in corneal disease. *Ophthalmology* 1988; **95**: 473–80.

26 Heyworth PLO, Lee JP. Persisting hypotropias following protective ptosis induced by botulinum toxin. *Eye* 1994; **8**: 511–5.

27 McNeer KW, Magoon EH, Scott AB. Chemodenervation therapy: technique and indications. In: Rosenhaum AL, Santiago AP, eds. *Clinical Strabismus Management*. WB Saunders, 1999.

28 Christiansen SP, Sandnas A, Prill R, Youle RJ, McLoon LK. Acute effects of the skeletal muscle-specific immunotoxin Ricin-mAb on extraocular muscles of rabbits. *Invest Ophthalmol Vis Sci* 2000; **41**: 3402–9.

Botulinum toxin treatment for squint

Information for patients attending the clinic for the first time

1 Q. What is the effect of botulinum toxin?

A. The effect of botulinum toxin is to cause a paralysis of the muscle into which it has been injected.

2 Q. How long has it been used?

A. It has been used as a form of treatment at this hospital since November 1982.

3 Q. Will it affect my general health?

A. The treatment is perfectly safe and there is no risk to general health. In particular there is no risk of developing botulism or food poisoning. There is no known risk to women who are pregnant or breastfeeding, but some patients prefer to postpone treatment till later.

4 Q. Who will I see when I attend the clinic?

A. Initially you will have an examination by an orthoptist. You will then see one of the doctors working with the consultant ophthalmologists. If the treatment is thought to be of value, you will be asked to sign a consent form and your name will be added to the list for that day.

5 Q. What is the procedure for the treatment?

A. Local anaesthetic drops which numb the eye are given prior to treatment. You will then have some wires attached to your forehead and these are connected to an amplifier and loudspeaker. This is to allow the exact site of the injection to be carefully monitored by recording the electrical activity of the muscle and this can be heard through the loudspeaker during the injection.

6 Q. What happens after I have had the injection?

A. You will be asked whether you prefer a pad on the eye or to wear your own glasses. The eye is numb after the drops and so should be protected for about 2 h in case something blows into your eye without your knowledge. Some patients have an ache in the eye after injection. If this is not better after an hour, take whatever medication you would normally take for a headache.

7 Q. When should I expect to see an effect from the treatment?

A. The effect is usually noticed about 2 days after the injection is given.

8 Q. How long does the effect last for?

A. The paralysis lasts for weeks, occasionally months and then wears off completely. You may notice a temporary reversal of the direction of the squint, followed by gradual straightening of the eyes as the paralysis wears off.

9   Q. What are the possible local side-effects?

A. Temporary reversal of the direction of the squint.

Temporary double vision. If this is significant and bothersome you should not drive unless
you cover one eye.

Temporary drooping of the eyelid on the side of the injection. This usually resolves after a few
weeks.

Slight bruising of the surface of the eye.

These will all get better without further treatment.

10   Q. When do I return to the clinic?

A. We like to see all our new patients 1 or 2 weeks after the injection. It is occasionally
necessary to give a further injection at that visit, if the first one does not produce an
adequate effect.

11 Other notes

If you have any reason to believe that you may be a carrier of hepatitis or the HIV virus, please
make sure that you tell the doctor who sees you in the clinic. The information is confiden-
tial but it is essential that we are informed.

If you are not clear about any aspect of this treatment, please ask the doctor who sees you to
explain further before signing the consent form.

Please keep this information sheet for future reference.

CHAPTER 17

Management of pain with botulinum toxin

TURO J. NURMIKKO

Introduction

It is not surprising that chronic pain is an attractive indication for botulinum toxin (Bt) treatment. From the early days of use of the toxin for cervical dystonia it has been clear that pain relief frequently accompanies improvement in motor function. In one of the first large series on Bt for cervical dystonia, Jankovic and Schwartz reported total relief of pain in 76% of their patients [1]. Other groups described sustained improvement of pain in 12/19 patients [2], or moderate to excellent reduction after 66% of treatments [3]. Pain improved in double blind controlled studies [4, 5] and in a recent large series of 133 patients with cervical dystonia [6]. Pain relief commonly outweighs the motor benefit [7].

Pain was not in itself the main outcome measure for any of these studies, and none of the studies employed sophisticated measures to detect changes in pain intensity. In contrast, Pacchetti *et al.* focused on the pain in 30 patients with painful dystonia due to levodopa treatment for Parkinson's disease [8]. Within 10 days of Bt injections pain diminished in every patient, with the improvement lasting for between 3 and 7 months [9].

Such a close relationship between pain relief and reduction in muscle tone appears to offer considerable scope for Bt treatment in any myalgia, as long as it is associated with increased muscle tone, e.g. tension in the neck, tension myalgia of the pelvic floor, acute lumbago, and nocturnal cramps and stiffness in the aged. Indeed some authors of review articles have forecast a promising future for this treatment [10,11]. Unfortunately, published evidence has not fulfilled these expectations. This may in part be due to the limitations of the methods used, and in part due to current lack of understanding of the mechanisms that generate and maintain pain.

In this chapter I will focus on the use of Bt to reduce or prevent pain in conditions in which pain, rather than abnormal muscle tone, dominates the picture. There is an implicit assumption that the pathophysiology is such that reduction of muscle tone can help the pain. As a first step I will set out the evidence that increased muscle tone generates the pain in common chronic conditions.

Mechanisms of muscle tension and muscle pain

Muscle pain occurs after strenuous exercise, direct trauma, inflammation and during sustained contractions. It frequently accompanies fever or exposure to excessive cold. The pain usually disappears in a matter of days or weeks if the original cause is eradicated, but some individuals experience chronic muscle pain for years. The prevalence of muscle pain in a Danish study was 37% in males and 65% in females—and most of the reported pains were transient [11]. The prevalence of fibromyalgia, a rheumatoid condition in which muscle pain dominates, is estimated at 2% [12]. The point prevalence of any headache, tension-type or migraine is 11% for men and 22% for women [13]. The annual incidence of whiplash injury is estimated at 1/1000 population: of which some 2–5% develop protracted soft-tissue pain [14,15].

Recent advances in pain research have unravelled several neural and muscular mechanisms that may serve as suitable targets for novel therapies. Animal models, experimental human pain models in volunteers and pathophysiological studies in patients with myofascial pain suggest that chronic muscle pain is associated with sensitization of muscular nociceptors, hyperexcitability of the second order nerve cells in the dorsal horn of the spinal cord, instability of the regional autonomic nervous system and alterations in segmental and general inhibitory systems [16].

Many of these studies emphasize the conceptually important differences between muscle spasm, muscle tension and muscle contracture, any of which may or may not be associated with pain [17]. In muscle spasm, muscle contraction is due to increased neuromuscular activity that can be identified with electromyography (EMG). Muscle spasms with these properties are encountered in peripheral and central neuropathic conditions, such as chronic sciatica, motor neurone disease and spasticity following stroke. Pain is likely to be caused by ischaemia and the forces that develop between cramping and normal muscles. Muscle contracture (different from the tendon and joint contractures commonly mentioned in the medical literature) is an altered state of muscle contractility which is unaccompanied by any electrical activity. Clinically, the 'taut band' described in myofascial conditions and fibromyalgia falls into this category, though there are a number of hereditary muscular conditions in which such bands are widespread. Irrespective of the primary cause of muscle dysfunction, it is likely that changes in the peripheral and central pain mediating processes are commonly associated with chronic contracture. This has been shown in whiplash injury and fibromyalgia [18,19].

Muscle tension is a term used loosely in the clinic to imply increased overall tone in one or several muscles. Whether or not it is associated with increased EMG activity remains a matter of debate—the likely explanation for this disagreement is that both increased and normal EMG activity can be recorded in patients with seemingly similar clinical features. A good example is tension-type headache. Because in most cases no abnormal EMG activity can be recorded, it has been suggested that the apparent muscle tension in these patients is due to the presence of taut bands rather than increase of muscle tone per se, and that pain reflects changes in the endogenous pain control systems [17,20].

The mechanism of increased muscle tone, irrespective of what it is called, is important in that only in muscle spasm is there increased activity at the neuromuscular junction that could provide a rational target for Bt therapy. Such an increase is seen in several chronic pain conditions such as nocturnal muscle cramps, dystonia and certain cases of spasticity.

However, there are equally many common painful conditions in which evidence of such activity is lacking or speaks against it. These include conditions associated with myofascial trigger points, stiffness in ageing and various rheumatoid disorders, and postural changes due to muscle weakness or neurological disease. In these conditions the increased muscle tone inferred by clinical examination is not caused by abnormal neural activity but by alteration in the muscle contractility apparatus [16]. Commonly used methods in the clinic (palpation, description of pain) are inadequate for this kind of differential diagnosis of the many types of muscle pain. In addition, all the other pathophysiological mechanisms mentioned above bear on the perception of pain. Thus patients with chronic pain need a substantial diagnostic work-up if Bt treatment is contemplated.

In the past, a popular explanation of pain reduction following various treatments is 'breaking the vicious cycle (of pain and muscle tension/spasm)'. According to this concept, pain increases γ-motorneurone activity which in turn increases α-motorneurone activity leading to muscle spasm. The spasm increases the pain and perpetuates the cycle [10]. Thus Bt could effectively break the cycle both by blocking activity at α-motor endings and by reducing muscle spindle activity, which in turn would decrease afferent input into the central nervous system [21,22].

There is, however, practically no evidence of the pain–spasm–pain cycle maintaining pain in any chronic condition. A number of elegant studies in patients and healthy volunteers show that pain does not lead to increased EMG activity. If anything, muscle pain tends to inhibit, not facilitate, voluntary and reflex contractile activity of the same muscle [17].

Muscle spasm associated with increased EMG activity *may* be painful, but usually is not [23–25]. Pain may arise indirectly through ischaemia or mechanical distortion of muscle fibres. By blocking increased activity at the motor endings Bt interferes with the pathophysiological mechanism maintaining the pain, usually without affecting the aetiology of the underlying problem. However, in some conditions such as anal fissure healing is prevented by ischaemia due to sustained contraction of the inner anal sphincter [26]. Bt acts as a disease modifying agent in anal fissure by reducing the chronic neurally mediated smooth muscle overactivity, relieving ischaemia and permitting healing.

There is growing interest within pain medicine towards targeted treatment. Bt seems particularly suitable for this approach, provided that the limitations of its mode of action are observed. Unfortunately the present lack of knowledge of the pathophysiology of most musculoskeletal conditions has hampered these developments.

Head and neck pain

A number of open label studies and anecdotal reports in the late 1990s suggested that Bt injections help in different types of headache and neck pain [27–30]. The assumption was that the major aetiological factor is excessive pericranial muscle tension, from whatever cause, and that pain relief correlates with muscle relaxation, an inference we know is not tenable. These papers suffer from lack of control treatments, short follow-up and small numbers of patients, and therefore have limited scientific value. More importantly, because various other injection therapies (saline or cortisone injections, or acupuncture) also benefit some patients, these reports could not differentiate the effects of the needle insertion, injection, volume or toxin. I shall therefore not discuss these papers further.

There are very few published randomized placebo-controlled studies on Bt for pain which warrant discussion here. They deal with migraine and daily tension-type headache, as well as headache associated with extension injury of the neck.

Migraine

Some patients receiving Bt for cosmetic purposes claimed their migraines improved as well. This sparked interest in using Bt for migraine. Following an open label study, 123 patients took part in a multicentre double blind, placebo controlled study in the US [31].

The study was carried out in 12 centres and had a design similar to most pharmacological trials of migraine prophylaxis. Each patient received one set of injections into the frontalis, temporalis and glabellar muscles. The active treatment groups received 25 mu or 75 mu botulinum toxin type A (BtA) (Botox®, Allergan®), the placebo group an equivalent volume of vehicle. The protocol required a 1 month baseline, an injection visit, three monthly postinjection visits and completion of a headache diary. The patients recorded the frequency, duration and intensity of migraine attacks, as well as other headaches and consumption of analgesics. All the patients except one had moderate or severe headaches.

The results were interesting and somewhat unexpected. The baseline frequency of migraine attacks was around five per month. Though the frequency of moderate-to-severe headaches fell in all groups there was a statistically greater reduction in the 25 mu BtA group than in the placebo group or the 75 mu BtA at 2 months and 3 months. A similar pattern was seen for migraines of all severity combined. At 3 months, more patients in the 25 mu BtA group than in the other groups reported two fewer migraines. Some 45% of the 25 mu BtA group reported a decrease in migraine frequency of at least 50% as opposed to 24% in the vehicle group, a statistically significant difference ($P=0.046$).

Adverse effects included blepharoptosis, diplopia and injection site weakness. They were mild and transient and were seen almost exclusively in the BtA groups. They were almost as common in the 25 mu BtA as in the 75 mu BtA group. Compared to placebo only the 75 mu BtA dose produced significantly more frequent adverse effects.

This study was inconclusive and is difficult to interpret. The main outcome measure was reduction in the number of moderate to severe migraines per month, and the difference between the 25 mu BtA and saline groups was relatively minor (1.88 vs. 0.98 migraines/month). During the preinjection month the patients had on average one migraine per week; the reduction of one extra attack per month over placebo must be weighed against similar results obtained with acupuncture [32] or beta-blockers, dihydroergotamine and sodium valproate [33]. Interestingly, migraine attack severity also improved more in this group than either the 75 mu BtA or placebo groups. This improvement was seen only at 1 and 2 months. At 3 months, the 75 mu BtA group experienced the most severe headaches (statistical significance not given).

The fact that the 75 mu BtA group did not show more improvement than the placebo group in any outcome measure (apart from subject global assessment at 2 months) speaks against a direct prophylactic effect of the toxin. There are no other reports of a therapeutic window in low dose Bt therapy.

Prophylactic Bt injections for migraine remain unproven. Despite the weak evidence, the very potential of this treatment in migraine will inevitably prompt a string of open label uncontrolled studies. For instance, one interesting open study [34] reported total remission of headache attacks in 38/77 (51%) patients with 'true' migraine, after a low-dose Bt injection into the pericranial muscles, mainly around the glabella and forehead. There was a partial response in many more (data not provided). It appears that less than 10% of those injected had no improvement. The mean follow up period was 4 months.

These surprisingly attractive figures are tempered by several observations. Ten of 13 subjects with migraine were completely relieved of their acute attack 1–2 h after the injection, an unlikely benefit from Bt. In addition, these patients were not naive to Bt before the study started; they were being treated with the toxin at cosmetic surgery, otolaryngology and movement disorder/dystonia clinics. They were recruited if they reported headaches, but it is not clear how many were known to respond to Bt before the trial, or whether benefit was sustained with repeated injections [34].

These results resemble the early successes of acupuncture, which could not be repeated in randomized controlled trials [32]. The authors present an interesting theory that involves the blockade of release of vasoactive substances from the free terminals of trigeminal fibres. In the light of its reported effect on migraine, such a possibility needs to be kept in mind, although most studies seem to indicate that Bt is specific for cholinergic neurones in the periphery, and blockade of corelease of other transmitters has not been reported [35,36].

Chronic tension-type and myofascial neck pain

Injections into the neck muscles to treat tension-type headache and neck ache have yielded controversial results. The first properly controlled trial with a reasonable but still small number of patients showed no difference between Bt and placebo [37]. In this study, 33 patients with chronic neck pain fulfilling the criteria for myofascial pain were divided into three groups to receive either saline, 50 mu, or 100 mu BtA (Botox®). The patients were manually examined for the presence of myofascial trigger points in the straight neck muscles, and their tenderness was quantified with pressure algometry. Other measurements included a Neck and Pain Disability Score and the patients' subjective assessment of improvement. None of these measures showed any difference between the groups.

The patients were then offered a second injection of 100 mu BtA. For reasons not discussed only 39% of the participants took up the offer. Several patients in this self-selected group became pain-free. However, as there was no control for the effects of concomitant medication and physiotherapy, the crucial question of superiority of Bt treatment over saline injections remains unanswered.

Another open label study reported that patients who receive targeted physiotherapy as well as Bt injections show improvement [38]. This is undoubtedly so, but without a placebo injection group we cannot know whether physiotherapy, BtA or needles was the pivotal factor in this improvement. In addition, there was no attempt to define the presence of true muscle spasms before treatment. When the same authors conducted a double blind study of Bt versus placebo in chronic neck pain without physical therapy they found no difference between treatment [39]. At present, there is little to support the policy of combining these costly therapies as opposed to conventional treatment with analgesics and self-exercises.

Neck muscle injections with or without concomitant temporal muscle injections were studied in two groups of patients, with chronic tension headache or with pain following a whiplash-type neck extension injury [40,41]. The first study randomized 41 patients with a headache history ranging from 1 to 10 years to receive either saline or 50 mu BtA (Botox®) into the temporal or cervical (splenius capitis, trapezius) muscles using EMG guidance [40]. The patients kept a daily headache diary for a month before the injections and 3 months afterwards. The outcome measures were the change in headache-free days, change in a categorical (0–6) headache score and change in a chronic pain index. Thirty-nine patients completed the study (22 in the Bt group and 17 in the saline group). The Bt group showed improvement in all outcome measures while there were no changes in the saline group; comparisons at 2 and 3 months postinjection were significant. Side-effects were not reported; the authors only concluded there were no serious adverse effects.

This study has only been published in abstract form [40]. Inevitably, the interpretation is limited by the scantiness of data provided. For example, the frequency and severity of headaches were not reported. The participants appear to have been military personnel aged 18–53 years; no data on their sick leaves or work performance were given. The mean increase of headache-free days was 6 days per month in the BtA group as opposed to 1 day in the saline group, but the impact of this on daily functioning is difficult to interpret without baseline data. Also, concomitant drug consumption was not reported.

Canadian investigators randomized 30 patients suffering from whiplash associated pain into two groups. One group received BtA (Botox®) and the other received saline injections into neck muscle trigger points determined by manual palpation [41]. The headaches were considered to fulfil the criteria of cervicogenic headache, and were often precipitated by external pressure over the neck or occiput. Headache intensity was measured using a Visual Analogue Scale (VAS), and range of motion of the neck using a composite score. The follow-up assessments were at 2 weeks and 4 weeks only. The authors did not report between group differences but instead carried out statistical analyses in the two groups separately, comparing pre- and postinjection measures. They dropped four patients from the final analysis. Temporary improvement was seen in the BtA group but not in the saline group [41].

This study does not help to decide whether Bt injections are any better than saline injections in whiplash associated headache. There were few patients, no intention-to-treat analysis, no direct comparison between groups, short follow-up, and insufficient outcome measures. The same study was published under a different title, this time focusing on combined neck pain, headache and shoulder pain [42]. The results were presented in a slightly different format but were obviously on a par with the first study. In this study the data may not have been normally distributed as the standard errors of the means of the pain scores in the saline group appear exceptionally large.

Another controlled study with a similar parallel group design randomized 21 patients to receive either saline (10 patients) or BtA 200 mu (Dysport®, 11 patients) into pericranial muscles [43]. The patients kept a diary for a month before the injection and for 3 months afterwards. There were no differences between the two groups in headache frequency, pain intensity, consumption of analgesics, scalp tenderness, clinical global impression or overall well being. A quality-of-life questionnaire (Everyday-Life Questionnaire) indicated greater improvement for placebo-treated patients.

This study was designed to evaluate pertinent features of headache but it suffers from the small number of patients enrolled. The authors argue that the negative outcome is no surprise as only in a proportion of patients with tension-type headache is there evidence of abnormal EMG activity in pericranial muscles [17,44]. This small study cannot be used to draw inferences on pathophysiology or possible lack of benefit from treatment. Interestingly, their data shows that the saline injections themselves can be very effective. Headache intensity in the saline group was reduced by 50% and frequency by 60% over a 3-month follow-up period [43].

One cannot conclude from any of the above studies whether or not Bt is more effective in chronic headache than saline injections (or any other injections, including acupuncture and other forms of 'dry needling'). The major problem in all published studies to date is the disregard of the pathophysiological mechanisms of headache on the one hand and the selective mode of action of Bt on the other. The advantages and disadvantages of Bt might be clearer if trials selected patients on the basis of presence (or not) of abnormal pericranial muscle EMG activity, had added a dry needle treatment and 'observation-only' arm, and recruited enough patients to allow robust statistical analysis.

While the flawed methodology in the above studies fails to provide evidence of efficacy of BtA treatment of chronic headache, it would be unwise to completely rule out benefit. Benefit is unlikely to result from the most prominent effect of Bt, blockade of cholinergic neurotransmission. Rather, it might affect some of the numerous neurotransmitters associated with pain transmission, some of which coexist in cholinergic nerve endings. We need to know more about the pathophysiology of tension-type headache and migraine so we can build a logical case based on facts rather than assumptions.

Other abstracts [45–47] have reported open label studies that do not add to our current understanding, and fail to impress for treatment results. A further study —available as a poster abstract only —on migraine prophylaxis involved 56 patients and 848 migraine attacks, and focused on injection sites. It narrowly suggested superiority of BtA over placebo when injected at frontal and temporal sites at the same time [48]. The significant difference, however, was in reduction of migraine pain severity and not migraine frequency or duration. These results have to be weighed against the disclosure of Allergan, Inc. at the Headache World 2000 Congress in London that the larger of the two proof-of-concept studies involving *in toto* more than 500 patients showed no significant difference between BtA and saline [49]. Obviously one should view claims of efficacy of Bt in headache with considerable reservation and await results from large randomized controlled trials, studies involving comparator treatments, and analyses of cost effectiveness before adding Bt treatment to one's armamentarium.

Low back pain

Low back pain remains one of the commonest health problems and significantly reduces quality of life. Estimates of prevalence of chronic mechanical low back pain range from 4.4 to 30% [50]. There are no estimates available for low back pain related to muscle dysfunction, perhaps because it would be too complicated to establish criteria for muscular low back pain for epidemiological surveys.

Where there is obvious postural change or a great deal of muscle tenderness, many clinicians invoke myofascial mechanisms as the cause, or at least consider that they contribute to the pain [51]. Structures potentially provoking chronic back pain include ligaments, muscles and fascia, outer layers of the annulus fibrosus, facet joints, the vertebral periosteum, blood vessels and nerve roots [52]. However, even with modern imaging techniques it is unusual to identify a specific cause in individual cases.

Porta compared deep back or neck muscle injections with BtA (Botox®) 80, 100 or 150 mu (depending on the muscle) against 80 mg methylprednisolone [53]. The patients had 'myofascial syndromes associated with spasm', and were chosen if they had trigger points or experienced pain on manoeuvre or stretching. Patients with a history of overt bone or disc disease or previous operations were excluded. Each patient received one injection into one of iliopsoas, piriformis or scalenus under computed tomography (CT) guidance, and then underwent a rigorous physiotherapeutic exercise programme. There was no difference between groups in pain relief at 1 month; however, at 2 months the Bt group had significantly less pain. No disability or quality-of-life measures were reported.

This study is interesting in that it involves a comparator drug, a rare example of the kind of study that is dearly needed. However, there are several weaknesses in the study design hampering interpretation of the results. There was no group that did not receive an injection, yet all patients received physiotherapy. Only two low back muscles and one neck muscle were chosen, and most injections were only carried out unilaterally. This suggests that these patients were unlikely to represent cases of common mechanical back pain or neck pain, in which pain is much more evenly distributed. In addition, it is a single author study in which the investigator recruited patients, gave the injections and reassessed the patients. Blinding may have been difficult because methylprednisolone tends to cause clouding in the syringe. Thus this study needs corroboration, preferably in a larger group of patients with clearly defined clinical inclusion criteria and a methodical approach to the choice of muscles to be injected. An independent assessor truly blinded to the interventions would provide a less easily criticised objective assessment.

Another placebo-controlled trial compared one set of paraspinal injections of 200 mu BtA (Botox®) against placebo in 28 patients with mechanical low back pain [54]. At 3 weeks 73% of the Bt group vs. 25% of the saline group showed more than 50% pain relief (as measured on a visual analogue scale, $P=0.012$); the figures at 8 weeks were 60% and 13%, respectively ($P=0.009$). Similar improvement was seen in functional ability, assessed by the Oswestry Disability Index.

A further randomized placebo-controlled trial has been published, but only in abstract form [55]. Seventy-two unoperated patients with chronic low back pain and muscle spasm enrolled at 10 separate centres and were randomized to receive placebo or 120, 180 or 240 mu BtA (Botox®) into the paraspinal muscles [54]. Outcome measures included pain, muscle spasm, physician and patient global assessment and overall disability. All patients groups improved, however, for muscle spasm and physician global assessment the high-dose group improved statistically more than the placebo group at 6 and 12 weeks.

None of these studies assessed muscle function with EMG, and muscle spasm was only evaluated arbitrarily by fingertip compression. It is not clear why Bt injection into the paraspinal muscles is effective in reducing low back pain. EMG studies suggest that in unoperated backs there is no increase in paraspinal activity [56], although not all authors agree [57]. It is of note that when Alo *et al.* [27] reported their results from an uncontrolled case series, it became evident that their technique was completely different from the ones above. Patients received up to three sets of injections of BtA (Botox® 90–300 mu) into both paraspinal and deep back muscles including the psoas, quadratus lumborum and piriformis, and the follow up period was much longer. The best results were seen at 6 months [27].

Though the published results seem favourable, a novice in this therapy will be bewildered by the enormous variability of patient recruitment, choice of muscles, dosage and follow up. Before we can provide firm recommendations for use of Bt in low back pain we need a much larger study using a protocol with detailed preinjection assessment, proof from EMG that excessive neuromuscular activity is present, standardized injection techniques and outcome measures including quality of life and functional ability. To date, no such study has been published.

Pain associated with dystonia and spasticity

Dystonias and most cases of spasticity are good examples of conditions in which the known action of Bt at the neuromuscular junction provides the rationale for treatment. A number of open label studies indicate that pain frequently associated with these conditions tends to improve, though the degree of such improvement is less clear. Again, there are few well designed and properly controlled studies, and inevitably this raises the question of how significant the addition of the toxin into injected saline is. A further problem is that pain itself does not feature high in these studies, possibly because not all patients have significant pain. A good case in question is the study by Snow *et al.* who specifically looked at this only to find out that their patients with multiple sclerosis (MS) and spasticity were not troubled by pain at all [58]. Most studies published on this topic are case series focusing on aspects other than pain; they evaluate pain only as a secondary outcome measure and use evaluation tools too crude for accurate conclusions. A particular problem is that the investigators have not distinguished spasticity-induced pain from central pain which is relatively common in both stroke and MS—the two groups most studied in this field. A recent prospective open label study by Wissel *et al.* [59] involving 60 patients selected pain and functional impairment as the primary outcome measure. Unfortunately, the study did not assess pain independently of function, and there was no third party investigator. Despite these weaknesses, the study showed improvement in the global score of combined pain and function after just one injection. In the 43 chronic cases, the mean reduction on a categorical scale of 0–4 was 0.9 ($P <$ 0.001) and, based on this result and patients' further ratings, the authors concluded that the amelioration of symptoms corresponded to 'moderate pain relief without improvement in function' [59]. Most of the patients remained on other antispasticity treatment, and the implicit conclusion has to be that the study supports the use of Bt as an add-on treatment for spasticity-induced pain.

Table 17.1 [2,4,5,60–64] lists double blind placebo controlled studies in dystonia and spasticity that have included pain as one of the outcome measures. Any conclusions are hampered by the small numbers of patients recruited and crude tools used to assess pain. Other studies make allusions to pain in the two conditions. Gelb and coworkers [65] comment on improvement in a subjective composite score of pain and dystonic

Table 17.1 Selection of published double-blind randomized controlled trials with pain as an endpoint.

Authors	Diagnosis	Number of patients with pain recruited	Study design	Pain improved	Method of measurement of pain relief used
Tsui et al. [60]	Cervical dystonia	16 BtA, 100 mu* / 17 placebo	Crossover	BtA, 14/16 / Placebo, 4/17 (P<0.02)	Pain relief vs. no pain relief (no scale)
Lorentz et al. [5]	Cervical dystonia	19 BtA, 150 mu* / 19 placebo	Crossover	BtA, 12/19 / Placebo, 1/18 (P<0.002)	Pain relief vs. no pain relief (no scale)
Blackie and Lee [2]	Cervical dystonia	16BtA, 960 mu‡ / 16 placebo	Crossover	BtA, 12/16 / Placebo, 2/16	Visual Analogue Scale / Mean Visual Analogue Scale fell from 6.1 to 3.3
Greene et al. [4]	Cervical dystonia	20BtA, 140–165 mu* / 18 placebo	Parallel group	BtA, 40% / Placebo 5% (P<0.003)	—
Lew et al. [61]	Cervical dystonia	31 BtB, 2500 mu / 31 BtB, 5000 mu / 30 BtB, 10000 mu / 31 placebo	Parallel group	2500 mu, 22% / 5000 mu, 21–22% / 10000 mu, 29–32% / Placebo, 0.5–5.0%	Visual Analogue Scale, TWSTRS Pain Subscale
Bakheit et al. [62]	Arm spasticity following stroke	22 BtA‡, 500 mu / 22 BtA‡, 1000 mu / 19 BtA‡, 1500 mu / 19 placebo	Parallel group	500 mu group, 46% / 1000 mu group, 30% / 1500 mu group, 40% / Placebo group, 43%	Categorical pain score 0–3 / Baseline pain levels not reported
Hyman et al. [63]	Hip adductor spasticity in MS (upper leg pain)	10 BtA‡, 500 mu / 14 BtA‡, 1000 mu / 10 BtA‡, 1500 mu / 13 placebo	Parallel group	500 mu group, no change / 1000 mu group, 1 improved / 1500 mu group, 4 improved / Placebo group, 7 improved	Number of pain free patients per group
Bhakta et al. [64]	Arm spasticity following stroke	26 who received either BtA‡, 1000 mu or placebo	Parallel group	Placebo group, no change / BtA group, −2 (NS)	Pain relief scale (0–10)

*Botox®; ‡Dysport®, Ipsen®.

BtA, botulinum toxin A; BtB, botulinum toxin B; mu, mouse unit; NS, not significant; TWSTRS, Toronto Western Spasmodic Torticollis Rating Scale.

posture; BtA 50–280 mu (Botox®) appeared superior to placebo irrespective of the dose used, whereas in poststroke limb spasticity there was no such effect [66]. A smaller study noted that in five patients BtA relieved frequent painful spasms [24].

The published evidence from randomized controlled trials suggests that in cervical dystonia Bt injections provide significant short-term alleviation of pain whereas in MS and stroke related spasticity such supportive evidence is scarce. In spasticity it is possible that the negative results obtained so far reflect deficiencies in study methodology [67] or lack of effect of the toxin. In spasticity there are likely to be several mechanisms that generate the pain, and it is unlikely that Bt with its pharmacologically narrow mode of action is able to block many of them. Future studies may show whether this treatment helps any subgroup of patients with spasticity, such as those with intermittent severely painful spasms.

Anal fissure (see also Chapter 15)

Most anal fissures are idiopathic with no identifiable underlying disease process. Fissures may also develop after trauma (usually obstetric or surgical), or be associated with Crohn's disease, ulcerative colitis, human immunodeficiency virus (HIV) infection, or syphilis [26].

The hallmark of chronic anal fissure is hypertonicity of the internal anal sphincter. This is associated with reduced local vascular perfusion. Small traumatic tears in the lining of the anal canal become chronic because the reduced blood supply is insufficient to promote healing [26]. Anal fissures cause pain especially after defecation, and the pain tends to improve as the tear heals. Current treatment aims to reduce sphincter tone and improve local blood supply.

There are several operations available for anal fissure. Surgeons currently favour lateral sphincterectomy because of its efficacy and relative safety. Yet, in long-term follow-up studies one-third of patients were incontinent of flatus and 5% complained of faecal soiling [26]. Other, less traumatizing treatment methods have therefore become popular.

Pharmacological approaches include nitric oxide donors (notably topical glyceryl trinitrate), calcium antagonists and Bt injections into the internal sphincter reduce anal pressure. Bt probably inhibits smooth muscle contractions by a presynaptic cholinergic mechanism, as in skeletal muscle.

In a randomized placebo controlled study involving 30 patients, the healing rate at 2 months following two injections of 20 mu BtA (Botox®) into the internal anal sphincter was 73% while in the placebo group it remained as low as 13% [68]. The same group went on to perform a comparative study with topical nitroglycerin [69]. In the latter study with a similar set-up, 50 patients were randomized to receive an intrasphincteric injection of 50 mu BtA (Botox®), or to receive 0.2% nitroglycerin ointment to be applied topically to the anus and anal canal twice a day for 6 weeks. At 1 month, 22/25 (88%) patients in the BtA group had healed fissures as opposed to 10/25 (40%) in the nitroglycerin group. At 2 months, these figures were 24/25 (96%) and 15/25 (60%), respectively. At 2 months, anal manometry demonstrated significantly more reduction in resting anal pressures in the BtA group (29%) than in the nitroglycerin group (14%). Adverse effects were only seen in the nitroglycerin group, who had transient headaches [69].

Recent open label studies suggest that most patients have improved at 3 months [70]. In a single long-term follow-up study, patients receiving either 15 or 20 mu BtA (Botox®), and some receiving 25 mu as a second injection, were assessed at 24 and 19 months, respectively. None of the patients who were healed at 2 months postinjection relapsed during this follow-up [71].

If corroborated, these very interesting results point to a longer term effect than could be assumed on the basis of chemodenervation. The exact pathogenesis of anal fissure is not known but probably involves dysregulation of autonomic and enteric neural stimulation of smooth muscle. Long-term relaxation of the sphincter may alter the regulatory drive enough to prevent recurrence. Alternatively, regeneration of the cholinergic terminals may be incomplete, preventing similar excessive contraction of the sphincter.

Achalasia

Achalasia is a primary oesophageal motility disorder characterized by the absence of peristalsis, an elevated pressure of the lower oesophageal sphincter, and incomplete relaxation of the sphincter during swallowing. Two-thirds of patients complain of chest pain [72]. Conventional treatments include balloon dilatation and myotomy aimed at relieving the functional obstruction of the distal oesophagus. Several groups have reported consistent results from intrasphincteric injection of Bt.

Following a pilot study, Pasricha et al. performed a double blind placebo controlled trial in 21 patients with achalasia [73]. Eleven received 80 mu BtA (Botox®) and 10 patients received saline injections into the lower oesophageal sphincter using endoscopy. After 1 week 9/11 of the Bt group had improved but only 1/10 in the saline group. There were statistically significant differences between groups in total symptom scores, and in pressure and width of the opening of the lower oesophageal sphincter. All 10 in the placebo group then received an injection of Bt with good initial effect. Some patients relapsed after the 1st month, but by 6 months 14/21 were still in remission [73].

Two other groups observed substantial benefit in larger groups of patients. Cuillere et al. reported clinical improvement in 60% of their patients at 6 months [74]. Another multicentre dose-finding study involved 118 patients who received varying doses of Bt intrasphincterically. About three-quarters reported initial symptom reduction. Patients who received two injections of 100 mu BtA (Botox®) 30 days apart showed the best results, with a remission rate of 60% after a mean of 12 months (range 7–24 months) [75]. Non-responders were generally those with more 'vigorous' achalasia. Oesophageal manometry showed significantly greater improvement in the Lower Oesophageal Sphincter Scores among responders.

These studies suggest that intrasphincteric BtA is a safe and effective treatment of achalasia in the short and medium term. Concerns relate to possible surgical problems that may arise if an operation is needed later [76]. The cost-effectiveness of this treatment is not clear [77].

Conclusions

At present, the evidence for the use of Bt injections to reduce pain is limited to a few positive results in conditions characterized by chronic muscle contraction (whether in smooth or skeletal muscle). Whether reduction in contraction or some other mechanism explains this benefit will require further research. In all these conditions the basic pathology involves aberration of the nervous regulation of the target organs, and it may well be that the effects of Bt will eventually be associated with neurogenic mechanisms as well [22,78,79].

Despite considerable interest expressed by some authors, evidence supporting Bt for headaches and various common musculoskeletal conditions is too meagre for firm conclusions. Problems in this promising field include a lack of understanding of the basic mechanisms that generate pain, and the traditional tendency of investigators to focus more on anatomy and assumed aetiology than on pathophysiology. We need well-designed controlled studies based on sound hypotheses to ascertain whether or not this powerful treatment has anything to offer to chronic pain patients. The widespread practice of lumping patients with a descriptive diagnosis (tension-type headache, myofascial pain, low back pain) together is likely to dilute any therapeutic effect trials might find with this treatment. Patient selection will be important. They should have muscle pain plus appropriate electrophysiological evidence of increased muscle contraction.

Investigators should adopt straightforward measures of pain and muscle tension separately, to identify candidates for double blind studies and to monitor the results. Simple clinical measures may suffice to score muscle activity in dystonia or spasticity, but the mechanism generating pain is often unclear and may involve some other organ. Future studies might show that Bt can induce plastic changes in the afferent pathways, similar to those seen in the peripheral motorneurones and central motor nuclei [80,81]. Bt may have effects in addition to blockade of release of acetylcholine into the synaptic cleft. If release of other peptides that coexist in the cholinergic terminals is also reduced, the toxin may prove useful in prevention of peripheral sensitization and ensuing protracted pain. Some very preliminary data suggest this may be possible, but we need much more basic research before drawing any firm conclusion.

There are several other potential indications for Bt therapy for pain relief, such as prevention of postoperative pain in muscles liable to spasm. A randomized controlled study showed that prophylactic Bt injections into adductor muscles reduce pain and speed recovery after adductor tenotomy in children with spastic cerebral palsy [82]. Similarly, patients with prolonged postoperative pain following cholecystectomy may be suitable for endoscopic injection of Bt into the sphincter of Oddi [83]. Other targets could be muscle cramps induced by chronic nerve irritation or hereditary muscle–cramp fasciculation syndromes, which are known to be associated with excessive EMG activity [24], and regional pain-provoking muscle spasms seen in MS and spinal cord injury.

In conclusion, there is potential to use Bt creatively in primarily painful conditions, but to date the potential has not been fully exploited. There are many uncontrolled studies and unjustifiable claims of efficacy. Controlled studies are far fewer, and have conflicting results. The bulk of existing evidence does not support the use of Bt in the treatment of the most common chronic pain conditions. We do not know whether there are subgroups of patients with chronic intractable pain who might benefit. The onus is on investigators to evaluate Bt critically and to focus studies to answer far more specific questions.

References

1 Jankovic J, Schwartz K. Botulinum toxin injections for cervical dystonia. *Neurology* 1990; **40**: 277–80.
2 Blackie JD, Lees AJ. Botulinum toxin treatment in spasmodic torticollis. *J Neurol, Neurosurgery Psychiatry* 1990; **53**: 640–3.
3 Anderson TJ, Rivest J, Stell R *et al*. Botulinum toxin treatment of spasmodic torticollis. *J Royal Soc Med* 1992; **85**: 524–9.
4 Greene P, Kang U, Fahn S *et al*. Double blind, placebo-controlled trial of botulinum toxin injections for the treatment of spasmodic torticollis. *Neurology* 1990; **40**: 1213–8.
5 Lorentz IT, Subramaniam SS, Yiannikas C. Treatment of idiopathic spasmodic torticollis with botulinum toxin A: a double blind study on 23 patients. *Mov Disord* 1991; **6**: 145–50.
6 Naumann M, Yakovleff A, Durif F. A randomized, double blind, crossover comparison of the safety and efficacy of original BOTOX® (botulinum toxin type A) in the treatment of cervical dystonia. *J Neurol* 2002; **249**: 57–63.
7 Brin MF, Fahn S, Moskowitz C *et al*. Localized injections of botulinum toxin for the treatment of focal dystonia and hemifacial spasm. *Mov Disord* 1987; **2**: 237–54.
8 Pacchetti C, Albani G, Martignoni E *et al*. 'Off' painful dystonia in Parkinson's disease treated with botulinum toxin. *Mov Disord* 1995; **10**: 333–6.
9 Guyer BM. Mechanisms of botulinum toxin in the relief of chronic pain. *Current Rev Pain* 1999; **3**: 427–31.
10 Porta M, Perretti A, Gamba M, Luccarelli G, Maurizio F. The rationale and results of treating muscle spasm and myofascial syndromes with botulinum toxin A. *Pain Digest* 1998; **8**: 346–52.
11 Drewes AM, Jennum P. Epidemiology of myofascial pain, low back pain, morning stiffness and sleep-related complaints in the general population. *J Musculoskeletal Pain* 1995; **3**: 68–72.
12 Wolfe F, Ros K, Anderson J, Russell IJ, Hebert L. The prevalence and characteristics of fibromyalgia in the general population. *Arthritis Rheum* 1995; **38**: 19–28.
13 Rasmussen BK, Jensen R, Schroll M, Olesen J. Epidemiology of headache in general population—a prevalence study. *J Clin Epidemiol* 1991; **44**: 1147–57.
14 Barnsley L, Lord SM, Bogduk N. Whiplash injuries. *Pain* 1994; **58**: 283–307.
15 Hamer AJ, Gargan MF, Bannister GC, Nelson RF. Whiplash injury and surgically treated disc disease. *Injury* 1993; **24**: 549–50.
16 Mense S. Nociception from skeletal muscle in relation to clinical muscle pain. *Pain* 1993; **54**: 241–89.

17 Simons DG, Mense S. Understanding and measurement of muscle tone as related to clinical muscle pain. *Pain* 1998; **75**: 1–7.

18 Johansen MK, Graven-Nielsen T, Olesen AS, Arendt-Nielsen L. Generalised muscular hyperalgesia in chronic whiplash syndrome. *Pain* 1999; **83**: 229–34.

19 Sorensen J, Graven-Nielsen T, Henriksson KG, Bengtsson M, Arendt-Nielsen L. Hyperexcitability in fibromyalgia. *J Rheumatol* 1998; **25**: 152–5.

20 Karst M, Rollnik JD, Fink M, Reinhard M, Piepenbrock S. Pressure pain threshold and needle acupuncture in chronic tension-type headache — a double blind placebo-controlled trial. *Pain* 2000; **88**: 199–203.

21 Rosales RL, Arimura K, Takenaga S, Osame M. Extrafusal and intrafusal effects in experimental botulinum toxin A injections. *Muscle Nerve* 1996; **19**: 488–96.

22 Giladi N. The mechanism of action of botulinum toxin type A in focal dystonia is most probably through its dual effect on efferent (motor) and afferent pathways at the injected site. *J Neurol Sci* 1997; **152**: 132–5.

23 Kutvonen O, Nurmikko T. Pain in spasmodic torticollis. *Pain* 1997; **69**: 279–86.

24 Bartolasi L, Priori A, Tomelleri G *et al*. Botulinum toxin treatment of muscle cramps: a clinical and neurophysiological study. *Ann Neurol* 1997; **41**: 181–6.

25 Richardson D, Sheean G, Werring D *et al*. Evaluating the role of botulinum toxin in the management of focal hypertonia in adults. *J Neurol, Neurosurgery Psychiatry* 2000; **69**: 499–506.

26 Bhardwaj R, Vaizey CJ, Boulos BP, Hoyle CHV. Neurogenic properties of the internal anal sphincter: therapeutic rationale for anal fissures. *Gut* 2000; **46**: 861–8.

27 Alo KM, Yland MJ, Kramer DL, Charnov JH, Redko V. Botulinum toxin in the treatment of myofascial pain. *Pain Clinic* 1997; **2**: 107–16.

28 Freund B, Schwartz M, Symington JM. The use of botulinum toxin for the treatment of temporomandibular disorders: preliminary findings. *J Oral Maxillofacial Surg* 1999; **57**: 916–20.

29 Freund B, Schwartz M, Symington JM. Botulinum toxin: new treatment for temporomandibular disorders. *Br J Oral Maxillofacial Surgery* 2000; **38**: 466–71.

30 Relja M. Treatment of tension-type headache by local injection of botulinum toxin. *European J Neurol* 1997; **4** (Suppl. 2): S71–3.

31 Silberstein S, Mathew N, Saper J, Jenkins S. Botulinum toxin type A as a migraine preventive treatment. For the BOTOX® Migraine Clinical Research group. *Headache* 2000; **40**: 445–50.

32 Manias P, Tagaros G, Karageorgiou K. Acupuncture in headache: a critical review. *Clin J Pain* 2000; **16**: 334–9.

33 Ferrari MD. Migraine. *Lancet* 1998; **351**: 1043–51.

34 Binder WJ, Brin MF, Blitzer A, Schoenrock LD. Botulinum toxin type A (BOTOX®) for treatment of migraine headaches: an open label study. *Otolaryngol — Head Neck Surg* 2000; **123**: 660–76.

35 Shaari CM, Sanders I, Wu B-E, Biller HF. Rhinorrhea is decreased in dogs after nasal application of botulinum toxin. *Otolaryngol — Head Neck Surg* 1995; **112**: 566–71.

36 Black JD, Dolly JO. Selective location of acceptors for botulinum neurotoxin A in the central and peripheral nervous systems. *Neuroscience* 1987; **23**: 767–79.

37 Wheeler AH, Goolkasian P, Gretz SS. A randomized, double blind, prospective pilot study of botulinum toxin injection for refractory, unilateral, cervicothoracic, paraspinal, myofascial pain syndrome. *Spine* 1998; **23**: 1662–6.

38 Wheeler AH, Goolkasia P. Open label assessment of botulinum toxin A for pain treatment in a private outpatient setting. *J Musculoskel Pain* 2001; **9**: 67–82.

39 Wheeler AH, Goolkasian P, Gretz SS. Botulinum toxin A for the treatment of chronic neck pain. *Pain* 2001; **94**: 255–60.

40 Smuts JA, Baker MK, Smuts HM *et al*. Botulinum toxin type A as prophylactic treatment in chronic tension type headache. *Cephalagia* 1999; **19**: 454.

41 Freund BJ, Schwartz M. Treatment of whiplash associated with neck pain with botulinum toxin botulinum toxin: a pilot study. *J Rheumatol* 2000; **27**: 481–4.

42 Freund BJ, Scwartz M. Treatment of chronic cervical-associated headache with botulinum toxin: a pilot study. *Headache* 2000; **40**: 231–6.

43 Rollnik JD, Tanneberger O, Schubert M, Schnbeider U, Dengler R. Treatment of tension-type headache with botulinum toxin type A: a double blind, placebo-controlled study. *Headache* 2000; **40**: 300–5.

44 Arena JG, Hannah SL, Bruno GM, Smith JD, Meador KJ. Effect of movement and position on the muscle activity in tension headache sufferers during and between headaches. *J Psychosomatic Res* 1991; **35**: 187–95.

45 Mauskop A, Basdeo R. Botulinum toxin is effective prophylactic therapy for migraines. *Cephalalgia* 2000; **20**: 422.

46 Relja MA. Treatment of tension-type headache with botulinum toxin: 1-year follow up. *Cephalalgia* 2000; **20**: 336.

47 Smuts JA, Barnard PWA. Botulinum toxin A in the treatment of headache syndromes. *Cephalalgia* 2000; **20**: 332.

48 Brin MF, Swope DM, O'Brien C, Abbasi S, Pogoda JM. Botox® for migraine: double blind, placebo controlled, region-specific evaluation. *Abstract Cephalalgia* 2000; **20**: 421–2.

49 Anonymous. Botox® in migraine prophylaxis. *Scrip* 2000; **24**: 2577.

50 Dionne CE. Low back pain. In: Crombie IK, Croft PR, Linton SJ, LeResche L, VonKorff M, eds. *Epidemiology of Pain*. Seattle: IASP Press, 1999: 283–97.

51 Travell JG, Simons DG. Myofascial pain and dysfunction. In: Travell JG, Simons DG, eds. *The Trigger Point Manual*, vol. 2. Baltimore: Williams & Wilkins, 1983.

52 Deyo RA. What can history and physical examination tell us about low back pain? *JAMA* 1992; **268**: 760–5.

53 Porta M. A comparative trial of botulinum toxin type A and methylprednisolone for the treatment of myofascial pain syndrome and pain from chronic muscle spasm. *Pain* 2000; **85**: 101–5.

54 Foster L, Clapp L, Eriksson M, Jabbari B. Botulinum toxin A and chronic low back pain. A randomized double controlled pain. *Neurology* 2001; **56**: 1290–3.

55 Knusel B, DeGryse R, Grant M *et al.* Intramuscular injection of botulinum toxin type A (BOTOX®) in chronic low back pain associated with muscle spasm. Abstract. 17th Annual Scientific Meeting, American Pain Society, San Diego, CA, 1998.

56 Arena JG, Sherman RA, Bruno GM, Young TR. Electromyographic recordings of low back pain subjects in six different positions: effect of pain levels. *Pain* 1991; **45**: 23–8.

57 Sihvonen T, Partanen J, Hanninen O, Soimakallio S. Electric behavior of low back muscles during lumbar pelvic rhythm in low back pain patients and healthy controls. *Arch Phys Med Rehab* 1991; **72**: 1080–7.

58 Snow BJ, Tsui JKC, Bhatt MH *et al.* Treatment of spasticity with botulinum toxin: a double-blind study. *Ann Neurol* 1990; **28**: 512–5.

59 Wissel J, Muller J, Dressnandt J *et al.* Management of spasticity associated pain with botulinum toxin A. *J Pain Symptom manage* 2000; **20**: 44–9.

60 Tsui JKC, Eisen A, Stoessl AJ *et al.* Double blind study of botulinum toxin in spasmodic torticollis. *Lancet* 1986; **ii**: 245–7.

61 Lew MF, Adornato BT, Duane DD *et al.* Botulinum toxin type B: a double-blind, placebo-controlled, safety and efficacy study in cervical dystonia. *Neurology* 1997; **49**: 701–7.

62 Bakheit AMO, Thilmann AF, Ward AB *et al.* A randomized, double-blind, placebo-controlled. Dose-ranging study to compare efficacy and safety of three doses of botulinum toxin type A (Dysport) with placebo in upper limb spasticity after stroke. *Stroke* 2000; **31**: 2402–6.

63 Hyman N, Barnes M, Bhakta BB *et al.* Botulinum toxin (Dysport) treatment of hip adductor spasticity in multiple sclerosis: a prospective, randomized, double blind, placebo controlled, dose ranging study. *J Neurol Neurosurg* 2000; **68**: 707–12.

64 Bhakta BB, Cozens JA, Chamerlain MA, Bamford JM. Impact of botulinum toxin A on disability and

career burden due to arm spasticity after stroke: a randomized double blind placebo controlled trial. *J Neurol Neurosurg Psychiatry* 2000; **69**: 217–22.

65 Gelb DJ, Lowenstein DH, Aminoff MJ. Controlled trial of botulinum toxin injections in the treatment of spasmodic torticollis. *Neurology* 1989; **39**: 80–4.

66 Simpson DM, Alexander DN, O'Brien CF *et al.* Botulinum toxin type A in the treatment of upper extremity spasticity: a randomized, double-blind, placebo-controlled trial. *Neurology* 1996; **46**: 1306–10.

67 Sheean G. Botulinum treatment of spasticity: why is it so difficult to show a functional benefit. *Curr Opin Neurol* 2001; **14**: 771–6.

68 Maria G, Cassetta E, Gui D *et al.* A comparison of botulinum toxin and saline for the treatment of chronic anal fissure. *N Engl J Med* 1998; **338**: 217–20.

69 Brisinda G, Maria G, Bentivoglio AR *et al.* A comparison of injections of botulinum toxin and topical nitroglycerin ointment for the treatment of chronic anal fissure. *N Engl J Med* 1999; **341**: 65–9.

70 Jost WH, Schrank B. Chronic anal fissures treated with botulinum toxin injections: a dose finding study with Dysport®. *Colorectal Dis* 1999; **1**: 26–8.

71 Maria G, Brisinda G, Bentivoglio AR *et al.* Botulinum toxin injections in the internal anal sphincter for the treatment of chronic anal fissure. *Ann Surg* 1998; **228**: 664–9.

72 Eckardt VF, Stauf B, Bernhard G. Chest pain in achalasia, patient characteristics and clinical course. *Gastroenterology* 1999; **116**: 1300–4.

73 Pasricha PJ, Ravich WJ, Hendrix TR *et al.* Intrasphincteric botulinum toxin for the treatment of achalasia. *N Engl J Med* 1995; **322**: 774–8.

74 Cuilliere C, Ducrotte P, Zerbib F *et al.* Achalasia: outcome of patients treated with intrasphincteric injection of botulinum toxin. *Gut* 1997; **41**: 87–92.

75 Annese V, Bassotti G, Coccia G *et al.* A multicentre randomized study of intrasphincteric botulinum toxin in patients with oesophageal achalasia. *Gut* 2000; **46**: 597–600.

76 Bonavina L, Incarnone R, Reitano M, Antoniazzi L, Peracchia A. Does previous endoscopic treatment affect the outcome of laparoscopic Heller myotomy? *Ann Chir* 2000; **125**: 45–9.

77 Panaccione R, Gregor JC, Reynolds RP, Preiksaitis HG. Intrasphincteric botulinum toxin versus pneumatic dilatation of achalasia: a cost minimization analysis. *Gastrointest Endosc* 1999; **50**: 492–8.

78 Hallett M. How does botulinum toxin work? [Editorial] *Ann Neurol* 2000; **48**: 7–8.

79 Hallett M. One man's poison—clinical applications on botulinum toxin. [Editorial] *N Engl J Med* 1999; **337**: 118–19.

80 Tarabal O, Caldero J, Ribera J *et al.* Regulation of motoneuronal calcitonin gene-related peptide (CGRP) during axonal growth and neuromuscular synapticplasticity induced by botulinum toxin. *European J Neurosci* 1996; **8**: 829–36.

81 Humm AM, Pabst C, Lauterburg T, Burgunder JM. Enkephalin and aFGF are differentially regulated in rat spinal motoneurons after chemodenervation with botulinum toxin. *Exp Neurol* 2000; **161**: 361–72.

82 Barwood S, Baillieu C, Boyd R *et al.* Analgesic effects of botulinum toxin A, a randomized, placebo-controlled clinical trial. *Dev Med Child Neurol* 2000; **42**: 116–21.

83 Banerjee B, Miedema B, Saiffudin T, Marshall JB. Intrasphincteric botulinum toxin type A for the diagnosis of sphincter of Oddi dysfunction: a case report. *Surg Laparosc Endosc Percutan Tech* 1999; **9**: 194–6.

CHAPTER 18

Cosmetic indications

BORIS SOMMER & NICK LOWE

Introduction

Botulinum toxin A (BtA) is becoming a very popular facial cosmetic treatment and is widely used to treat hyperfunctional lines including glabellar lines, horizontal forehead lines, crow's feet and mesolabial folds [1–11]. Carruthers and Carruthers first reported its value in improving glabellar frown in 1992 [12]. It has been used extensively since then in clinical practice, alone and in conjunction with other cosmetic procedures.

BtA is a potent drug that blocks presynaptic acetylcholine release and causes transient and dose-dependent muscle weakness. Because facial lines result in part from the repetitive contraction of the underlying facial muscles and their action on the skin, the reduction in facial muscle tone by BtA helps eliminate facial lines at their source.

Review of botulinum toxin in cosmetic indications

Despite its extensive use in clinical dermatological practice, there are still relatively few controlled dose-ranging studies that have been published on BtA for aesthetic use. All of the studies have been conducted using the product Botox®.

Glabellar lines

A dose–response study [13] enrolled 46 women and tested different BtA doses injected into the glabellar region. Five injection sites were injected in each patient with a total dose per glabellar area of 5.0, 12.5, 20.0, 25.0 and 50.0 mu Botox®. The authors concluded that an effective starting dose for female glabellar lines is between a total dose of 12.5–20.0 mu or 2.5–4.0 mu per injection site. A 1-year two-stage study [14] examined the safety and efficacy of repeat treatment with BtA for glabellar lines. In the first stage, 537 patients were treated in a randomized, blinded fashion with either placebo or 20 mu BtA (Botox®). In the second stage, 373 of these subjects received two open-label treatments with BtA. All injections were separated by a 4-month follow-up period. At every follow-up visit in the first stage, subjects treated with BtA showed significantly greater reductions in glabellar line severity, both at rest and at maximum frown, and significantly greater improvements in self-assessed appearance than subjects treated with placebo ($P < 0.001$). These benefits not only persisted in the second stage but, among the

258 subjects who received a third BtA treatment, benefit increased with successive treatments.

Crow's feet

A dose ranging, open label, crossover study [15] tested placebo against 6 mu, 12 mu or 18 mu BtA (Botox®) injected into the periorbital or crow's feet area. All doses of BtA improved the appearance of the patients' moderately severe crow's feet more than placebo. There was no difference in the degree of improvement or in the rate of adverse effects between the different doses. The lack of a dose–response effect suggests that the lowest dose produced the maximum benefit possible and that increasing the dose could effect no further improvements. A second injection of the same dose lasted longer than the first injection, with half the patients still above baseline 16 weeks after the second injection. This finding is consistent with other published reports of BtA in crow's feet.

Platysmal bands

Kane [16] injected 50 patients with platysmal bands with excellent subjective improvement using open-label doses between 5 and 20 mu BtA (Botox®) per platysmal band. This was not specifically a dose-ranging study and the dose injected depended on the perceived severity of the platysmal bands. It is not clear which dose gave the best effect.

Practical treatment

Anatomy of the facial muscles

Botulinum toxin (Bt) paralyses the muscles by inhibiting acetylcholine release, thereby blocking the neuromuscular end plate. It is important to have a good knowledge of the functional anatomy of facial muscles (Figs 18.1 and 18.2). Special features of the facial muscles include:
- Depending on the region treated, it can be difficult to distinguish between different muscle groups. Individual muscles can be heavily interwoven or merge, and there are many anatomical variants. Textbook illustrations do not always correspond to the actual anatomy. The classical anatomy of the facial muscle groups is summarized in Table 18.1 [17].
- Facial expression depends upon the balance of agonist–antagonist interactions so that paralysis of one muscle will cause imbalance which will be especially noticeable if it is asymmetric.

Spread of the toxin to surrounding tissues depends in part on the toxin concentration and volume injected. Paralysis of an injected muscle can spread to adjacent muscles. Gravity may influence the direction of spread.

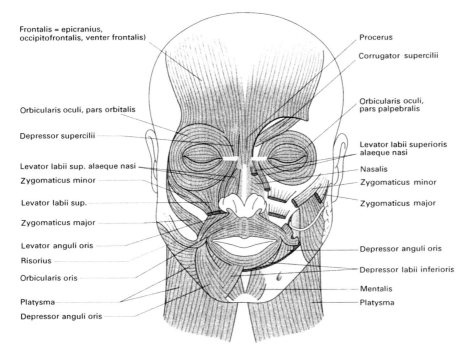

Fig. 18.1 Facial musculature. Reproduced with permission from [17].

Techniques for using botulinum toxin A

Procedural checklist

1. Find out what the patient wants, and why.
2. Take a full history, including allergies, medications currently being taken, and other possible contraindications.
3. Examine the skin, facial expression and general health.
4. Explain the likely results of treatment.
5. Explain the potential risks and side-effects.
6. Explain the alternatives to BtA treatment.
7. Have patient sign the consent form.
8. Photograph the patient.
9. Decide the treatment regime.
10. Dilute the toxin.
11. Position the patient.
12. Prepare the target area.
13. Inject the toxin.
14. Record the treatment details.

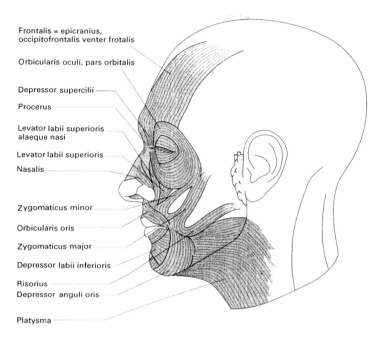

Frontalis = epicranius,
occipitofrontalis venter frotalis

Orbicularis oculi, pars orbitalis

Depressor supercilii

Procerus

Levator labii superioris
alaeque nasi

Levator labii superioris

Nasalis

Zygomaticus minor

Orbicularis oris

Zygomaticus major

Depressor labii inferioris

Risorius
Depressor anguli oris

Platysma

Fig. 18.2 Facial musculature. Reproduced with permission from [17].

15 Give the patient post-treatment instructions.
16 Perform a follow-up examination.

Assessing the patient's expectations

Always consider what the patient wants, and whether this is realistic or achievable. Remember that in cosmetic indications the patient's expectations define the goal, and patients may need guidance as to what is possible. When considering Bt therapy, discuss each of the target regions individually with the patient.

Case history and skin status

Skin status Examine the age, elasticity and texture of the skin, the presence or absence of sun damage, existing skin diseases, and/or precancerous conditions.

Which wrinkles really bother the patient? In many cases, the patient's subjective complaints do not correspond objectively to their physical features. Some patients, for example, only want to have frown lines improved although their crow's feet are much more prominent. It is essential to ask, 'What bothers you the most?' or 'Which problem zone do you want to have treated'?

Table 18.1 Facial musculature.

Muscle	Origin	Insertion	Function
Epicranial muscles			
Frontalis	Skin of the eyebrows	Galea aponeurotica	Draws eyebrow upward, wrinkles forehead to express emotion, e.g. frowning, astonishment
Corrugator supercilii	Nasal process of frontal bone	Skin above eyebrow	Makes vertical forehead lines (frown lines)
Orbicularis oculi			
Pars palpebralis	Medial palpebral ligament	Lateral palpebral ligament	Blinking, eyelid closure
Pars orbitalis	Anterior lacrimal crest	Concentrically around the orbit	Squinting
Pars lacrimalis	Posterior lacrimal crest, lacrimal sac	Pars palpebralis	Enlarges lacrimal sac
Muscles of the nose			
Procerus	Skin over nose	Skin between eyebrows	Wrinkles nose, makes transverse nasal folds
Nasalis			
Pars transversa	Skin over canine tooth	Bridge of nose	Narrows nostril
Pars alaris	Skin over incisors	Side of nose	Narrows nostril
Muscles of the mouth			
Orbicularis oris	Forms the perioral ring	—	Closes and protrudes the lips
Pars marginalis			
Pars labialis			
Levator labii superioris	Above infraorbital foramen	Orbicular muscle	Raises corners of mouth
Levator labii superioris alaeque nasi	Medial to orbital wall	Cartilage of ala nasi and upper lip	Raises upper lip and dilates nostril (nasal flaring)
Zygomaticus major	Outer aspect of zygomatic bone	Angle of mouth	Draws angle of mouth backward and downward
Zygomaticus minor	Zygomatic bone near maxillary suture	Orbicularis oris and levator labii superioris	Draws upper lip upward and laterally
Levator anguli oris	Canine fossa of maxilla	Angle of mouth	Draws angle of mouth upward
Risorius	Parotid fascia	Angle of mouth	Draws angle of mouth laterally (smile)
Buccinator	Pterygoimandibular raphe, maxilla, mandible	Orbicularis oris at angle of mouth	Puffs up cheeks
Depressor anguli oris	Lower edge of mandible	Angle of mouth	Draws angle of mouth downward (expresses sadness)
Depressor labii inferioris	Lower edge of mandible, platysma	Lower lip	Draws lower lip downward (used in drinking)
Mentalis	Alveolar wall of incisors of lower jaw	Skin of chin	Wrinkles skin of chin
Superficial muscles of neck			
Platysma	Base of mandible, parotid fascia	Pectoral fascia	Tenses the skin of the neck

426

Complete or partial paralysis of the target muscles? The desired degree of paralysis determines the dose. Higher doses give more complete paralysis. Many patients, especially women, prefer full paralysis of areas such as the glabella, whereas others prefer partial paralysis because they are afraid of ending up with a mask-like face.

Put simply, facial wrinkles can be caused by gravity (gravity lines), sleeping habits (sleep lines), and muscle contraction. BtA therapy is indicated for treatment of wrinkles caused by muscle contraction. Gravity lines and sleep lines do not improve after Bt therapy.

No-one has a perfectly symmetrical face. Facial asymmetries are usually minor and normally go unnoticed in everyday situations. It is therefore important to point them out, especially when they are more pronounced. BtA therapy can make facial asymmetries more prominent, especially when multiple simultaneous treatments are performed.

Explaining the expected results of treatment

It is impossible to predict the final result precisely, but predictions become increasingly accurate with experience. Patients usually ask the physician to eliminate a particular wrinkle. It is important to make them understand what BtA can and cannot do, and this is easy to demonstrate. Place a thumb on the wrinkle and pull the skin slightly to the side to show how the wrinkle will respond to Bt therapy.

Explaining the potential risks and side-effects

No severe complications have been reported in the literature after cosmetic use of Bt. There have been isolated cases of mild nausea, headaches, and flu-like symptoms. Local symptoms such as pain at the injection site, reflex erythema, bruising, and transient hypoesthesia may well occur.

Other specific risks and side-effects of Bt therapy in cosmetic uses are detailed in Table 18.3 (p. 431).

Patient consent and explaining the alternatives to botulinum toxin A treatment

For medicolegal reasons, each patient must be told about the available treatment alternatives, even if Bt therapy is the best treatment option or if it is to be used together with other procedures such as soft-tissue augmentation or skin resurfacing. The patient consent form must clearly state that the patient has been informed about alternative treatments, about the potential risks and side-effects of BtA therapy, and that Bt has not yet been licensed for treatment of hypertrophic facial expression muscles. Remember to tell the patient that once the toxin has worked there is no antidote, and any side-effects can only be treated symptomatically. They will wear off.

Photographic documentation

Before Bt injections, the physician should always take photographs to show the target muscles both relaxed and fully contracted. Document the therapeutic effect as well.

Establishing the treatment regime

Before drawing up any toxin from the vial, work out which muscles to treat, and the doses and volumes of toxin needed. We recommend sketching the treatment regime directly onto the patient record sheet or on a separate sheet of paper. Add up the units required for each injection. Record the total dose on the patient record sheet and use it to guide preparation of the toxin. Some experienced physicians first inject the toxin 'intuitively' and then record the number of units injected, but we do not recommend this approach.

Dilution of the toxin

Decide the best dilution before starting the procedure. Higher concentrations diffuse less, giving more focused paralysis and a more prolonged effect. We usually dilute 1 vial Botox® or Dysport® with 2–2.5 mL 0.9% saline.

Follow-up examination

Remind the patient that muscle weakening does not begin until at least 1–2 days after treatment, and sometimes takes as much as 12 days. If this reminder is forgotten, the patient may worry and call the doctor unnecessarily.

Explain the expected duration of effect and what to do as the treated muscles recover. After cosmetic treatment with Bt the effects usually persist for about 4 months before muscle activity is gradually restored. This varies between patients and facial areas treated.

Practical tips for injection

- *Tensing the target muscle before an injection reduces the discomfort.*
- *Bt can be injected either with or without electromyographic (EMG) guidance.* Most physicians give cosmetic injections without EMG guidance, whereas others always use it. Table 18.2 summarizes the pros and cons of EMG-guided injections.
- *Local anaesthesia.* Patients often do not need local anaesthesia. If required, apply an ice pack to the target area before and after injections to prevent pain and bruising at the injection site. Alternatively, use a local anaesthetic cream (e.g. EMLA® or Ametop®).
- *Use smallest cannula available.* The tiny quantities of lyophilized toxin hardly change

Table 18.2 Pros and cons of electromyographic (EMG) guidance.

Pros	Cons
Provides audible confirmation of needle position, ensures more precise localization	EMG recorders and needles are expensive
Patient understands the treatment better	Prolongs procedure
Novices learn more easily	More complicated
Useful for locating hard-to-find muscles	No proven advantage over freehand injections
Useful for locating muscle subsections that remain responsive after initial treatment	
Increases patient compliance and the 'aura curae' effect	

the flow properties of the diluent. Use the smallest available cannula (30 or 32 gauge) to reduce injection site pain and bruising.

• *Keep syringe scale visible.* This tip may sound obvious, but can be very helpful for the novice. Make a habit of keeping the scale on the syringe visible regardless of where the injection is made or in which direction the tip of the needle is pointed.

• *Watch out for blood vessels.* Avoid the temporal artery and vein when injecting cranio-lateral to the orbit. Determine the exact location of the vessels under good lighting before starting treatment.

• *Respect anatomic boundaries.* When making injections near structures, such as the orbicular septum, monitor the position and direction of the needle carefully to prevent damage to septae and ligaments. Inserting the needle too close to, or perforating the septum, disproportionately increases the risk of unwanted paralysis of the levator palpebrae muscle. Keep the tip of the needle pointed away from eye.

Contraindications

ABSOLUTE CONTRAINDICATIONS TO COSMETIC USE

• Neuromuscular transmission disorders (myasthenia gravis, Lambert–Eaton syndrome).

• Known hypersensitivity to any ingredient in the formulation.

• Local infection or recent trauma at the injection site.

• Pregnancy and lactation.

RELATIVE CONTRAINDICATIONS TO COSMETIC USE

• Coagulation disorders or use of anticoagulants.

• Lack of patient cooperation.

• Unstable mental state.

• Unrealistic expectations.

• Unrealistic fear of systemic botulism.

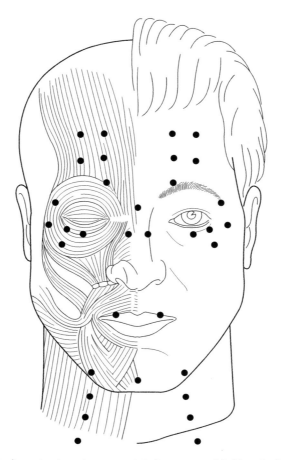

Fig. 18.3 Typical injection points in various cosmetic indications (modified from [17]).

Specific indications and dose range

DOSES: A HEALTH WARNING

Please read the warning on p. 35 about doses of Bt. There are three preparations available. *Dysport®* and *Botox®* are type A toxins (BtA), *NeuroBloc®/MYOBLOC™* is type B (BtB). Even though the doses for each are quoted in mouse units (mu), the three preparations have different dose schedules: one mu of *Dysport®* is **not** the same as one mu of *Botox®*, and neither is equivalent to one mu of *NeuroBloc®/MYOBLOC™*.

Table 18.3 and Fig. 18.3 give details of anatomical areas most frequently injected and recommended dose ranges [17]. Please note: older patients need lower doses. Clinical examples of BtA use in glabellar lines and in a patient with crow's feet before and after BtA, are given in Fig. 18.4a–d.

Table 18.3 Practical treatment in cosmetic applications, including hypertrophic lines of the face.

Anatomic region	Cosmetic indication	Involved muscles	Injection sites and techniques	Notes	Dose range BOTOX®	Dose range Dysport®	Risks, complications
Glabella	Frown lines	Corrugator supercilii orbicularis oculi procerus	Injection into procerus, the medial and lateral aspects of the corrugator muscles (depending on findings) and medial aspects of orbicularis oculi. If massage is applied, only gentle and away from the eye	Injection varies according to findings in individual patient	20–35 mu depending on gender and muscle hypertrophy	80–175 mu depending on gender and muscle hypertrophy	Levator ptosis, bruising, mild reversible headaches
Forehead	Horizontal forehead lines	Venter frontalis of occipitofrontalis muscle	Injection into frontalis muscle along an imaginary line between eyebrows and hairline. Gentle massage needed after injection	In elderly patients with some degree of brow ptosis, brow depressors to be treated also	14–20 mu depending on gender and muscle hypertrophy	70–100 mu depending on gender and muscle hypertrophy	Brow ptosis Elevation of lateral end of the eyebrow ('cockeyed brow')
Periorbital region	Crow's feet, syn. Lateral canthal rhytides, squint lines	Orbital part of orbicularis oculi	Two or three injections per side, c. 1 cm lateral to the orbital marginal	The most medial injection site is lateral to a line extending through the outer canthus	14–15 mu depending on muscle hypertrophy and intended clinical endpoint	20–75 mu depending on muscle hypertrophy and intended clinical endpoint	Drooping of lower eyelid with accentuation of 'bags' under the eyes Diplopia in paralysis of m. rectus lateralis oculi
Suborbital region	'Open-eye look' in younger patients	Orbital and palpebral parts of orbicularis oculi	Strictly subcutaneous injection of very small doses	Most medial injection in medpupillary line	1–2 mu per injection site, max. two sites per side	3–8 mu per injection site, max. two sites per side	Laxity of lower eyelid, ectropion

Continued on p. 432

Table 18.3 *Continued*

Anatomic region	Cosmetic indication	Involved muscles	Injection sites and techniques	Notes	Dose range BOTOX®	Dose range Dysport®	Risks, complications
Nose	Nasoglabellar lines nasal scrunch, 'bunny lines'	Nasalis	Injection of very small doses	Do not massage	2–5 mu depending on gender and muscle hypertrophy	8–20 mu depending on gender and muscle hypertrophy	Drooping of angle of mouth Upper lip: partial incompetence
Perioral region	Perioral folds upper lip wrinkling, lower lip wrinkling. 'Marionette lines'	Upper lip: orbicularis oris Lower lip: depressor anguli oris	Upper lip: very small doses around perioral folds Lower lip: injection of the origin of M. depressor anguli oris at edge of mandible	Upper lip: minimal doses	Upper lip: 1–2 mu per injection site, max. four sites Lower lip: 2–5 mu per side. max. two sites	Upper lip: 4–10 mu per injection site, max. four sites Lower lip: 5–20 mu per side	of orbicularis oris muscle Lower lip: asymmetrical smile
Chin	Mental creases, popply chin	Mentalis	Injection just above tip of chin	Stay well away from lower lip	4–10 mu depending on muscle hypertrophy and intended clinical endpoint	15–50 mu depending on muscle hypertrophy and intended clinical endpoint	Asymmetry of mouth movement
Neck	Platysmal bands	Platysma	Manually hold the target platysmal band	Injection superficially only	4–5 mu per injection site. max. dose 30–60 mu per session	20–25 mu per injection site. max. 120–300 mu per session	Dysphagia Change in pitch of voice, weakness of levator muscles of the neck

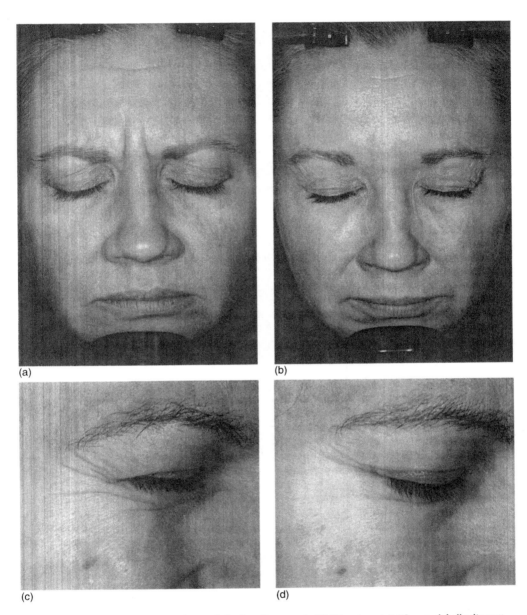

Fig. 18.4 Two patients before and after botulinum toxin (BtA) treatment. (a) Severe glabellar lines at maximum frown. (b) Same patient 2 weeks after Botox®; 20 units total to corrugator procerus complex at maximum frown. (c) Patient with mainly upper quadrant crow's feet before treatment. (d) Same patient 1 week after 12 units Botox® to the area. Improvement is already seen.

433

Conclusion

The cosmetic use of BtA is now well established as monotherapy or part of combination therapy for facial lines. In early 2001, BtA (Botox®) was approved for treating glabellar lines in Canada and in April 2002 its use was approved by the FDA. We anticipate that other countries will approve it within the next year. As we stress in this chapter, providing that the injecting physician follows guidelines for dose, dilution and sites of injection, then there is a wide safety margin for cosmetic indications. It is important for any physician planning to use BtA as a cosmetic treatment to be fully trained. We need more research to examine optimum dosing schedules, especially for lower face muscles.

References

1 Carruthers A, Carruthers JDA. The use of botulinum toxin to treat glabellar frown lines and other facial wrinkles. *Cosmet Dermatol* 1994; **7**: 11–15.

2 Guyuron B, Huddleston SW. Aesthetic indications for botulinum toxin injection. *Plast Resonstr Surg* 1994; **93**: 913–18.

3 Keen M, Blitzer A, Aviv J et al. Botulinum toxin A for hyperkinetic facial lines. results of a double blind, placebo-controlled study. *Plast Reconstr Surg* 1994; **94**: 94–9.

4 Carruthers JDA, Carruthers JA. Treatment of glabellar frown lines and other facial wrinkles. In: Jankovic J, Hallett M, eds. *Therapy with botulinum toxin.* New York: Marcel Dekker, 1994: 577–95.

5 Lowe NJ, Maxwell A, Harpe H. Botulinum toxin A exotoxin for glabellar folds: a double blind study, placebo controlled study. *J Am Acad Derm* 1996; **35**: 569–72.

6 Blitzer A, Binder W, Aviv J, Keen MS, Brin M. The management of hyperfunctional facial lines with botulinum toxin. *Arch Otolaryngol Head Neck Surg* 1997; **123**: 389–92.

7 Guerrissi GO. Intraoperative injection of botulinum toxin A into orbicularis oculi muscle for the treatment of crow's feet. *Plast Reconstr Surg* 2000; **105**: 2219–28.

8 Fagien S. Botox for the treatment of dynamic and hyperkinetic facial lines and furrows: adjunctive use in facial aesthetic surgery. *Plast Reconstr Surg* 1999; **103**: 701–3.

9 Jankovic J, Brin MF. Therapeutic uses of botulinum toxin. *N Engl J Med* 1991; **324**: 1186–94.

10 Garcia A, Fulton J. Cosmetic denervation of the muscles of facial expression with botulinum toxin. *Dermatol Surg* 1996; **22**: 39–43.

11 Pribitkin EA, Greco TM, Goode RL et al. Patient selection in the treatment of glabellar wrinkles with botulinum toxin type A injection. *Otolaryngol Head Neck Surg* 1997; **123**: 321–6.

12 Carruthers JDA, Carruthers JA. Treatment of glabellar frown lines with botulinum A exotoxin. *J Dermatol Surg Oncol* 1992; **18**: 17–21.

13 Hankins CL, Strimling R, Rogers GS. Botulinum A toxin for glabellar wrinkles. *Dose Response Dermatol Surg* 1998, **11**: 1183–7.

14 Carruthers JA, Lowe NJ, Menter MA et al. One-year, two-period study of the safety and efficacy of botulinum toxin yype A in patients with glabellar lines. Presented at the American Academy of Dermatology, Washington, D.C., 2001.

15 Lowe NJ, Lask G. Bilateral. Double blind, randomized, paired evaluation of three doses of botulinum toxin type A and placebo in patients with crow's feet. Presented at the American Academy of Dermatology, Washington, D.C., 2001.

16 Kane MA. Platysmal band treatment with botulinum toxin A. *Plast Reconstr Surg* 1999; **103**: 656–65.

17 Sommer B, Sattler G, eds. *Botulinumtoxin in der ästhetischen Medizin.* Berlin: Blackwell Wissenschaft, 2001.

Common sites for cosmetic use of BtA

1. Glabellar frown lines

General considerations should include the following.
- Wrinkles, lines or furrows between the brows.
- When deep and prominent, glabellar frown lines may project unintended emotions such as anger, fear or worry.
- Treatment options:
  filling agents
  botulinum toxin A (BtA)
  laser resurfacing.

BtA treatment

- Sites of injection determined by brow shape

- Arched, female-type brow requires less toxin

- Horizontal, male-type brow has greater muscle mass and requires more toxin

- Brow asymmetry or ptosis?

- Individuals vary—examine!

- 4 units of Botox per O

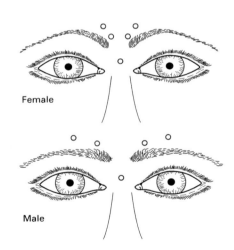

Female

Male

- Dose is adjusted for each site; brow type; muscle mass
- Patient should be in sitting position with chin down
- Chill the area to be injected
- The injection site should always be above the supraorbital rim and medial to the mid-pupillary line
- Post injection, the patient should frown as much as possible during the next 2–3 h

2. Crow's feet

General considerations should include the following.
- Wrinkles extending laterally from the periorbital area.
- Ususally associated with photoageing.
- Produced by contraction of orbicularis oculi.
- Treatment options:
  surgery
  resurfacing
  botulinum toxin A (BtA).

BtA treatment

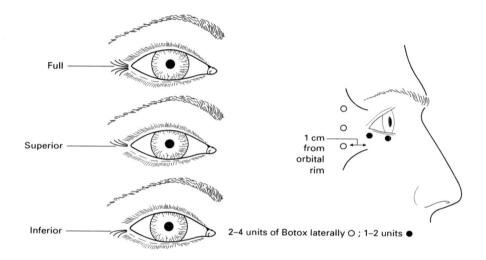

2–4 units of Botox laterally O ; 1–2 units ●

- Patient is asked to smile maximally
- Note the extent of the crow's feet
- 6–18 mu Botox® are injected laterally
- 1–2 mu Botox® injected into lower lateral lid

3. Horizontal forehead lines

BtA treatment
- Approach should be conservative:
  8–20 mu Botox® in four to eight divided doses
- Avoid the following areas
  immediately above the eyebrow;
  area above the lateral eyebrow
- Injection sites should be firmly massaged post injection

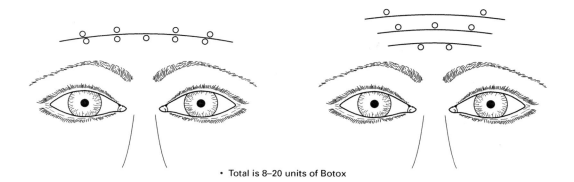

- Total is 8–20 units of Botox

APPENDIX

Muscles and recommended dose ranges of botulinum toxins for adults

*NeuroBloc®/MYOBLOC™ doses for arm and leg muscles in italics and marked with an asterisk are kindly provided by WE MOVE (http://www.wemove.org). Most of them are not based on clinical trials and do not necessarily reflect authors' personal experiences.

Note: As Bt doses may be lower in dystonia than in spasticity, separate dosing tables are provided for upper and lower limb treatments of spasticity and dystonia.

Facial and oromandibular muscles: DYSTONIA

Muscle	Action	Injection site (number of injections)	Dose (mu)		
			Botox®	Dysport®	NeuroBloc®/ MYOBLOC™
Orbicularis oculi	Eye closure	Periocular injections (3–6) per side	20 (10–25) HFS/Bleph per side	80 (40–160) HFS 150 (100–180) Bleph per side	250–1000 HFS* 750–2500 Bleph* per side
Zygomaticus minor Zygomaticus major Levator anguli oris Levator labii superioris Risorius Depressor anguli oris Depressor labii inferioris	Various effects on facial expression	Muscle belly (1–2)	2.5 (2.5–7.5)	10 (10–30)	125–250*
Mentalis	Chin skin spasm	Muscle belly (1–2)	5 (2.5–10.0)	20 (10–40)	125–250*
Orbicularis oris	Mouth closure	Perioral injections (careful)	5 (2.5–5.0)	20 (10–40)	250–500*
Platysma	Various effects on facial expression and head movement	Along platysmal bands (several)	5 (2.5–10) per band	20 (10–30) per band	500–2500 total*
Masseter Temporalis	Jaw closure	Muscle belly (2–4)	25 (15–50)	100 (60–200)	1000–3000*
Medial pterygoid	Jaw closure	Transoral or percutaneous (1–2)	15 (5–40)	60 (20–160)	1000–3000*
Lateral pterygoid	Jaw opening	Transoral or percutaneous (1–2)	15 (10–40)	60 (40–160)	1000–3000*
Digastric	Jaw opening	Ventral third of the muscle (1–2)	5 (2.5–20)	20 (10–80)	250–750*

Bleph, Blepharospasm; HFS, hemifacial spasm. (For cosmetic use, see Chapter 18.)

Cervical muscles: DYSTONIA

Muscle	Action	Injection site (number of injections)	Dose (mu) Botox®	Dysport®	NeuroBloc®/ MYOBLOC™
Sternocleidomastoid	See Table 8.3	Upper half of muscle (2–3)	20–50	80–200	1000–3000
Splenius capitis	See Table 8.3	Upper third of muscle (2–3)	50–100	200–400	1000–5000
Semispinalis capitis	See Table 8.3	Deep injections (3.0–5.0 cm) along muscle strand beneath the splenius muscle (2–4)	20–40	80–160	750–5000
Levator scapulae	See Table 8.3	Anterior to upper fibers of trapezius (1–2)	10–30	40–120	1000–4000
Trapezius (upper portion)	See Table 8.3	At the upper border of the shoulder and posterior neck (2–6)	20–50	80–200	1000–5000
Scalenus complex	See Table 8.3	Muscle belly in the floor of the posterior triangle two fingers anterior to the anterior border of trapezius (1–2)	10–20	40–80	1000–3000

Shoulder girdle: SPASTICITY

Muscle	Action	Injection site (number of injections)	Dose (mu) Botox®	Dysport®	NeuroBloc®/ MYOBLOC™
Trapezius	Scapular elevation and rotation	Upper border of shoulder and posterior neck (2–6)	50–75	200–300	1000–5000*
Supraspinatus	Abduction of arm from 0–15°	Supraspinous fossa of scapula (1–2)	20–40	40–160	–
Infraspinatus	External rotation of arm	Infraspinous surface of scapula (1–2)	40–60	120–200	160–240*
Subscapularis	Internal rotation of arm	Under lateral border of scapula (1–2)	30–50	120–200	1000–3000*
Deltoid	Arm adduction from 15–90°	Anterior, middle and posterior fibres (2–4)	50–75	200–300	–
Teres major	Adducts, internally rotates and extends arm	Lateral aspect lower scapula (1–2)	30–50	120–200	1000–3000*
Teres minor	Adducts and externally rotates arm	Lateral aspect scapula above (1)	30–40	120–160	–
Latissimus dorsi	Adducts, retracts and internally rotates arm	Find in posterior fold of axilla while asking patient to pull down elevated arm (2–3)	50–80	200–300	2500–5000*
Serratus anterior	Protracts arm	Lateral aspect of upper eight ribs (2–3)	60–70	250–275	–
Pectoralis complex	Adducts and internally rotates arm	Anterior axillary fold (2–4)	50–75	200–300	2500–5000*

Shoulder girdle: DYSTONIA

Muscle	Action	Injection site (number of injections)	Dose (mu) Botox®	Dysport®
Supraspinatus	Abduction of arm from 0–15°	Supraspinous fossa of scapula	20–40	40–160
Infraspinatus	External rotation of arm	Infraspinous surface of scapula	40–60	160–240
Deltoid	Arm abduction from 15–90°	Inject anterior, middle and posterior fibres	50–75	200–300
Teres major	Adducts, medially rotates and extends arm	Lateral aspect lower scapula	20–30	80–120
Teres minor	Adducts and laterally rotates arm	Lateral aspect scapula above	20–30	80–120
Pectoralis major	Adducts and medially rotates arm	Anterior axillary fold	30–75	120–300

Arm muscles: SPASTICITY

Upper arm

Muscle	Action	Injection site (number of injections)	Dose (mu) Botox®	Dysport®	NeuroBloc®/ MYOBLOC™
Biceps brachii	Supination and elbow flexion	Anterior aspect of upper arm. Inject both heads (2)	75–100	300–400	2500–5000*
Triceps brachii	Elbow extension	Three heads on post aspect of arm (3)	75–100	300–400	–
Coracobrachialis	Flexes and adducts upper arm	Medial to upper humerus between it and neurovascular bundle (1–2)	30–40	120–160	–
Brachialis	Flexes elbow	Lower anterior humerus medial and lateral of biceps tendon (1–2)	30–50	120–200	1000–3000*

441

Extensor aspect of forearm: SPASTICITY

Muscle	Action	Injection site (number of injections)	Dose (mu)			
			Botox®	Dysport®	NeuroBloc®/ MYOBLOC™	
Brachioradialis	Elbow flexion	Radial side upper forearm	30–60	120–250	1000–3000*	
Supinator	Supinates forearm	Extensor aspect of arm below radial neck—deep	30–40	120–160	—	
Extensor carpi radialis longus	Extends and abducts hand at wrist	Posterior to brachioradialis on back of forearm	30–40	120–160	—	
Extensor carpi radialis brevis	Extends and abducts hand at wrist	Posterior and medial to ECR longus	20–30	75–120	—	
Extensor carpi ulnaris	Extends wrist and elbow and adducts hand	Most medially placed extensor muscle. Halfway down ulna shaft	30–40	120–160	—	
Extensor digitorum communis	Extends wrist and fingers	Middle of back of forearm distal to radial tuberosity	20–40	80–160	—	
Extensor digiti minimi	Extends 5th finger	Medial to Ext. digitorum	10–30	40–120	—	
Extensor pollicis longus	Extends all joints of thumb	Midway down back of forearm	15–30	40–120	—	
Extensor pollicis brevis	Extends CMC and MCP joints of thumb	Distal third of forearm. Palpate by moving CMC and MCP joints	15–25	40–100	—	
Adductor pollicis longus	Adducts thumb and hand	Proximal to Ext. pollicis brevis on back of forearm. Palpate action	10–30	40–120	—	
Extensor indicis	Extends index finger	Found medial of most lateral tendon of ext. digit communis	10–30	40–120	—	

CMC, carpal metacarpal; ECR, extensor carpi radialis; Ext, extensor; MCP, metacarpophalangeal.

Flexor aspect of forearm: SPASTICITY

Muscle	Action	Injection site (number of injections)	Dose (mu) Botox®	Dysport®	NeuroBloc®/ MYOBLOC™
Pronator teres	Pronates forearm and flexes elbow	Medial border of anterior cubital fossa—medial to brachial artery	30–40	120–160	1000–2500*
Flexor carpi radialis	Flexes wrist and elbow	Upper forearm just below bicipital aponeurosis and medial to pronator teres	30–50	120–200	1000–3000*
Flexor carpi ulnaris	Flexes and adducts hand at wrist	Upper forearm medial aspect of flexor surface below bicipital aponeurosis. Medial to FCR. Observe action of wrist flexion	20–40	80–160	1000–3000*
Flexor digitorum superficialis	PIP joint flexor and MCP joint flexor	Middle of forearm halfway down to either side of palmaris tendon	20–50	80–200	1000–3000*
Flexor digitorum profundus	Flexes all finger joints	Upper third of forearm. Deep muscle above lateral border of ulna	20–50	60–200	1000–3000*
Flexor pollicis longus	Flexes all joints of thumb	Mid forearm over anterior aspect of radius	15–30	60–120	1000–2500*
Pronator quadratus	Pronates forearm	Approach muscle from extensor aspect of forearm just proximal to wrist and advance through interosseous membrane	20–30	80–120	1000–2500*

MCP, metacarpophalangeal; PIP, posterior interphalangeal.

Arm muscles: DYSTONIA

Extensor aspect of forearm

| Muscle | Action | Injection site (number of injections) | Dose (mu) | | NeuroBloc®/ |
			Botox®	Dysport®	MYOBLOC™
Supinator	Supinates forearm	Extensor aspect of arm below radial neck—deep	10–30	40–120	—
Extensor carpi radialis	Extends and abducts hand at wrist	Posterior to brachio radialis on back of forearm	10–30	40–120	500–1500*
Extensor carpi ulnaris	Extends wrist and elbow and abducts hand	Most medially placed extensor muscle. Halfway down ulna shaft	10–30	40–120	500–1500*
Extensor digitorum communis	Extends wrist and fingers	Middle of back of forearm distal to radial tuberosity	5–15 (per fascicle)	20–40 (per fascicle)	—
Extensor pollicis longus	Extends all joints of thumb	Midway down back of forearm	5–20	20–80	—
Extensor pollicis brevis	Extends CMC and MCP joints of thumb	Distal third of forearm. Palpate by moving CMC and MCP joints	5–20	20–80	—
Adductor pollicis longus	Adducts thumb and hand	Proximal to extensor pollicis brevis on back of forearm. Palpate action	10–25	40–100	500–1500*
Extensor indicis proprius	Extends forefinger	Found medial of most lateral tendon of extensor digit communis	5–15	20–60	500–1000*

CMC, carpal metacarpal; MCP, metacarpophalangeal.

Flexor aspect of forearm: DYSTONIA

Muscle	Action	Injection site (number of injections)	Dose (mu)		
			Botox®	Dysport®	NeuroBloc®/ MYOBLOC™
Pronator teres	Pronates forearm and flexes elbow	Medial border of anterior cubital fossa—medial to brachial artery	15–30	60–120	500–1500*
Flexor carpi radialis	Flexes wrist and elbow	Upper forearm just below bicipital aponeurosis and medial to pronator teres	20–50	80–200	500–2500*
Flexor carpi ulnaris	Flexes and adducts hand at wrist	Upper forearm medial aspect of flexor surface below bicipital aponeurosis. Medial to FCR. Observe action of wrist flexion	15–40	60–160	500–2500*
Flexor digitorum superficialis	PIP joint flexor and MCP joint flexor	Middle of forearm halfway down to either side of palmaris tendon	10–20 (per fascicle)	40–80 (per fascicle)	250–1500*
Flexor digitorum profundus	Flexes all finger joints	Upper third of forearm. Deep muscle above lateral border of ulna	10–20 (per fascicle)	40–80 (per fascicle)	250–1500*
Flexor pollicis longus	Flexes all joints of thumb	Mid forearm over anterior aspect of radius	10–20	40–80	1000–2500*
Pronator quadratus	Pronates forearm	Approach muscle from extensor aspect of forearm just proximal to wrist and advance through interosseous membrane	15–25	60–100	500–1500*

MCP, metacarpophalangeal; PIP, posterior interphalangeal.

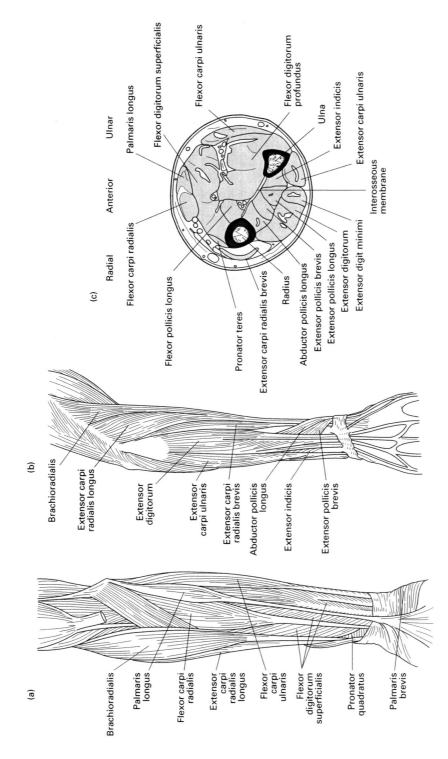

Fig. A1 Lower arm muscles: (a) anterior, (b) posterior and (c) cross section.

Trunk muscles: SPASTICITY

Muscle	Action	Injection site (number of injections)	Dose (mu)		
			Botox®	Dysport®	NeuroBloc®/MYOBLOC™
Psoas major	Flexes hip	Approach posteriorly advancing spinal needle between transverse processes at L2, L3 and L4	150–200 (50–60 at each site)	600–800 (200–250 at each site)	3000–7500*
Quadratus lumborum	Flexes vertebral column laterally	Posterior approach lateral to vertebral column	100	400	—

Leg muscles: SPASTICITY

Thigh flexors and knee extensors

Muscle	Action	Injection site (number of injections)	Dose (mu)		
			Botox®	Dysport®	NeuroBloc®/MYOBLOC™
Iliopsoas	Hip flexion	Groin, lateral to femoral artery and nerve (two points)	100–150	400–800	3000–7500*
Rectus femoris	Hip flexion and knee extension	Four points along the middle of quadriceps muscle mass	100–150	400–600	2500–5000*
Vastus lateralis, intermedius and medialis	Knee extension	Two points in lateral aspect of thigh: one deep centrally in lower half of thigh and one to two medially	100–150	400–600	5000–7500*

Thigh adductors and knee flexors: SPASTICITY

Muscle	Action	Injection site (number of injections)	Dose (mu)		
			Botox®	Dysport®	NeuroBloc®/ MYOBLOC™
Adductor muscles (adductor magnus, longus, brevis)	Adduct thigh	Large muscles in upper medial thigh. Inject into upper third of thigh	100–200	400–800	5000–10000*
Gracilis	Adducts thigh and flexes knee. Medially rotates flexed leg	Postero-medial edge of thigh several points of injection down medial thigh	80–120	300–400	—
Semimembranosus	Flexes knee. Medially rotates flexed leg and extends hip	Medial muscles in posterior thigh – multiple injection sites	80–100	300–400	3000–7500*
Semitendinosus	Same as semimembranosus	Medial muscles in posterior thigh – multiple injection sites	80–100	300–400	3000–7500*
Biceps femoris	Flexes knee, rotates leg externally and extends hip	Lateral muscle in posterior thigh – multiple injection sites	100–150	400–600	2500–7500*
Popliteus	Flexes knee and internally rotates lower leg at beginning of flexion	Deep over back of medial tibial condyle. Down to bone medial aspect of popliteal fossa and then withdraw	30	120	—

Lower leg — antero lateral compartment: SPASTICITY

Muscle	Action	Injection site (number of injections)	Dose (mu)		
			Botox®	Dysport®	NeuroBloc®/ MYOBLOC™
Tibialis anterior	Dorsiflexes and inverts foot	Front of shin, lateral to tibia	75–120	300–500	2500–5000*
Extensor digitorum longus	Dorsiflexes toes and foot	Lateral to tibialis anterior in front of and border of fibula	50–80	200–300	2000–4000*
Extensor hallucis longus	Extends great toe	Between tibialis anterior and extensor digitorum longus in middle of shin	50–60	200–250	2000–4000*
Peroneus longus	Everts and plantar flexes foot	Lateral aspect of shin anterior to fibula	50–80	200–300	—

Lower leg — posterior compartment: SPASTICITY

Muscle	Action	Injection site (number of injections)	Dose (mu) Botox®	Dysport®	NeuroBloc®/ MYOBLOC™
Gastrocnemius (medial and lateral head)	Plantar flexes foot and flexes knee	Superficial muscle of medial aspect of calf	80–200	300–800	3000–7500*
Soleus	Plantar flexes foot	Back of calf, midway down between muscle bellies of gastrocnemius	50–100	200–400	2500–5000*
Flexor hallucis longus	Flexes great toe (IP + MTP joints) maintains longitudinal arch	Under soleus mid calf immediately posterior to peroneus longus and fibula	30–50	120–200	1500–3500*
Flexor digitorum longus	Flexes toes 2–5 (IP + MTP joints) and maintains longitudinal arch	Behind medial border of tibia in its upper mid area. Inject near origin just behind tibia	30–80	120–300	2500–500*
Tibialis posterior	Plantar flexes and inverts foot	Mid calf, deep behind tibia and in depression between tibia and fibula	50–100	200–400	3000–7500*
Flexor hallucis brevis	Flexes first MTP joint	Plantar aspect of foot under first metatarsal	10–20	40–80	—
Flexor digitorum brevis	Flexes first IP joint and lateral four MTP joints	Plantar aspect of foot at base of metatarsals	10–20	40–80	—

IP: interphalangeal; MTP: metatarsophalangeal.

Leg muscles: DYSTONIA

Lower leg—anterolateral compartment

Muscle	Action	Injection site (number of injections)	Dose (mu) Botox®	Dysport®	NeuroBloc®/ MYOBLOC™
Tibialis anterior	Dorsiflexes and inverts foot	Front of shin, lateral to tibia	75–120	300–500	2500–5000*
Extensor digitorum longus	Dorsiflexes toes and foot	Lateral to tibialis anterior in front of and border of fibula	50–80	200–300	–
Extensor hallucis longus	Extends great toe	Between tibialis anterior and extensor digitorum longus in middle of shin	20–50	80–200	2000–4000*
Peroneus longus	Everts and plantar flexes foot	Lateral aspect of shin anterior to fibula	40–80	160–300	2500–5000*

Lower leg—posterior compartment

Muscle	Action	Injection site (number of injections)	Dose (mu) Botox®	Dysport®	NeuroBloc®/ MYOBLOC™
Gastrocnemius	Plantar flexes foot and flexes knee	Superficial muscle of medial aspect of calf	50–100	200–400	3000–7500*
Soleus	Plantar flexes foot	Back of calf, midway down between muscle bellies of gastrocnemius	50–100	200–400	2500–5000*
Flexor hallucis longus	Flexes great toe (IP + MTP joints) and maintains longitudinal arch	Under soleus mid calf immediately posterior to peroneus longus and fibula	20–50	80–200	1500–3500*
Flexor digitorum longus	Flexes toes 2–5 (IP + MTP joints) and maintains longitudinal arch	Behind medial border of tibia in its upper mid area. Inject near origin just behind tibia	30–50	120–200	2500–5000*
Tibialis posterior	Plantar flexes and inverts foot	Mid calf, deep behind tibia and in depression between tibia and fibula	50–100	200–400	2500–7500*
Flexor hallucis brevis	Flexes first MTP joint	Plantar aspect of foot under first metatarsal	10–20	40–80	
Flexor digitorum brevis	Flexes first IP joint and lateral four MTP joints	Plantar aspect of foot at base of metatarsals	10–20	40–80	2500–5000*

IP, interphalangeal; MTP, metatarsophalangeal.

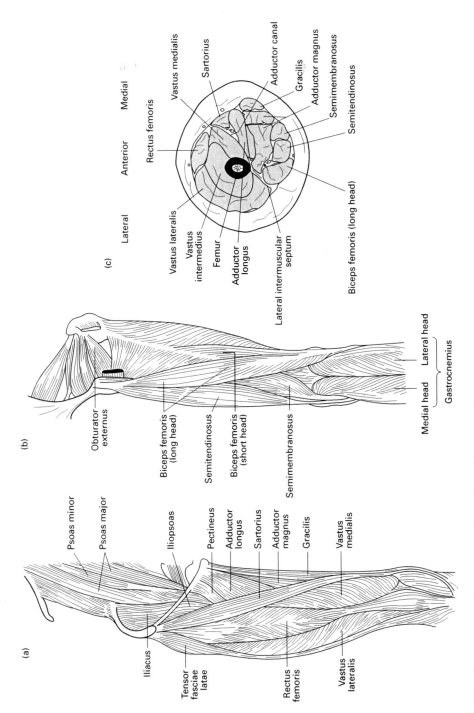

Fig. A2 Upper leg muscles: (a) anterior, (b) posterior and (c) cross section.

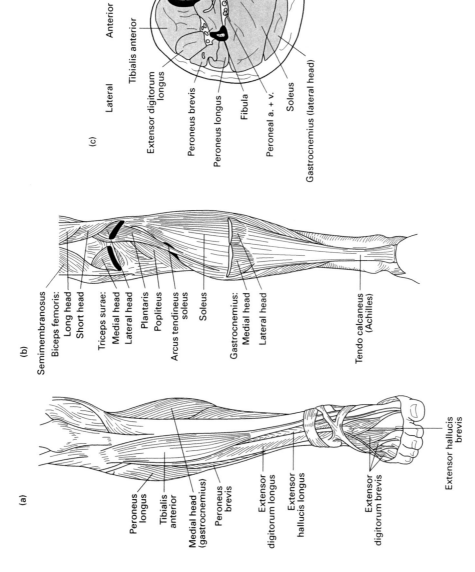

Fig. A3 Lower leg muscles: (a) anterior, (b) posterior and (c) cross section.

(a)

Peroneus longus
Tibialis anterior
Medial head (gastrocnemius)
Peroneus brevis
Extensor digitorum longus
Extensor hallucis longus
Extensor digitorum brevis
Extensor hallucis brevis

(b)

Semimembranosus
Biceps femoris:
   Long head
   Short head
Triceps surae:
   Medial head
   Lateral head
Plantaris
Popliteus
Arcus tendineus soleus
Soleus
Gastrocnemius:
   Medial head
   Lateral head
Tendo calcaneus (Achilles)

(c)

Lateral
Anterior
Medial
Tibia
Flexor digitorum longus
Tibialis posterior
Posterior tibial a. + v.
Tibial n.
Gastrocnemius (medial head)
Tibialis anterior
Extensor digitorum longus
Peroneus brevis
Peroneus longus
Fibula
Peroneal a. + v.
Soleus
Gastrocnemius (lateral head)

Children (cerebral palsy): SPASTICITY

Target muscle	Botox® (mu)		Dysport® (mu)	
	Per target muscle/ kg body weight	Total per muscle	Per target muscle/ kg body weight	Total per muscle
Small muscles Adductor pollicis brevis Hand and finger flexors Brachialis Brachioradialis	1–3	10–50	5–10	50–150
Large muscles Gastrocnemius Soleus Tibialis posterior Adductor muscles Gracilis Hamstrings Rectus femoris Iliopsoas Biceps brachii	3–6	30–100	10–30	100–500

Index

INDEX